aacn

American Academy of
Ambulatory Care Nursing

CORE
CURRICULUM for

AMBULATORY
CARE
NURSING

D0813786

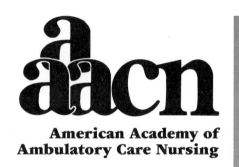

**American Academy of
Ambulatory Care Nursing**

CORE
CURRICULUM for

AMBULATORY
CARE
NURSING

Edited by

JOAN ROBINSON, MS, RN, CNAA

Health Care Services Consultant
Ann Arbor, Michigan

W.B. SAUNDERS COMPANY
A Harcourt Health Sciences Company
Philadelphia London New York St. Louis Sydney Toronto

W.B. SAUNDERS COMPANY

A Harcourt Health Sciences Company

The Curtis Center
Independence Square West
Philadelphia, Pennsylvania 19106-3399

Library of Congress Cataloging-in-Publication Data

AAACN core curriculum for ambulatory care nursing / edited by Joan Robinson.

p. ; cm.

Includes bibliographical references and index.

ISBN 0-7216-8628-1

1. Nursing. 2. Ambulatory medical care. I. Title: Core curriculum for ambulatory care nursing. II. Robinson, Joan, 1941- III. American Academy of Ambulatory Care Nursing.
  [DNLM: 1. Ambulatory Care. 2. Nursing Care. 3. Specialties, Nursing. WY 150 A1105 2001]

RT42 .A195 2001

610.73—dc21   00-067054

Vice President and Publishing Director: Sally Schrefer
Senior Editor: Michael S. Ledbetter
Senior Developmental Editor: Laurie K. Muench
Project Manager: Karen A. Edwards
Book Designer: Teresa Breckwoldt

CORE CURRICULUM FOR AMBULATORY CARE NURSING   ISBN: 0-7216-8628-1

Printed in the United States of America

Last digit is the print number: 9   8   7   6   5   4   3   2   1
GW/FF

CONTRIBUTORS

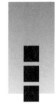

Nancy M. Albert, MSN, RN, CCRN, CNA
Clinical Outcomes Researcher/Clinical
  Nurse Specialist
Kaufman Center for Heart Failure,
  Cleveland Clinic Foundation
Cleveland, Ohio

Ida M. Androwich, PhD, RNC, FAAN
Professor, Community and Administrative
  Nursing
Niehoff School of Nursing, Loyola
  University Chicago
Maywood, Illinois

Cindy Angiulo, MSN, RN, Cm
Assistant Administrator, Patient Care
  Services
University of Washington Medical Center
Seattle, Washington

JoAnn Appleyard, PhD, RN
Medical Group Administrator
Kaiser Permanente
South San Francisco, California

Nancy Bair, MSN, RN
Nurse Manager, Clinical Nurse Specialist
Cleveland Clinic Foundation
Cleveland, Ohio

Carolyn A. Benson, MS, RNC, NP
Nurse Practitioner, Neurology Clinic
UMass Memorial Medical Center,
  University Campus
Worcester, Massachusetts

Linda Brixey, RN
Program Manager, Clinical Education
Kelsey-Seybold Clinic
Houston, Texas

Rose Browne, MSN, RN-C
Medical Care Line Manager
VA NY Harbor Health Care System,
  Brooklyn Campus
Brooklyn, New York

Ellen Butensky, MSN, RN, C-PNP
Pediatric Nurse Practitioner/Predoctoral
  Student
University of California at San Francisco
San Francisco, California

Marianne Buzby, MSN, RN, CPNP
Pediatric Nurse Practitioner
The Children's Hospital of Philadelphia
Philadelphia, Pennsylvania

Dorothy A. Calabrese, MSN, RN, CURN, CNP
Nurse Practitioner/Clinical Nurse
  Specialist—Urology/Oncology
Cleveland Clinic Foundation
Cleveland, Ohio

Debra Ann Clementino, JD, MS, RN
Attorney
Plunkett & Cooney, P.C.
Lansing, Michigan

David R. Crumbley, MSN, BS, RN, CWCN
Clinical Nurse Specialist
United States Navy
Roosevelt Roads, Puerto Rico

Linda D'Angelo, MSN, MBA, RN
Chief Operating Officer
Coordinated Care Services
Urbana, Illinois

Mary G. Daymont, MSN, RN
Regional Director, Hospital Services
  Management
Kaiser Permanente
Rockville, Maryland

Pamela S. Del Monte, MS, RN
Clinical Coordinator—Specialties
Kaiser Permanente
Springfield, Virginia

Gail DeLuca, MS, RN, CS, FNP
Instructor, Family Nurse Practitioner
Loyola University Chicago
Chicago, Illinois

Elizabeth Dickey, MPH, RN, FNP
Practice Management Consultant
Tucson, Arizona

Linda Edwards, MHS, RN, CDE
Diabetes Foundation Coordinator
Kaiser Permanente
Denver, Colorado

Maureen Espensen, BSN, RN
Manager, ASK-A-NURSE & Physician
  Referral Services
Rockford Health System
Rockford, Illinois

Kate G. Felix, PhD, RN, CNAA
Administrator
Kaiser Permanente
Denver, Colorado

Carrol Gold, PhD, RN
Associate Professor, Community/Mental
  Health/Administration/Dietetics
Niehoff School of Nursing, Loyola
  University Chicago
Chicago, Illinois

Sheila A. Haas, PhD, RN
Professor and Dean, Niehoff School of
  Nursing
Loyola University Chicago
Chicago, Illinois

Diana P. Hackbarth, PhD, RN
Professor, Community Health Nursing
Loyola University Chicago
Chicago, Illinois

Clare Hastings, PhD, RN
Chief, Nursing and Patient Care Services
National Institutes of Health Clinical Center
Bethesda, Maryland

Margaret B. Hough, MHSA, BSN, RN
Manager, Clinical Nursing Services
University of Michigan Health System
Ann Arbor, Michigan

Lisa Harvatine Ingalls, MSN, RN, CRNP
Pediatric Nurse Practitioner
Milton S. Hershey Medical Center
Hershey, Pennsylvania

Debra L. Janikowski, MSN, RN, CNA
Captain, Nurse Corps, United States Navy
Director of Nursing, Naval Hospital
Camp Lejeune, North Carolina

Patricia Jassak, MS, RN, AOCN
Administrative Director
Illinois Masonic Medical Center
Chicago, Illinois

E. Mary Johnson, RN, BSN, Cm, CNA
Credentialing Consultant, Division of
  Nursing
Cleveland Clinic Foundation
Cleveland, Ohio

Margaret Ross Kraft, MS, RN
Decision Support Coordinator/Program
  Analyst
Hines VA Hospital
Hines, Illinois

Candia Baker Laughlin, MS, RN, Cm
Director, Patient Care Services
University of Michigan Health System
Ann Arbor, Michigan

Margaret Fisk Mastal, PhD, MSN, RN
Chief Operating Officer
Health Services for Children with Special
  Needs, Inc.
Washington, DC

Bobbie McCarthy, RN
Clinic Nurse Int. Med.
Camp Lejeune Naval Hospital
Camp Lejeune, North Carolina

Karole Mourek, PhD, RN
President
Consulo, Inc.
Riverside, Illinois

Suzanne Nelson, MS, RN, C, CNA
Manager, Department of Pediatrics
Ochsner Clinic
New Orleans, Louisiana

Cindy Noa, MS, RN, CNAA
Chief, Immunization Section
Illinois Department of Public Health
Springfield, Illinois

Linda S. Paskiewicz, PhD, CNM, RN
Assistant Professor
Loyola University Chicago
Chicago, Illinois

Rebecca Linn Pyle, MS, RN
Medical Office Administrator
Kaiser Permanente Health Plan
Westminster, Colorado

Joan Robinson, MS, RN, CNAA
Health Care Services Consultant
J. Robinson Consulting
Ann Arbor, Michigan

Patricia A. Rutowski, MSN, RN, CS
Nurse Practitioner
University of Michigan
Ann Arbor, Michigan

Assanatu I. Savage, BSN, RNC, MA
Lieutenant, Nurse Corps, United States
   Navy
Camp Lejeune Naval Hospital
Camp Lejeune, North Carolina

Chris Schaefer, MSN, RN, CDE
Diabetes Care Manager
Kaiser Permanente
Denver, Colorado

Linda Schneider, BSN, RN
Clinical Level IV
The Children's Hospital of Philadelphia
Philadelphia, Pennsylvania

Jan Sheldon, MS, RN, ANP
Adult Nurse Practitioner, Ambulatory Care
Hines VA Hospital
Hines, Illinois

Jane W. Swanson, MS, RN, CNAA
Nursing Doctoral Student
University of Texas Medical Branch
Galveston, Texas

Mary Szyszka, MSN, RN, AOCN
Clinical Support Specialist
Amgen, Inc.
Thousand Oaks, California

Catherine Turner, MSN, FNP, RN
Commander, United States Navy
Naval Hospital
Cherry Point, North Carolina

Carol Jo Wilson, PhD, RN, CS, FNP
Assistant Professor
Loyola University Chicago
Chicago, Illinois

Marcia Winston, MSN, RN, CRNP
Certified Pediatric Nurse Practitioner,
   Division of Pulmonary Medicine
The Children's Hospital of Philadelphia
Philadelphia, Pennsylvania

REVIEWERS

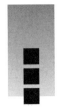

Tania Adkins, MSN, RN
Supervisor, Patient Care Services
Sutter Gould Medical Foundation
Modesto, California

Karen Biancolillo, MBA, BSN, RN
Nurse Manager, Ambulatory Care Clinics
VA NY Harbor Health Care System,
   Brooklyn Campus
Brooklyn, New York

Julie K. Briggs, MHA, BSN, RN
Administrative Director, Emergency
   Services
Good Samaritan Community Healthcare
Puyallup, Washington

Pamela Cittan, MSA, RN
Nurse Manager, Health Center Manager IV
University of Michigan Health System
Livonia, Michigan

Pamela S. Del Monte, MS, RN
Clinical Coordinator, Specialities
Kaiser Permanente
Springfield, Virginia

Telia Emanuel, MHA, RN
Administrator, Patient Care Services
Florida Health Care Plans
Daytona Beach, Florida

Sally Faggella, RN
Coordinator, Pediatrics
Harvard Vanguard Medical Associates
Chelmsford, Massachusetts

Sheila A. Haas, PhD, RN
Professor and Dean, Niehoff School of
   Nursing
Loyola University Chicago
Chicago, Illinois

Margaret B. Hough, MHSA, BSN, RN
Manager, Clinical Nursing Services
University of Michigan Health System
Ann Arbor, Michigan

Debra L. Janikowski, MSN, RN, CNA
Captain, Nurse Corps, United States Navy
Director of Nursing, Naval Hospital
Camp Lejeune, North Carolina

Lorry Johnson, MS, RN, CNA
Administrator, Nursing Services
Rice Medical Center
Stevens Point, Wisconsin

Reena Kakka, PharmD, BS
Clinical Pharmacist
Stanford Hospitals and Clinics
Stanford, Connecticut

Shirley Kedrowski, MSN, RN
Project Manager, Ambulatory Care
Stanford Hospitals and Clinics
Stanford, California

Nancy R. Kowal, MSN, RN, C, ANP
Pain Consultant
University of Massachusetts Memorial
   Health Care System
Worcester, Massachusetts

Kathleen Krone, MS, RN
Project Consultant, Psychiatric/Mental
   Health Nursing
University of Michigan Health System
Ann Arbor, Michigan

Helen Leavy, PhD, MSN, CCRN, TNS
Charge Nurse, Telephone Triage
University of New Mexico Health Sciences
   Center
Albuquerque, New Mexico

Ann Lockhart, MN, RN
Administrator, Ambulatory Nursing
   Services
Ochsner Clinic
New Orleans, Louisiana

Anita Markovich, MSN, MPA, RN
Clinical Director, Ambulatory Care
Practice Director, Primary Care Network
Lourdes Hospital
Binghamton, New York

Cathy J. Martin, MSN, RN
Ambulatory Care Director, Clinical Services
Kelsey-Seybold Clinic
Houston, Texas

Cheryl L. Martin, MS, RN, C
Clinical Administrator
Westchester Medical Center
Valhalla, New York

Margaret Fish Mastal, PhD, MSN, RN
Chief Operating Officer
Health Services for Children with Special
    Needs, Inc.
Washington, DC

Penny Meeker, BS, RN
Director, Communications Center and
    Patient Advisory Nurse Department
Carle Clinic Association
Urbana, Illinois

Maryalice Morro, MSN, RN
Head, Health Promotion
Naval Hospital Charleston
Charleston, South Carolina

Cindy Noa, MS, RN, CNAA
Chief, Immunization Section
Illinois Department of Public Health
Springfield, Illinois

Laura Shouse, BSN, RN, CEN
Director, Physician Operations
Sutter Gould Medical Foundation
Modesto, California

Vicki Siebs, MSN, RN
Director of Nursing
Saint Luke's Shawnee Mission Medical
    Group/Saint Luke's South Primary Care
Overland Park, Kansas

Carralee Sueppel, MSN, RN, CURN
Urology Nurse Consultant, Continence Care
    Nurse
Physician's Clinic of Iowa—Urology
Cedar Rapids, Iowa

Jane W. Swanson, MS, RN, CNAA
Nursing Doctoral Student
Universtiy of Texas Medical Branch
Galveston, Texas

Carol Hricz Townsend, MSN, GNP, CS
Geriatric nurse Practitioner
Gainesville Clinic at VA
Gainesville, Florida

Cathy Turner, MSN, FNP, RN
Commander, United States Navy
Naval Hospital
Cherry Point, North Carolina

Sally Walker, RN
Director, Telephone Triage Services of
    Covenant Health System of Iowa
Covenant Medical Center
Waterloo, Iowa

Kristin Hardy Wicking, MSN, RN
Adjunct Faculty/Clinical Instructor
Palomar College
San Diego, Callifornia

PREFACE

■ ■ This first edition of *Core Curriculum for Ambulatory Care Nursing* is intended as a state-of-the-art document on ambulatory care nursing. The text addresses the challenge of identifying the context of patient care delivery and the content of the nursing role dimensions, specifying in greater detail those unique to ambulatory care nursing. The American Academy of Ambulatory Care Nursing (AAACN) has stated that ambulatory care nursing takes place on an episodic basis, is less than 24 hours in duration, and occurs in a variety of settings. The focus of ambulatory care nursing services encompasses cost-effective ways to assist patients in promoting wellness, preventing illness, and managing acute and chronic disease to effect the most attainable positive health status, over the life span (AAACN, 2000). As patient care continues to move to ambulatory care settings, the demand for nurses to work in ambulatory care organizations is growing.

Core Curriculum for Ambulatory Care Nursing will serve as a resource to advance the art and science of ambulatory care nursing practice. This text will be valuable to nurses who wish to work in ambulatory care settings and to those who wish to demonstrate their expertise in ambulatory care nursing practice. The impetus for this text was the decision of the American Nurses Credentialing Center to offer an Ambulatory Care Nursing Certification Examination in 1999.

The audience for this text includes nurses preparing for certification in the specialty practice of ambulatory care nursing. In addition, other nurses will find the text invaluable. Managers in ambulatory care settings can use this text as a unit resource. Staff educators can use this text as a resource for clinicians and the basis of orientation and continuing education. The text will answer questions and provide insights for nurses transitioning into ambulatory care and/or nurses transitioning within ambulatory care subunits. Schools of nursing preparing future nurse clinicians can use this text to enhance an understanding of a unique nursing role and new practice environment.

The organization of the text is based on the Ambulatory Care Nursing Conceptual Framework, which was developed by an AAACN "think tank" in 1998 (Haas, 1998). The AAACN Think Tank identified areas of knowledge and skill in ambulatory care nursing practice and how the areas related to each other. This conceptual framework depicts the scope of ambulatory care nursing practice. It identifies the nurse and the patient population as the two major concepts. The framework recognizes three roles of the ambulatory care nurse: organizational/systems role, clinical role, and professional role. The three sections of the text correspond to the three roles. The core concepts, knowledge, and skill dimensions for each role are developed within the sections.

Section One contains ten chapters that describe the core knowledge and skills of the organizational/systems role. Section Two contains eleven chapters. Ten practice areas with two to four patient prototypes per chapter are used to illustrate the clinical role dimensions. The use of specific patient prototypes demonstrates the clinical role dimensions of the nurse and the typical patient care demands/needs encountered by the ambulatory care nurse. The final chapter in the clinical section is an expanded chapter on telehealth nursing practice. Each of the preceding clinical chapters discusses the role dimension of telephone nursing practice from a specific practice perspective. This final chapter addresses the overall parameters of telehealth nursing practice and significant issues affecting practice in this growing ambulatory care nursing practice area. Section Three speaks to the core knowledge and skill dimensions that are part of the professional role.

The chapters are presented in outline format for easy review and reference. References are available for each chapter. Although effort has been made to provide a current validated knowledge base, this text is not intended to be a sole reference source. Readers are advised to recognize the dynamic nature of knowledge in health care and to tap additional resources, including those available for other specialty organizations.

This text is a collaborative effort of many contributing authors and reviewers representing various practice settings and regions of the United States. The goal of having diverse contributors was to provide an inclusive view of the roles of the ambulatory care nurse. The reader may see occasional language differences based on various settings and parts of the country. For example, some authors refer to clients whereas others refer to patients. Many thanks go to all the authors and reviewers that have made this text possible. Thanks also to the leadership of the AAACN who have provided the vision for this text.

Joan Robinson

REFERENCES

American Academy of Ambulatory Care Nursing (2000): *Ambulatory care nursing administration and practice standards.* Pitman, NJ: Author.

Haas S (1998): Ambulatory care nursing conceptual framework. *AAACN Viewpoint* 20(3):16-17.

ACKNOWLEDGMENTS

The development of this publication is the result of the expertise and hard work of a large number of people who served as authors and reviewers. It has been a privilege to work with each one of them in the development of this text. They have been responsive and committed to the need for this core curriculum.

In addition, I would like to thank individuals who have been helpful and supportive through the development of this text from a vision to a reality. I thank Sheila Haas who provided both vision and practical support from the proposal for the text and the conceptual framework to this end product. I thank Cynthia Nowicki for her encouragement, advice, and sustained humor as we addressed little snags along the way. I thank Lisa Astorga for providing her expertise in incorporating and tracking the chapters and revisions into the text and her positive attitude throughout. I thank Patrica Hettwer for her painstaking efforts to pull the concept words for a glossary to assist the reader. I thank my husband, David, for his ongoing support and encouragement throughout this project. Lastly, I thank the leadership of the AAACN and particularly the Board Liaisons, Candia Laughlin and Kathleen Krone, for the privilege of serving as editor for this important work.

Joan Robinson

CONTENTS

THE ORGANIZATIONAL/ SYSTEMS ROLE OF THE AMBULATORY CARE NURSE

1 Ambulatory Care Nursing Specialty Practice

SHEILA A. HAAS, PhD, RN

OBJECTIVES

Study of the information presented in this chapter will enable the learner to:

1. Discuss the characteristics of ambulatory care nursing practice.

2. Differentiate ambulatory care nursing practice from other forms of specialty nursing practice.

3. Discuss the ambulatory care nursing conceptual framework.

4. Enumerate opportunities for nurses in ambulatory care nursing.

5. Discuss ambulatory care standards.

■■ Ambulatory care nursing is a unique realm of nursing practice. It is characterized by rapid, focused assessments of patients, long-term nurse/patient/family relationships, and teaching and translating prescriptions for care into doable activities for patients and their caregivers. Ambulatory care nursing is a specialty practice area that is characterized by nurses responding rapidly to high volumes of patients in a short span of time while dealing with issues that are not always predictable. Because ambulatory care nursing spans all populations of patients and care ranges from wellness/prevention to illness and support of the dying, there is a need for an ambulatory care nursing conceptual framework that specifies: (1) the concepts unique to ambulatory care nursing, and (2) how these core concepts are linked in ambulatory care nursing practice. Ambulatory care nursing provides multiple opportunities as well as challenges for nurses. It offers great interdisciplinary as well as autonomous practice opportunities. It demands that ambulatory care nurses develop processes and procedures that meet the needs of ambulatory care patients. Ambulatory care standards define the structure and process of ambulatory care nursing.

CHARACTERISTICS OF AMBULATORY CARE NURSING PRACTICE

Characteristics are unique features of ambulatory care nursing practice.

    A. Differences between ambulatory care nursing and inpatient nursing practice are often overlooked.

   B. Assumptions are made that practice styles, policies, and approaches used in inpatient care apply equally in ambulatory care, when in fact they often do not.
   C. Ambulatory care focuses on the individual patient, with some population-based care protocols versus population-focused public health practice.
   D. Focus groups (Haas, 1994) of experienced ambulatory care nurses identified the following characteristics of nursing practice in ambulatory care:
   1. Nursing autonomy.
   2. Patient advocacy.
   3. Skillful rapid assessment.
   4. Holistic nursing care.
   5. Client teaching.
   6. Wellness and health promotion.
   7. Coordination and continuity of care.
   8. Long-term relationships with patients and families.
   9. Telephone triage, instruction, and advice.
   10. Patient and family control as major caregivers, users of the health care systems, and decision-makers regarding compliance with care regimen.
   11. Collaboration with other health care providers.
   12. Case management.
   E. Challenges and characteristics of ambulatory care nursing evolve from each of the following:
   1. Control of care by patient and family.
   2. Timing pressure where visits are short and assessment time is compressed.
   3. The need for collaboration where roles are less clear.
   4. Use of communication devices as alternatives to face-to-face encounters for clinical practice.
   5. Desire to standardize care delivered.

DEFINITION OF AMBULATORY CARE NURSING

The definition of ambulatory care nursing must delineate the scope and unique dimensions of ambulatory care nursing practice and differentiate ambulatory care nursing from other areas of specialty nursing practice.
   A. Traditional definition of ambulatory care nursing.
   1. Ambulatory care nursing defined by practice setting such as HMO, physician group practice, and hospital/clinic.
   2. Ambulatory care nurse would see patients who were generally nonacute and able to walk in for appointments.
   3. Ambulatory care nursing defined by length of care episode (less than 24 hours).
   B. Today, ambulatory care nursing is defined in terms of:
   1. Wellness or functional goals.
   2. Patient expectations.
   3. Setting and encounter.

C. Definition of ambulatory care nursing (AAACN/ANA, 1997).
   1. Ambulatory care nursing includes clinical, management, educational, and research activities.
   2. Ambulatory care nurses work with patients who seek care for health promotion, health maintenance, or health-related problems.
   3. Ambulatory care patients provide their own care or have family or significant others as caregivers.
   4. Ambulatory care nursing encounters are episodic and are less than 24 hours in duration. Encounters may occur singly or in a series lasting days/weeks/months/years.
   5. Ambulatory care nursing sites are community-based in hospitals, schools, workplaces, or homes.
   6. Ambulatory care nursing encounters may occur face-to-face or via telephone or other communication device.
   7. Ambulatory care nursing services focus on cost-effective ways to maximize wellness and to prevent illness, disability, and disease.
   8. Ambulatory care nursing services also support patients in management of chronic disease to effect more positive health states throughout the lifespan up to and including a peaceful death (AAACN/ANA, 1997).

DEVELOPMENT OF AN AMBULATORY CARE NURSING CONCEPTUAL FRAMEWORK

To guide the education/orientation of nurses who wish to work in ambulatory care and to assist nurses wishing to demonstrate their expertise in ambulatory care, a simple, concise blueprint of ambulatory care nursing practice is essential.

A. A conceptual framework is a diagram that specifies:
   1. Essential major concepts and skills in an area of practice.
   2. Relationships between major content and skill areas.
B. An ambulatory care nursing conceptual framework can assist in:
   1. The design of ambulatory care delivery models.
   2. Development of educational materials for ambulatory care nursing.
   3. Development of testing materials for certification.
   4. Development of orientation programs for ambulatory care nursing.
   5. Development of performance appraisal instruments for ambulatory care nurses.
C. American Academy of Ambulatory Care Nursing (AAACN) Ambulatory Care Conceptual Framework was developed by an AAACN expert member "think tank" in 1998.
   1. AAACN Think Tank Group used a nominal group approach to delineate major areas of practice, knowledge, and skills.
   2. The Group identified 61 core areas of knowledge and skills.
   3. Group members specified how these 61 areas were related to each other and the ambulatory care nurse role.
   4. The 61 areas were categorized under three roles that are a part of every

ambulatory care nurse's practice. Ambulatory care nurses practice within the organization/system's role when they manage and coordinate resources and workflow in their setting; they practice within the professional role as they continuously practice according to standards, evaluate the outcomes of practice, develop themselves and other staff; and finally, they practice in the clinical role as they provide care within each of the clinical dimensions.

   a. Organizational/systems role.

     (1) Practice/office support.

     (2) Health care fiscal management (reimbursement and coding).

     (3) Collaboration/conflict management.

     (4) Informatics (i.e., management of information and data that become information).

     (5) Context of care delivery/models.

     (6) Care of the caregiver.

     (7) Priority management/delegation/supervision.

     (8) Ambulatory culture/cross cultural competencies.

     (9) Ongoing political/entrepreneurial skills.

     (10) Structuring customer-focused systems.

     (11) Workplace regulatory compliance (EEOC, OSHA).

     (12) Advocacy interorganizational and in community.

     (13) Legal issues.

     (14) Workload

   b. Professional role.

     (1) Evidence-based practice.

     (2) Leadership inquiry and research utilization.

     (3) Clinical quality improvement.

     (4) Staff development.

     (5) Regulatory compliance (risk management).

     (6) Provider self-care.

     (7) Ethics.

   c. Clinical nursing role.

     (1) Patient education.

     (2) Advocacy.

     (3) Care management.

     (4) Assess, screen, triage.

     (5) Telephone nursing practice.

     (6) Collaboration/resource identification and referral.

     (7) Clinical procedures, independent/interdependent/dependent.

     (8) Primary, secondary, and tertiary prevention.

     (9) Communication/documentation.

     (10) Outcome management.

     (11) Protocol development/usage.

5. Core knowledge and skill dimensions that are a part of the clinical role are also related to the patient populations served.

   a. Think Tank members defined ambulatory patient populations in categories of well, acute, chronic, and terminally ill.

b. Think Tank members defined characteristics of ambulatory patient populations:
   (1) Patient/family/significant other initiates encounter/visit.
   (2) Patient/family/significant other lives in the community.
   (3) Patient/family/significant other collaborates with ambulatory interdisciplinary team regarding treatment regime.
   (4) Patient/family/significant other manages and provides health care between visits.
   (5) Patient/family/significant other controls health care decisions and has choices.
   (6) Patient/family/significant other can have long-term relationships with ambulatory care providers.
c. Think Tank members recognized that ambulatory care patient populations may also be defined in terms of:
   (1) Age (e.g., pediatrics, gerontology).
   (2) Health states or illness categories, (e.g., primary care, cardiac clinic, diabetes clinic, oncology clinic).
   (3) Type of reimbursement (e.g., capitation versus fee-for-service).
   (4) Source of reimbursement (e.g., Medicare, Medicaid, private insurance, federal employee, TriService).
d. Ambulatory Care Nursing Conceptual Framework (ACNCF) (Figure 1-1).
   (1) Within the roles (clinical, organizational, and professional) specified in the Ambulatory Care Nursing Conceptual Framework depicted in Figure 1-1, the nurse modifies the nursing process to meet the needs of patient populations.
   (2) Ambulatory patient population health status:
      (a) Well or essentially healthy.
      (b) Acutely ill but otherwise healthy (e.g., patient with ear infections, appendicitis).
      (c) Chronically ill (e.g., patient with diabetes, heart disease); chronically ill persons can have acute illness and/or exacerbations of chronic disease, (e.g., the diabetic with the flu who also has hypoglycemia).
      (d) Terminally ill, (e.g., patient with end-stage liver failure).
      (e) Ambulatory patients can exhibit more than one of these states simultaneously.
      (f) Ambulatory nurses must be cognizant of all operative health states for patients encountered.
   (3) The ACNCF in Figure 1-1 assumes the patient's health status to be dynamic and to change between encounters such that persons with an acute illness at one encounter may be well at the next and that a chronically ill patient may have an acute exacerbation at intervals.
   (4) The ACNCF in Figure 1-1 represents characteristics of a patient's health status at the encounter and for the duration of care initiated at the encounter.

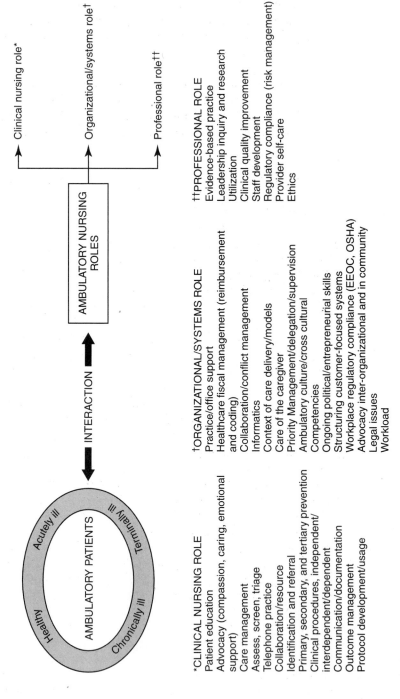

Clinical nursing role*

Organizational/systems role†

Professional role††

AMBULATORY NURSING ROLES

INTERACTION

AMBULATORY PATIENTS

Healthy

Acutely ill

Terminally ill

Chronically ill

*CLINICAL NURSING ROLE
Patient education
Advocacy (compassion, caring, emotional support)
Care management
Assess, screen, triage
Telephone practice
Collaboration/resource
Identification and referral
Primary, secondary, and tertiary prevention
Clinical procedures, independent/interdependent/dependent
Communication/documentation
Outcome management
Protocol development/usage

†ORGANIZATIONAL/SYSTEMS ROLE
Practice/office support
Healthcare fiscal management (reimbursement and coding)
Collaboration/conflict management
Informatics
Context of care delivery/models
Care of the caregiver
Priority Management/delegation/supervision
Ambulatory culture/cross cultural
Competencies
Ongoing political/entrepreneurial skills
Structuring customer-focused systems
Workplace regulatory compliance (EEOC, OSHA)
Advocacy inter-organizational and in community
Legal issues
Workload

††PROFESSIONAL ROLE
Evidence-based practice
Leadership inquiry and research
Utilization
Clinical quality improvement
Staff development
Regulatory compliance (risk management)
Provider self-care
Ethics

FIGURE 1-1 ■ Ambulatory Care Nursing Conceptual Framework (Adapted from Haas, S [1998]. Ambulatory care nursing conceptual framework. *Viewpoint* 20[3]: 16-17.)

(5) The ACNCF in Figure 1-1 assumes that the overall goals of ambulatory care nurses are:
  (a) To foster and maintain health.
  (b) To prevent illness.
  (c) To diagnose illness early and treat effectively.
  (d) To prevent complications and initiate rehabilitation early to regain optimal functioning.
(6) The ACNCF in Figure 1-1 assumes that persons at all stages of health-illness in this continuum could benefit from nursing interventions at all three levels of prevention (Leavell & Clark, 1965): primary prevention, secondary prevention, and tertiary prevention.
  (a) The three levels of prevention are the classic framework for organizing health promotion and disease prevention used by nurses and physicians.
  (b) Primary prevention includes health promotion (HP) interventions and specific protections (SP); it may be directed at individuals, groups, or populations; targeted at well populations or those already ill (e.g., HP = nutrition education, or sex education; SP = use of seat belts, avoidance of allergens, or inoculations).
  (c) Secondary prevention involves early diagnosis and prompt treatment to avoid disability (e.g., screening, biopsies, medication, surgery).
  (d) Tertiary prevention involves rehabilitation to return maximum use of remaining capacities (speech, occupational, physical therapy).
(7) Addressing simultaneously the concurrent needs of patients across the wellness-illness continuum is required of ambulatory care nurses, for example:
  (a) In the clinical role.
    (i) Patient education dimension: the nurse understands that although chronically ill, patients still require wellness education.
    (ii) Case management dimension: the nurse recognizes that cost effectiveness is maximized if case management protocols are implemented for chronically or terminally ill, but case management protocols can also enhance recovery, prevent complications, and decrease costs in acute illnesses.
  (b) In the organizational role.
    (i) Management dimension: The nurse understands that reimbursement for some interventions may differ if the patient is acutely ill versus well at the time of the encounter.
    (ii) Care of the caregiver dimension: Although ambulatory nurses are attuned for caregivers of chronically or terminally ill patients, they also work with caregivers of

acutely ill patients who need counsel, advice to see them through an exhausting acute illness.

(c) In the professional role.

(i) Evidence-based practice dimension: The nurse understands that protocols can be applied to health promotion for well populations as well as treatment interventions for the chronically or terminally ill.

(ii) Staff development dimension: Ambulatory care nurses are responsive to needs of staff for development in areas of new therapies and pharmacologic agents for acute or chronically ill patients but also aware of needs for staff development in use of therapies and drugs for palliative care of the terminally ill.

6. All AAACN members had opportunity to review the ambulatory care nursing conceptual framework and provide feedback on how well it represented the reality of ambulatory care nursing practice.

7. The ambulatory care nursing conceptual framework was used to organize the content for this Core Curriculum text.

8. Benefits of use of the ambulatory care nursing conceptual framework include:

a. Provides clarity of the nursing role dimensions versus role dimensions of other health care providers.

b. Reflects the uniqueness of the ambulatory care nursing role.

c. Provides a resource for developers of performance standards and competency measures.

d. Acts as a catalyst for further refinement of the role.

CHANGE CREATES OPPORTUNITIES FOR NURSES IN AMBULATORY CARE

A. Movement of U.S. health care system from specialty-based acute care to primary care-oriented ambulatory care offers diverse opportunities for ambulatory care nurses.

1. Primary care clinic nurses.

2. Nurse practitioners and nurse midwives.

3. Nurse educators for wellness, health promotion, and disease prevention.

B. Movement from fee-for-service to capitated payment systems offers opportunities.

1. Nurse case managers.

2. Telephone nursing practice.

a. Cost-effective: decreases number of patient visits.

b. Increases patient satisfaction.

c. Enhances rapidity of response to patient problems.

3. Nurse specialist (e.g., breast care, gastroenterology, wound care, skin care).

C. Movement of acute-care into ambulatory settings offers opportunities.

1. Ambulatory oncology care.

2. Ambulatory surgery, nurse anesthetists, and post-anesthesia recovery.
3. Ambulatory pediatrics.
4. Day hospitals for psychiatric patients.
5. Nurse managed clinics (anticoagulation clinics, wound care clinics, incontinence clinics).

D. There is potential for regulations to require use of RNs in ambulatory care, for example, need for RNs to monitor/evaluate conscious sedation patients.

E. Increasing demand for nurse managers in ambulatory settings.
   1. Demand for nurse managers in areas where strict adherence to quality standards is paramount.
   2. Physician group practice management.
   3. Supervision of assistive personnel.
   4. Supervision of telephone practice centers.
   5. Supervision of high-risk, high-volume procedure areas.

F. Preparation for these emerging opportunities includes:
   1. Patient teaching methods and strategies for health promotion as well as disease prevention and disease treatment.
   2. Understanding of community resources.
   3. Expertise with specific patient populations.
   4. Care management skills.
   5. Telephone nursing practice knowledge and skills.
   6. Experience with acute care nursing modalities (critical care, OR, PACU).
   7. Understanding of health care payment methods.

G. Resources to assist in preparation for opportunities:
   1. Formal coursework in undergraduate and graduate nursing programs.
   2. Continuing education programming offered through professional organizations such as AAACN, ONS, AORN.
   3. Readings in professional journals.
   4. Programming available on Internet/cable TV.

H. Nurses currently working in ambulatory care will also provide opportunities through:
   1. Design changes in nursing practice systems in ambulatory care.
   2. Alterations in role and job descriptions for ambulatory care nurses.
   3. Enhanced ambulatory care nursing experiences for nursing students.

AMBULATORY CARE NURSING ADMINISTRATION AND PRACTICE STANDARDS

A. Standards promote effective management of increasingly complex ambulatory care nursing roles and responsibilities in a changing health care environment.
   1. The AAACN Ambulatory Care Nursing Administration and Practice Standards are in their fourth edition.
   2. The first edition of the AAACN Telephone Nursing Practice Administration and Practice Standards was published in 1997.
   3. The AAACN Standards are the result of collaborative effort of nurses from an array of ambulatory settings in a variety of geographic locations.

    4. Ambulatory care nursing values are reflected in the AAACN standards. The AAACN values* are:

      a. Shared responsibility among patients, families, and other members of the health care team in all phases of the episode of health care.

      b. Education to enable patients and families to understand and make informed decisions.

      c. Continuity of care.

      d. Excellence in care that balances patient needs, cost-effectiveness, outcomes, and appropriate resource utilization.

      e. The opportunity to serve as a patient advocate.

B. Definitions. Used as the common foundation in the development of standards.[†]

    1. *Standard*—is an authoritative statement developed and disseminated by a professional organization or governmental or regulatory agency by which the quality of practice, services, research, or education can be judged.

    2. *Patient*—an individual who requests or receives nursing services. Also called client, consumer, member, or customer in many settings.

    3. *Family*—family members are defined by the patient in his/her own terms and may include individuals related by blood or marriage, or in self-defined relationships. (This definition is intended to include the family in nursing care as appropriate. It is *not* intended as a legal definition of family.)

    4. *Nursing staff*—staff members who participate in delivering nursing care. These staff are either registered nurses or are supervised by a registered nurse.

    5. *Health care team*—includes the patient, family, and other members of the health care system who are involved in the development and implementation of the care plan.

    6. *Nursing services*—organized services delivered to groups of patients by nursing staff. Includes nursing care as well as services to support or facilitate direct care, such as referral and coordination of care.

C. Components of each standard.

    1. Standard statement.

    2. Rationale: a concise statement of the underlying reason for the standard.

    3. Measurement criteria: specific, measurable indicators that can demonstrate compliance with the standard.

D. Assumptions.

    1. Ambulatory care nurses use AAACN standards and nursing practice standards developed by professional nursing organizations such as the

---

*From American Academy of Ambulatory Care Nursing (2000). *Ambulatory Care Nursing Administration and Practice Standards.* Pitman, NJ: Anthony J. Jannetti.

†From American Academy of Ambulatory Care Nursing (2000). *Ambulatory Care Nursing Administration and Practice Standards.* Pitman, NJ: Anthony J. Jannetti.

■ BOX 1-1
■ **AMBULATORY CARE NURSING ADMINISTRATION AND PRACTICE STANDARDS**

Standard I. Structure and Organization of Ambulatory Care Nursing
Ambulatory care nursing is based on a philosophy committed to the delivery of efficient, cost-effective, and quality nursing care.

Standard II. Staffing
The foundation of an adequate staffing plan is determined by patient care indicators, organizational outcomes, and the quality of work life of the professional ambulatory care nurse.

Standard III. Competency
Professional ambulatory care nurses demonstrate knowledge and skills necessary to complete their assigned responsibilities.

Standard IV. Ambulatory Nursing Practice
The nursing process is the foundation used by professional ambulatory care nurses in making clinical decisions as they assess and identify patient health status, establish outcomes, plan, implement, and evaluate the care they provide.

Standard V. Continuity of Care
Ambulatory care nurses facilitate continuity of care utilizing the nursing process, interdisciplinary collaboration, and coordination of all appropriate health care services, including available community resources.

Standard VI. Ethics and Patient Rights
Ambulatory care nurses recognize the dignity, diversity, and worth of individuals and families, respect individual cultural, spiritual, and psychosocial differences, and apply philosophical and ethical concepts that promote access to care, equality, and continuity of care.

Standard VII. Environment
Professional ambulatory care nurses participate in a coordinated system-wide process that creates and maintains a safe, comfortable, and hazard-free therapeutic environment for patients, visitors, and staff.

Standard VIII. Research
Professional ambulatory care nurses conduct and participate in clinical and health care systems research. Valid research findings are disseminated and used to improve patient care and organizational effectiveness.

Standard IX. Quality Management
The quality management process is coordinated and integrated with that of the organization and includes the continuous assessment, evaluation, and improvement of the quality and appropriateness of ambulatory care nursing. Ambulatory care nursing leaders set expectations, provide resources and training, foster communication and coordination, and participate in improvement activities.

From American Academy of Ambulatory are Nursing (2000): *Ambulatory care nursing administration and practice standards.* Pitman, NJ: Anthony J. Jannetti.

■ BOX 1-2
■ **TELEPHONE NURSING PRACTICE ADMINISTRATION AND PRACTICE STANDARDS**

Standard I. Structure and Organization of Telephone Nursing
Telephone nursing practice is based on a philosophy committed to the goals of delivering quality, cost-effective, and safe nursing care. Maintaining a balance of focus between these goals is critical. Cost-effectiveness is achieved by the provision of quality nursing care services through telephone encounter(s) with patients or their families.

Standard II. Staffing
Sufficient numbers of qualified registered nursing staff are available to meet the quantity and complexity of patients' needs for telephone encounters.

Standard III. Competency
Telephone nurses demonstrate the knowledge and skills necessary to provide safe and effective telephone nursing care and service.

Standard IV. Use of the Nursing Process in Telephone Nursing Practice
Registered nurses use the nursing process as a framework to determine and provide the delivery of health care through telephone encounters with patients and their families.

Standard V. Continuity of Care
Telephone nurses facilitate continuity of care through the nursing process, interdisciplinary collaboration, and coordination of appropriate health care services, including available community resources.

Standard VI. Ethics and Patient Rights
Telephone nursing practice recognizes the dignity and worth of individuals; respects cultural, spiritual, and psychosocial differences; and applies philosophical and ethical concepts with patients' rights to ensure quality and continuity of care.

Standard VII. Environment
Telephone nursing practice is conducted in a hazard-free, safe, comfortable, and efficient environment for staff. Staff are protected from harassment from any source of any type. If there is the potential for telephone nurses to also see patients in walk-in situations, the environment is safe for patients and the face-to-face nurse interactions.

Standard VIII. Research
Telephone nurses participate in clinical and health care systems research. Research findings are used to improve telephone nursing practice, patient care, organizational effectiveness, individual nursing competency, and quality performance.

Standard IX. Quality Management
The quality management process is coordinated and integrated with the overall organization's quality improvement program. The quality management process includes: continuous assessment, evaluation, and improvement of the quality and appropriateness of telephone nursing practice. Telephone nursing leaders set both individual and group expectations, provide resources and training, foster communication and coordination, and participate in quality improvement activities. Telephone nursing leaders will identify and apply current telephone nursing practice benchmarks to organizational goals and expectations.

From American Academy of Ambulatory Care Nursing (1997): *Telephone nursing practice administration and practice standards.* Pitman, NJ: Anthony J. Jannetti.

American Nurses' Association (ANA), Oncology Nursing Society (ONS), Emergency Nurses Association (ENA), and Association of Operating Room Nurses (AORN) for care specific to patient populations.

2. Ambulatory care nurses also use Clinical Practice Guidelines developed by federal agencies such as the Agency for Health Care Policy and Research (AHCPR) to guide care for specific patient populations. AHCPR guidelines can be obtained via the Internet at http://www.ahcpr.gov/clinic/ngcfact.htm

E. Purposes for use of Ambulatory Care Nursing and Administration Practice Standards:
1. Provide guidance for the structure and processes in delivery of ambulatory care nursing.
2. Serves as a guide for provision of quality patient care.
3. Facilitates professional nursing development.
4. Facilitates evaluation of professional nursing performance.
5. Stimulates participation in research and use of research findings.
6. Serves as a guide for quality management.
7. Serves as a guide for ethics and patient advocacy.

F. Content addressed in standards:
1. Environment.
2. Resources (human and material).
3. Competency.
4. Quality of care.
5. Collaboration.
6. Ethics.
7. Research.
8. Education.
9. Nursing practice.
10. Performance evaluation.

G. Nine AAACN Ambulatory Care Nursing Administration and Practice Standards (Box 1-1).

H. Nine AAACN Telephone Nursing Practice and Administration Standards (Box 1-2).

REFERENCES

American Academy of Ambulatory Care Nursing (2000): *Ambulatory care nursing administration and practice standards.* Pitman, N.J: Anthony J. Jannetti.

American Academy of Ambulatory Care Nursing and American Nurses' Association (1997): *Nursing in ambulatory care: the future is here.* Washington, DC: American Nurses Publishing.

American Academy of Ambulatory Care Nursing (1997): *Telephone nursing practice administration and practice standards.* Pitman, N.J.: Anthony J. Jannetti.

Haas S (1998): Ambulatory care nursing conceptual framework. *Viewpoint* 20(3):16-17.

Leavell H, Clark E (1965): *Preventive medicine for the doctor in his community: an epidemiologic approach.* New York: McGraw-Hill.

2 The Ambulatory Care Practice Arena

CLARE HASTINGS, PhD, RN

OBJECTIVES

Study of the information presented in this chapter will enable the learner to:

1. Describe the domain of ambulatory care nursing practice.

2. Discuss the characteristics of patients seen in ambulatory care and the implications for nursing practice.

3. Compare nursing practice in ambulatory and acute inpatient settings.

4. Identify and describe current practice settings for ambulatory care nursing.

5. Discuss challenges faced by nurses moving from inpatient to ambulatory care settings and describe strategies to facilitate the transition.

■■ Nurses in ambulatory care practice in a diverse and changing environment. As health care increasingly moves out of the acute care hospital and into the community and home settings, nurses looking to ambulatory care as a practice setting find a broad array of possible settings, roles, and opportunities. It is important for nurses practicing in ambulatory care to be aware both of the diversity in roles and practice settings as well as the common themes that are present across ambulatory practice settings. This chapter will provide nurses in ambulatory care with an overview of the broad domain of ambulatory practice and clarify the common factors that occur in all ambulatory care settings. The differences between ambulatory and inpatient practice and the often unexpected challenges faced by nurses transitioning from traditional inpatient roles to ambulatory care will also be discussed. An understanding of the effect of the practice setting on nursing practice is important to enable nurses to effectively contribute to the health care team. Significant content in this chapter is abstracted with permission from the monograph *Nursing in Ambulatory Care: The Future is Here* (American Academy of Ambulatory Care Nursing and American Nurses' Association, 1997).

THE DOMAIN OF AMBULATORY NURSING PRACTICE

The domain of ambulatory nursing practice is defined as the overall scope of nursing practice in the ambulatory arena. It includes attributes of the environment in which practice occurs, patient requirements for care, and specific nursing role dimensions.

  A. The movement of health care out of the hospital.

    1. Fueled by changes in reimbursement.

      a. Prospective payment for inpatient services has compressed hospital length of stay and pushed care into the ambulatory setting.

      b. Growth of HMOs and managed care has created incentives for keeping patients out of the hospital.

      c. Growth of population-based and capitated care has placed increased emphasis on preventive services, which are often provided in the ambulatory setting.

      d. Growth of 23-hour short stay units has increased use of outpatient observation or short-stay status as alternatives to an inpatient admission.

    2. Further speeded by changes in technology.

      a. Minimally invasive surgical techniques that shorten recovery time.

      b. Improved methods for short-term anesthesia that shorten recovery time which allow more procedures to be performed on an outpatient basis.

      c. Innovations in vascular access and intravenous pump technologies that allow patients to remain out of the hospital during long-term intravenous therapy.

    3. Early discharge creates the requirement for ambulatory follow-up, often in combination with home health visits.

      a. Enhanced surgical techniques have shortened stays, but recovery still must be monitored, drains removed, wound healing assessed.

      b. Shortened hospital stays mean that pre- and post-intervention patient education and support must be done on an ambulatory basis.

    4. Advances in the care of chronically ill patients.

      a. A growing elderly population requires ongoing ambulatory treatment, monitoring, and follow-up for chronic illness.

      b. Ambulatory infusion centers are used as alternatives to inpatient care.

      c. Outpatient invasive testing and treatment centers allow much of the ongoing care for severe chronic illness (heart disease, cancer, renal failure) to be provided in an ambulatory care setting.

      d. Nurses are becoming involved in multidisciplinary disease management teams for the chronically ill.

  B. Descriptions of the domain of ambulatory nursing.

    1. Early literature on ambulatory nursing role changes in the 1970s. (Johnston, 1980; Marzalek, 1980).

      a. Appearance of anecdotal descriptions noting the differences between inpatient and ambulatory nursing.

      b. Descriptions of underutilization and downward substitution of nurses.

      c. New efforts to understand ambulatory nursing as a distinct specialty practice area in nursing.

2. Verran's Taxonomy of Ambulatory Care Nursing Practice (Verran, 1981).
   a. First attempt to systematically describe the role of professional nurses in ambulatory care.
   b. First time that a distinct domain of practice for ambulatory nursing was proposed.
   c. Taxonomy formed the basis for several studies of the role dimensions of nurses in ambulatory care (Tighe, et al., 1985; Hastings and Muir-Nash, 1989; Bunting, 1994).
   d. Taxonomy also became the basis for attempts to classify nursing care requirements in ambulatory care and measure nursing intensity (Hastings, 1987; Parrinello, Brenner, and Vallone, 1988).
3. American Academy of Ambulatory Care Nursing.
   a. Only professional nursing organization with a focus on nursing practice in ambulatory care.
   b. Clearinghouse for information and consensus on the role of nursing in ambulatory care.
   c. Published Standards of Administration and Practice (AAACN, 2000), telephone practice standards (AAACN, 1997), and the monograph *Ambulatory Care Nursing: The Future is Here* (AAACN and ANA, 1997).
4. Recent research and conceptual development.
   a. Ambulatory nursing role dimensions (Hackbarth, et al., 1995).
   b. Ambulatory nursing in the context of the interdisciplinary team (Hastings, 1997).
   c. Impact of ambulatory nurses on outcomes in specific settings (Eck, Picagali, and Boyle, 1997; Mayer, 1996).

C. Current consensus on role dimensions in ambulatory nursing (Haas, 1998). Components include:
   1. Assessment and triage.
   2. Prevention.
   3. Clinical procedures.
   4. Collaboration.
   5. Care management.
   6. Patient education.
   7. Advocacy.
   8. Telephone practice.
   9. Communication and documentation.
   10. Outcome management.
   11. Protocol development and use.

AMBULATORY PATIENT CHARACTERISTICS

A. Ambulatory patients aren't ambulatory any more.
   1. Patients may not walk in and walk out.
   2. Increasing numbers of patients have chronic illnesses managed at home with complex treatment regimens and medical equipment.

3. Movement of elective surgeries to the ambulatory setting means patients have to be recovered after invasive procedures and anesthesia.
4. Ambulatory sites may also provide service to patients who are actually inpatients at another facility.
5. Ambulatory services are often delivered over the telephone.

B. Ambulatory patients are as diverse as inpatients in their clinical presentation.
1. Acutely ill requiring triage and possible emergency care.
2. Acutely ill requiring support, diagnosis, and treatment.
3. Chronically ill with an acute exacerbation.
4. Chronically ill requiring ongoing monitoring and assistance with self-management.
5. In need of a clearly defined treatment or procedure, including recovery, monitoring, and discharge instructions.
6. In need of education, reassurance, and support.
7. In need of preventive services and self-care education.

C. Ambulatory patients are informed consumers.
1. Media coverage and the availability of comparative quality of care data have created a skeptical and informed consumer group.
2. Many people have access to the Internet; they come already knowing much about their condition, its prognosis, and current treatment.
3. As health care begins to adopt systematic assessment of patient satisfaction, patients themselves have become more willing to come forward with complaints and provide feedback.
4. Because of the growth in consumerism, nurses in ambulatory care are very likely to encounter situations in which patients question the rationale or quality of care.

D. Each patient has a constituency of family members and/or concerned others who may become involved with care and care decisions.
1. Ambulatory care is community-based, often involving care that must be continued in the home between ambulatory visits.
2. With the increase in early hospital discharge and self-managed chronic disease, it is necessary to involve others as caregivers in the home.
3. Involving family members or other significant individuals can enhance the effectiveness of patient education, and increase the likelihood of adherence to the plan of care.

COMPARISON OF NURSING PRACTICE IN INPATIENT ACUTE CARE AND AMBULATORY CARE

Inpatient acute care is defined as hospital-based care in which patients are admitted overnight for diagnosis, treatment of an acute problem, or treatment of an acute exacerbation of a chronic problem. Ambulatory care is defined as outpatient care in which patients stay less than 24 hours and are discharged to their normal residential situation after care.

■ TABLE 2-1
■ ■ **Differences Between Nursing Role in Ambulatory and Inpatient Settings**

Aspect of Role	Inpatient Practice	Ambulatory Practice
Treatment episode	Inpatient admission	Visit or phone encounter
Observation mode	Direct and continuous	Episodic, often using patient as informant
Management of treatment plan	By nurse, with input from patient and family	By patient and family, with input from the nurse
Primary intervention mode	Direct	Consultative
Organizational presence of nursing	Nurse-managed department	May or may not be formal structure for nursing
Workload variability and intensity	Determined by bed capacity and admission criteria	Theoretically determined by scheduling system

Adapted from Hastings C (1987): Classification issues in ambulatory care nursing, *J Ambulatory Care Manage* 10(3):50-64.

A. Summary of differences between the nursing role in ambulatory and inpatient settings (Table 2-1).
   1. The key to the difference between nursing care in inpatient and ambulatory settings lies in differences in the underlying assumptions about the relationship (or "contract") between the patient and the nurse (Hastings, 1987).
   2. Distinct differences exist in the level of accountability for care and control over the treatment plan assumed by both the patient and the nurse in the two settings.
   3. Although it is a requirement that RNs be present at all times in the inpatient setting to provide or coordinate patient care, this requirement does not universally exist in ambulatory care.
   4. Differences in the focus of nursing practice in the two types of settings have led to different evolutions in the structure of care delivery and understanding of staffing requirements (see Chapter 10).
B. Patient contacts in the hospital setting.
   1. Patients are admitted to the hospital because of the requirement for nursing care. This fact is behind the requirement that all hospitalized patients be under the care of a registered nurse while they are admitted.
   2. Accountability for managing care is transferred to the nurse when the patient is admitted.
      a. This includes even those activities in which the patient was competent, such as medication administration.
      b. Nurse assumes total accountability for care and observation during admission.
C. Patient contacts in the ambulatory setting.

1. Ambulatory visits usually initiated by patient for the purpose of seeking medical care.
2. Most prevalent site for ambulatory care is still the physician office.
3. Between provider visits, patients are expected to manage their own self-care and treatments prescribed by the provider, and seek additional help if needed.
4. Need for nursing in ambulatory care is not universal as it is in the hospital setting.
   a. Must define patients or groups of patients requiring nursing care.
   b. Must define level of care to be provided.
   c. No universal professional or regulatory standards exist on this issue.
D. Differences in the definition of treatment episode.
   1. Episode of care in acute care nursing is the hospital admission.
      a. Episode has defined beginning and end points (admission and discharge).
      b. Treatment period is continuous with an admission.
   2. Episode of care in ambulatory care is a visit or phone encounter.
      a. Treatment is episodic rather than continuous.
      b. Treatment period may include multiple episodes.
      c. Treatment period often has poorly defined beginning and end point.
E. Differences in observation mode.
   1. In acute care, the nurse has the opportunity to continuously observe the patient and collect assessment data.
      a. Variations in disease process and treatment effectiveness can be directly observed.
      b. Physical assessment can be used to corroborate patient-reported findings on an ongoing basis.
   2. In ambulatory care, opportunity for direct observation and physical assessment is minimal.
      a. Nurse must rely on patient report and description of symptoms, self-care, and results.
      b. Nurse must have a comprehensive understanding of patient condition and treatment to effectively probe for additional data.
      c. Nurse must often rely on the report of family members if patient is unable to describe situation.
      d. The assessment is compressed into a much shorter time frame.
      e. There are often gaps in critical information needed to make judgements about diagnosis and care.
F. Differences in management of the treatment plan.
   1. In acute care, control over implementation of the treatment plan resides primarily with the nurse, with the patient playing the role of active participant.
      a. Determining the approach.
      b. Timing of care.
      c. Modifications and adaptations to improve effectiveness or tolerance of treatment.

2. In ambulatory care control over implementation of the treatment plan resides primarily with the patient (and family), with the nurse serving in a consultative role.
   a. Approach is described and recommended during the visit, with possible demonstration by patient or family members.
   b. Timing is prescribed.
   c. Actual implementation occurs under the control of the patient, when the nurse is not present.
   d. Adaptations and modification are made by the patient, often not in consultation with health care providers.
   e. Changes in implementation may be made without a detailed understanding of the rationale for treatment and implications of making changes.

G. Differences in nursing interventions.
   1. Until recently there was a clearly discernable difference in the types of interventions and locus of control over interventions between hospital and ambulatory care nursing.
      a. Historically hospital-based care was initiated by the nurse, and related to either monitoring, treatment, or self-care activities that the patient would be unable to perform.
      b. Hospital-based interventions are often technologically complex and involve hands-on care.
      c. In contrast, interventions by ambulatory care nurses historically tended to be patient-initiated, focused on health care advice or instructing patients how to manage care at home or prepare for tests and procedures.
   2. Recent changes in the health care system have blurred the boundaries of inpatient and outpatient care.
      a. Patients with complex conditions and treatment regimens are being cared for in outpatient and day hospital settings.
      b. There has been a dramatic growth in 23-hour short stay units.
      c. Complexity of ambulatory surgery has increased.
      d. Increasingly, outpatients are being seen on inpatient units for evaluation and triage (oncology and labor and delivery, for example).

H. Differences in the organizational position of nursing.
   1. Traditionally, inpatient nursing staff are part of an organized department of nursing with a defined nurse executive with a voice at the governing body level.
   2. Traditionally, ambulatory nurses work within a variety of structures.
      a. Often report to a non-nursing administrator.
      b. May be hired directly by physicians in a group practice.
      c. Except for large hospital-based or group practices, may not have a defined nursing administrative structure.
      d. Even in the same organization, nurses in different ambulatory roles may have different reporting and supervisory relationships.

I. Differences in workload variability and intensity.

1. In acute care, the inpatient unit has a defined capacity that is based on bed size.
   a. Although acuity and census may fluctuate, there is at least a theoretical limit to the number of patients who may be cared for.
   b. Unit admission and discharge criteria set a level of care, which predicts what types of patients may be seen.
2. In ambulatory care, workload is theoretically predicted by the appointment system.
   a. Every ambulatory nurse knows that the appointment system is easily bypassed by walk-ins and urgent visits.
   b. No-show patients and resulting overbooking practices also add to problems predicting workload.

CURRENT PRACTICE SETTINGS FOR AMBULATORY CARE NURSES

Practice setting is defined as the type of organizational delivery system in which the nurse practices.

A. The context for ambulatory nursing practice.
   1. Nurses practice within a broad continuum of ambulatory care settings (Figure 2-1).
   2. The ambulatory health care system spans primary care, when the patient first seeks care through acute care and chronic follow-up and palliative care.
   3. Nurses care for patients in every phase of preventive care, health maintenance, diagnosis, treatment, and follow-up, as the patients move in and out of acute care settings.
B. Ambulatory care nurses practice within several distinct organizational settings.
   1. Characteristics of the setting are determined by its organizational structure, its patient population, its financial and reimbursement structure, and the organization of its primary providers (usually physicians).
   2. Within each type of setting, there are also differences based on size, regional location, affiliation with a network or health system, and regional differences in health finance administration.
   3. Dimensions of clinical nursing practice are similar across settings, however the frequency of performance of certain dimensions varies a great deal by setting (Haas, Hackbarth, Kavanaugh, and Vlasses., 1995).
   4. Major categories of practice setting include:
      a. University hospital outpatient departments.
      b. Community hospital outpatient departments.
      c. Solo and group medical practices.
      d. Health maintenance organizations clinics and services.
      e. Government health systems (federal, state, and local).
      f. Community and freestanding centers such as:
         (1) Occupational health centers.

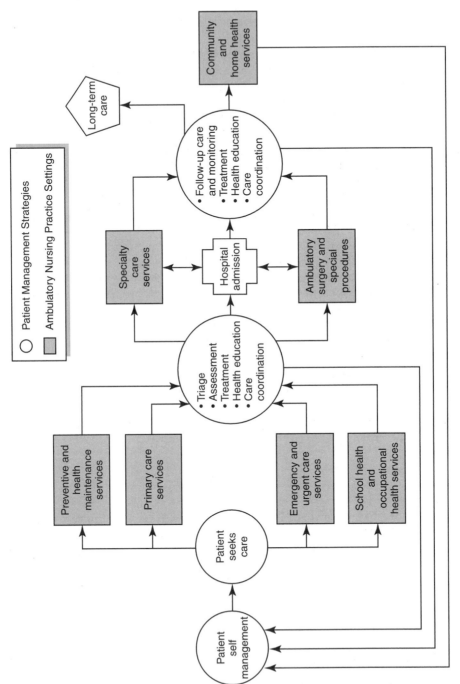

FIGURE 2-1 ■ Context for Ambulatory Care Nursing Practice (Developed by Clare Hastings. Adapted from AAACN/ANA [1997]: *Nursing in ambulatory care: the future is here*, Washington, DC: American Nurses Publishing.)

(2) School health clinics.

(3) Shelters for the homeless.

(4) Surgery/special procedure centers.

(5) Urgent care centers.

C. University hospital outpatient departments.

　1. History and development.

　　a. Teaching hospital outpatient clinics have been used since the early 1900s to provide teaching opportunities for medical students, residents, and other health care providers.

　　b. Traditionally, care was provided free or at minimal charge to those primarily in the local community.

　　c. May also include specialty clinics based on the expertise of medical faculty members that pull referrals from a greater distance.

　2. Ambulatory nursing role.

　　a. Nurses have been active collaborators in the development of teaching hospital clinics and programs.

　　b. Nurses are often the only constant for patients receiving chronic illness care through cycles of rotating residents.

　　c. Nurses in academic medical centers were among the first to begin to describe the role of the nurse in ambulatory care.

　　d. Teaching hospital clinics are often the site for innovations in nursing care, including nurse-run clinics and other forms of collaborative practice.

　　e. Because of the teaching focus, many teaching clinics are plagued by long waits, poor access to urgent care, and difficulties obtaining medical records.

　　f. Recently, financial pressures and changing reimbursement have forced many academic medical centers to reorganize their teaching clinics, streamline operations and improve patient support services (Billi, 1995).

D. Community hospital outpatient centers.

　1. History and development.

　　a. Began as an outgrowth of the dispensary movement in the 1800s to serve the urban poor.

　　b. As financial incentives and pressures changed, became more focused on adjunctive services, such as ambulatory surgery and short stay units.

　　c. Not financially or operationally competitive as a large source of primary care services.

　2. Ambulatory nursing role.

　　a. Usually small programs with limited numbers of nursing staff.

　　b. Focus on the use of ancillary staff and use of RNs as working managers.

　　c. As more high tech programs were implemented, use of RNs increased.

E. Medical group practices.

1. History and development.
   a. Medical group practices are an outgrowth of the economic pressures on solo physician private practices.
   b. Movement of patients out of the hospital and rapid growth of large multi-specialty practices has increased the intensity of services provided in the medical group practice setting (Curran, 1995).
2. Ambulatory nursing role.
   a. Nursing role is focused on facilitating the care of patients and the work of the physicians.
   b. Physicians are usually the employer and often the supervisor of nurses.
   c. Role components include triage and access management, managing and coordinating care, providing technical support for complex clinical procedures, and patient education.

F. Health maintenance organizations (HMOs).
1. History and development.
   a. Since the 1970s, the number of pre-paid comprehensive health plans that provide all services to members based on a fixed fee per month has grown.
   b. This organizational structure created a whole new set of incentives and needs for care management.
   c. Emphasis on reducing use of hospital days and utilization in general stimulated development of processes to triage patients and direct them to different level of care.
   d. Incentives to reduce hospital utilization also led to a new focus on prevention and health maintenance.
2. Ambulatory nursing role.
   a. Extensive involvement in assessment and triage.
   b. First sites to identify telephone triage as a specific nursing function.
   c. Nurses also involved in health maintenance activities, technical procedures (such as outpatient chemotherapy), and care management.

G. Federal health systems.
1. History and development.
   a. Include federally mandated programs to serve specific populations.
      (1) Department of Defense programs for active duty and retired military personnel.
      (2) Veterans Administration programs.
      (3) U.S. Public Health Service programs, including Indian Health Service hospitals, clinics, and community health centers.
   b. Systems represent large networks of organizations operating on a fixed budget.
   c. Until recently most services provided free of charge to members of enrolled populations.
2. Ambulatory nursing role.
   a. Nursing practice supported by a longstanding tradition of well-trained unlicensed assistive personnel (Navy corpsmen and Army medics).

    b. Nursing role has developed rapidly in recent years, involving nurses in health assessment and promotion/disease prevention, patient education, and the provision of complex procedures in the outpatient setting.

    c. Federal health systems have been sites for development of innovative models and approaches to nurses providing primary ambulatory care services.

H. Community and freestanding centers.

    1. Program types include:

      a. Surgery centers.

      b. Diagnostic centers.

      c. Local health departments.

      d. Free and grant-supported experimental clinics.

      e. College health centers.

      f. Occupational health offices in large employers.

    2. Ambulatory nursing role.

      a. Many centers small in size and scope.

      b. Nurses assume multiple roles.

      c. Many such sites have been experimental sites for piloting nurse-run clinics.

TRANSITIONING INTO AMBULATORY CARE NURSING

A. Why nurses are making the transition to ambulatory care.

    1. Increased emphasis on ambulatory care as a care delivery site.

    2. Expansion of complex services offered in ambulatory care, with resulting needs for nursing support.

    3. Nurses seeking alternative practice settings to the hospital.

      a. Opportunities for greater professional autonomy.

      b. Opportunities for increased collaboration with physicians.

      c. Scheduling and lifestyle advantages.

      d. Expectations that ambulatory care will provide a low-stress work environment.

B. Transition challenges.

    1. Change in locus of control.

      a. Experience of diminished control.

        (1) Over the general treatment regimen.

        (2) Over the timing and method of implementation.

        (3) Especially noticed by nurses transitioning from critical care.

      b. Combined with general sensory overload.

        (1) Large numbers of patients arriving for care.

        (2) Large numbers of providers.

      c. Lack of a shift start and end, with resulting requirement that the nurse stays to see to the needs of all patients in the setting.

      d. Changes in expected workload.

      e. Difficulty planning time and controlling pace of work.

    2. Changes in data available.

    a. Requirement that clinical decisions be made with less than usual amount of data.

    b. Unavailability of continuous observation that allows nurse to pick up subtle changes in patient condition.

    c. Reliance on new methods of assessment and integration of information.

        (1) Nuances of patient self-reporting.

        (2) Rapid observation and synthesis, combined with probing and assessment skills.

3. Changes in scope of services provided.

    a. Scope dictated by both needs of the patient and the purpose of the visit.

        (1) May not be able or required to meet all assessed needs at a given visit.

        (2) May use referral or recommendation as opposed to direct intervention.

        (3) May create conflict in a newly transitioned nurse used to meeting the total needs of each patient.

    b. May apply health assessment standards based on inpatient experience.

        (1) Not appropriate for ambulatory visits.

        (2) Creates an unnecessary burden on both the nurse and the patient.

        (3) Critical transition task is to learn how to assess only the essential data for purpose of visit and patient need.

    c. Scope of services may vary substantially from visit to visit.

        (1) For one visit the nurse may briefly review the patient record and assign the patient to an unlicensed staff member.

        (2) For another patient, the nurse may do a complete assessment and provide education and counseling or direct care.

    d. Important that population assessment be done.

        (1) Establish overall needs for nursing care within the population.

        (2) Identify major visit types and level of nursing care required for each.

        (3) Establish process by which patients may gain access to nurse as needed.

4. Changes in collaborative relationships.

    a. Relationships among health team members change.

    b. Focus of nursing care shifts.

        (1) Away from the medical plan of care and implementing that plan.

        (2) Toward a more consultative role with patients, families, and physicians.

    c. Nurse seen more as coordinator and manager of care and less as direct implementer.

        (1) Creates opportunities for collaborative practice with physicians.

        (2) Identified by nurses practicing in ambulatory care as a valued aspect of role.

    d. Nurse becomes a conduit between physician directing care and patient managing care at home.

    e. Requires demonstration of key competencies to be accepted as a colleague in patient management by physicians.

        (1) Clinical competence.

        (2) Confidence in decision-making.

        (3) Ability to communicate effectively.

  5. Diversity in practice assignments.

    a. Often a shock for nurses transitioning from single specialty inpatient units.

    b. Due to episodic nature of care, some specialty programs may meet only once or twice per week.

    c. Nurse may be assigned in multiple locations to fill out the week.

    d. Requires broad competency to manage care for diverse groups of patients.

    e. For experienced ambulatory nurses this variability is the "spice" in their roles.

    f. For the new nurse it may seem like chaos.

C. Strategies to support a successful transition.

  1. Nurses transitioning to ambulatory care need full orientation to the setting and the practice styles for each area assigned.

  2. Although clinical competency is not usually the major issue, the new nurse will need assistance adapting practice approaches to the new setting.

  3. Attention should be paid to signs that the new staff member is becoming overwhelmed with multiple demands.

REFERENCES

American Academy of Ambulatory Care Nursing and American Nurses' Association (1997): *Nursing in ambulatory care: the future is here.* Washington, DC: American Nurses Publishing.

American Academy of Ambulatory Nursing Administration (1997): *Telephone nursing practice administration and practice standards.* Pitman, N.J.: Anthony J. Jannetti.

American Academy of Ambulatory Nursing Administration (2000): *Ambulatory care nursing administration and practice standards.* ed 5. Pitman, N.J.: Anthony J. Jannetti.

Billi JE, Wise CG, Bills EA, Mitchell RL (1995): Potential effects of managed care on specialty practice at a university medical center. *JAMA* 333(13): 979-984.

Bunting LK (1994): Role of the ambulatory care nurse in the Indian Health Service. Unpublished master's thesis, Johns Hopkins School of Nursing, Baltimore, MD.

Curran C (1995): An interview with Linda D'Angelo. *Nurs Econ* 13(4): 193-196.

Eck SA, Picagali D, Boyle S (1997): Improving health outcomes in underserved women. *Viewpoint* 19(4): 1, 4-5, 9.

Haas S (1998): Ambulatory care nursing conceptual framework. *Viewpoint* 20(3): 16-17.

Haas SA, Hackbarth DP, Kavanaugh JA, Vlasses E (1995): Dimensions of the staff nurse role in ambulatory care. Part II: Comparison of role dimensions in four ambulatory settings. *Nurs Econ* 13(3):152-165.

Hackbarth DS, Haas S, Kavanaugh JA, Vlasses E (1995): Dimensions of the staff nurse role in ambulatory care. Part I: Methodology and analysis of data on current staff nurse practice. *Nurs Econ* 13(2):89-98.

Hastings C, Muir-Nash J (1989): Validation of a taxonomy of ambulatory nursing practice. *Nurs Econ* 7(3):142-149.

Hastings C (1987): Classification issues in ambulatory care nursing. *J Ambulatory Care Manage* 10(3):50-64.

Hastings C (1997): The context for ambulatory care nursing. Washington, DC: The Washington Hospital Center, internal document.

Hastings C (1997): The changing multidisciplinary team. *Nurs Econ* 15(2):106-108, 105.

Johnston M (1980): Ambulatory care into the 80's—Looking ahead to a decade of dilemmas. *Am J Nurs* 80:70-79.

Marzalek E (1980): Ambulatory nursing: At the crossroads? *Nurs Health Care* 1:245-255.

Mayer GG (1996): Case management as a mindset. *Quality Management in Health Care* 5(1):7-16.

Parrinello KM, Brennan PS, Vallone B (1988): Refining and testing a nursing patient classification instrument in ambulatory care. *Nurs Admin Q* 13(1):54-65.

Tighe MG, Fisher SG, Hastings C, Heller BA (1985): Study of the oncology nurse role in ambulatory care. *Oncol Nurs Forum* 12(6):23-27.

Verran J (1981): Delineation of ambulatory care nursing practice. *J Ambulatory Care Manage* 4(2):1-13.

3 Context of Ambulatory Care

MARGARET FISK MASTAL, PhD, MSN, RN

OBJECTIVES

Study of the information presented in this chapter will enable the learner to:

1. Describe the concept of health and its evolution in the 20th and into the 21st century.
2. Discuss the application of current health concepts in the ambulatory care environment.
3. Apply principles and practices of customer-focused care in ambulatory care practice.
4. Integrate cultural differences into ambulatory nursing care practice.
5. Describe nursing care delivery models in ambulatory settings.

■■ The concept of health has changed over the course of the 20th century, evolving from reactive responses to illness and disease to proactive initiatives that focus on the health and wellness of both the individual and populations. In ambulatory settings, this shift gave rise to emphasizing the context of care as well as different practice patterns. Traditional nursing roles shifted from an emphasis on technological skills to a broader focus, one that requires diverse professional, expert knowledge and competencies.

This chapter initially provides an overview of how the concept of health evolved over the 20th and into the 21st century, discusses the evolution of the managed care environment, and the impact of changes on the ambulatory care environment and professional nursing practice. Significant environmental changes address the rationale of and the behaviors appropriate to a consumer-focused environment, including care that is culturally competent. Last, it describes the major nursing models currently in operation in ambulatory settings, models categorized as those that: (1) facilitate access; (2) provide direct health care services; and (3) those that manage or coordinate care across the continuum of care.

CONCEPT OF HEALTH AND ITS EVOLUTION IN THE 20TH CENTURY

Over the past centuries, health as a concept has evolved from a focus on treating disease to include an emphasis on disease prevention and health promotion. In this century, as health care industry activities shifted from hospital-centered to the outpatient setting, evolving notions of health have been integrated into the ambulatory environment. Rooted in Nightingale's holistic approaches to nursing care, modern nursing in ambulatory care settings is poised to support optimal health for all.

A. Health and health promotion.

   1. Health and health promotion are fundamental concepts of nursing.

   2. "Nursing involves practices that are restorative, supportive and promotive in nature . . . promotive practices mobilize healthy patterns of living, foster personal and family development, and support self-defined goals of individuals, families, and communities." (American Nurses' Association Social Policy Statement, 1995, p. 11).

B. Defining health promotion—definitional changes over time.

   1. *Medieval era*—defined by isolation and quarantine of those with communicable diseases.

   2. *19th century*—defined by emerging control and adjustment of environmental factors.

      a. Sanitation of waste, adequate housing, hygiene.

      b. Hand washing practices emphasized (initiated by Isaac Semmelweis).

      c. Vector control practices initiated—eradication of rats, fleas, mosquitoes, etc.

      d. Influence of Florence Nightingale experienced—emphasis on clean environments, nutrition, etc.

      e. Lillian Wald spotlights health care for women and children at the Henry Street Settlement.

   3. *Early 20th century*—prevention of disease becomes a focus.

      a. Focus on the individual as responsible for own health care.

      b. Development of immunizations, antibiotics, tranquilizers, and antidepressants.

   4. *Latter part of the 20th century*—perspectives begin to expand.

      a. Lalonde Report: Marc Lalonde, Canadian Health Minister, 1974.

         (1) Health is affected by multiple factors (human biology, lifestyle, the organization of health care, and the social and physical environment).

         (2) Initiated a shift from the focus of treating disease to one of disease prevention and health promotion (McDonald and Bunton, 1992).

      b. World Health Organization (1978): publicized the Alma Ata declaration, committing the WHO organization to work for health for all world citizens by the year 2000.

         (1) Expanded the conceptualization of primary care to primary health care.

         (2) Primary health care defined as "essential health care . . . made universally accessible to individuals and families in the community . . . through their full participation and at a cost that the community and country can afford" (WHO, 1978, p. 3).

      c. Institute of Medicine (1978): issued the first definition of primary care.

(1) Conceptualized primary care as personal health services rather than public health services.

(2) Primary care should be "accessible, comprehensive, coordinated and continual care delivery by accountable providers of *personnel* health services" (IOM, 1978).

(3) Placed increasing emphasis on prevention, removing barriers to care, coordination, continuity, and the inclusion of patients and families in the decision-making process (Hackbarth, 1995).

d. U.S. Surgeon General's report "Health Promotion and Disease Prevention" (1979): disease prevention and health promotion were declared separate, but equal concepts.

(1) Disease prevention was defined as protection from environmental threats.

(2) Health promotion was considered in terms of positive lifestyle changes (DHHS, 1991).

e. U.S. Surgeon General's report *Promoting Health/Preventing Disease: Objectives for a Nation* in 1980.

(1) Identified specific, quantifiable objectives for promoting health and preventing disease.

(2) Objectives were organized around 15 priority areas (e.g., blood pressure and cancer screening, timely immunizations, smoking cessation, reduction of alcohol use, etc.) (DHHS, 1991).

f. Ottawa Charter (1986): evolved from a meeting of the World Health Organization, Health and Welfare Canada, and the Canadian Public Health Association.

(1) Broadly defined health as individuals' ability to achieve physical, mental, and social well-being by their abilities to identify and realize aspirations, satisfy their needs, and change or cope with the environment.

(2) Broadly defined health promotion as a process enabling people to increase their control over abilities to improve health.

(3) Perceived health as a resource for daily life, not the objective of living.

(4) Described health as a positive concept that emphasizes social and personal resources as well as physical capacities, that goes beyond healthy lifestyles to well-being.

(5) Outlined five major health promotion actions.

   (a) Build health public policy.

   (b) Create supportive environments.

   (c) Develop personal skills.

   (d) Strengthen community action.

   (e) Re-orient health services (WHO, 1987).

g. Healthy People 2000: created a platform for action to help Americans fulfill their health potential (Morgan and Marsh, 1998).

(1) Outlined three broad goals.

   (a) Increase the span of healthy life.

(b) Reduce health disparities.

(c) Achieve access to preventive services.

(2) Established 300 measurable objectives.

(3) Described health promotion strategies in terms of:

(a) Actions related to individual lifestyle.

(b) Personal choices are made in a social context (e.g., physical activity, use of substances, family planning, mental health, and abusive or violent behaviors) (DHHS, 1991).

h. Healthy People 2010 was initiated at a meeting of the Healthy People 2000 Consortium in New York City, November 1996 (DHHS, 1999).

(1) Builds on prior health initiatives, the Surgeon General's Reports of 1979 and 1980, and the Healthy People 2000 movement, as an instrument to improve health for the first decade of the 21st century.

(2) Overarching purpose: "promoting health and preventing illness, disability, and premature death" (DHHS, 2000, p. 1).

(3) Assumption: the context of change will change the practice of medicine and health care such as (DHHS, 1999):

(a) Advances will occur in preventive therapies, vaccines, pharmaceuticals, assistive technologies, and computer technologies.

(b) New relationships between public health departments and health care organizations will be defined.

(c) U.S. demographic changes (e.g., older and more racially diverse) will create new demands on the health care system.

(d) Global forces (fluctuating food supplies, emerging infectious diseases, environmental interdependence) will present new public health challenges.

(4) Goals of Healthy People 2010 (DHHS, 2000, pp. 8-16).

(a) *Goal 1: Increase the quality and years of healthy life.* Evaluation will include measuring changes in the following indicators:

(i) *Life expectancy*—is the average number of years people born in a given year are expected to live based on a set of age-specific death rates.

(ii) *Health-related quality of life*—subjective, personal sense of physical and mental health and the ability to react to factors in the physical and social environments.

(iii) *Global assessments*—personal ratings of one's own health status.

(iv) *Years of healthy life*—average amount of time spent in less than optimal health as a result of chronic or acute limitations.

(b) *Goal 2: Eliminate health disparities among different segments of the population.* Evaluation will occur by measuring the decrease in health status gaps that exist because of:

(i) Gender.

(ii) Race and ethnicity.

(iii) Income and education.

(iv) Disability.

(v) Rural or urban location.

(vi) Sexual orientation.

(5) 2010 objectives (467 objectives in 28 focus areas) will be distinguished from Healthy People 2000 by having:

(a) Broadened preventive, scientific base.

(b) Improved surveillance and data systems.

(c) Heightened awareness and demand for preventive health services and quality health care.

(d) Integrated the changes in demographics, science, technology, and disease spread that will affect health in the 21st century.

(6) Healthy People 2010 will be the United States' contribution to the World Health Organization (WHO) "Health for All" strategy.

(7) The U.S. effort will be characterized by key partnerships, that is, collaboration between and among federal, state, local, and private sectors as well as community participation (DHHS, 2000).

5. The shift in perspectives about health over the latter part of the 20th century and the possibilities that present for the 21st century have significant implications for nurses.

C. The role of nursing in health promotion—evolved from a focus on treatment of disease and illness to one of disease prevention and promotion.

1. Current status.

a. The focus of nursing intervention has shifted to health-related lifestyle modifications.

b. In contrast to the newly developed health focus, the traditional nursing process is a scientific method that is related to the medical model (i.e., the assessment, diagnosis, planning, intervention and evaluation processes require labeling a person's problem and recommending or advising some universal lifestyle modification).

c. Further, the current nursing focus does not generally address societal responsibilities (Rush, 1997).

d. Dispensing health education advice often assumes that the person is ignorant about healthy habits.

2. Future: expanding nurse's health horizons to include the sociopolitical and cultural environments (Morgan and Marsh, 1998).

a. Nurses need to include environmental factors and challenges (including culture and finances) in assessing health needs before engaging in health promotion activities.

b. Adopt the health advocacy role.

(1) Consider economic, political, social, and cultural factors; look upstream where the real problems lie (Butterfield, 1990).

(2) Address factors that cause poor health.

(3) Initiate social and political activism against social, environmental, economic, and other factors that impair optimum health (e.g., poverty, homelessness, illiteracy, violence, or unemployment).

   D. The ambulatory health care environment.
      1. Is the site in the community where care is usually initiated.
      2. Is the optimal milieu for providers to initiate and integrate current concepts of health into the delivery of health care services.

HEALTH CARE CONCEPTS IN THE AMBULATORY ENVIRONMENT

The outpatient setting is uniquely poised to integrate current health care concepts into the delivery of care. Ambulatory services, the traditional site of primary care in America, focus on health promotion and disease prevention as well as the treatment of acute and minor illness and chronic disease. Over the latter quarter of the 20th century, the scope of ambulatory care services has expanded significantly. Care has emerged from an emphasis on the single physician dispensing health care for an individual patient to a group of providers facilitating access to a broad array of diverse, comprehensive, integrated services designed to meet community needs.

   A. Primary care is regarded as *essential* health care and is the cornerstone for ambulatory health services (Shi and Singh, 1998, p. 222).
      1. Not all settings where patients walk in are considered primary care (e.g., a hospital Emergency Department is not considered primary care).
      2. Definitions vary slightly depending on differing viewpoints but the one generally accepted definition comes from the Institute of Medicine (IOM).
         a. "Primary care is the provision of integrated, accessible health care services by clinicians who are accountable for addressing a large majority of *personal* health care needs, developing a sustained partnership with patients, and practicing in the context of family and community." (Institute of Medicine, 1996).
         b. IOM Definitional concepts—the definition embodies a number of concepts including:
            (1) *Comprehensiveness*—means that care addresses any health concern at any stage across the individual's life span.
            (2) *Coordinating*—refers to the function that ensures that the care (any combination of therapies and services) occurs to meet the individual's needs holistically.
            (3) *Continuity*—refers to the care that is received over time is delivered or coordinated by a single provider or team of health care professionals.
            (4) *Accessible*—the concept refers to the ease with which consumers can initiate interaction with a clinician about the health problem/s. It includes activities to eliminate barriers raised by geography, financing, culture, race, language, etc.
            (5) *Accountability*—the concept embodies both the provider and the consumer.
               (a) The clinical system is accountable for providing quality care,

effecting consumer satisfaction, using resources efficiently, and acting in an ethical, culturally competent manner.

    (b) Consumers are accountable for their health and to use health care resources judiciously.

  c. A second definition of primary care focuses on community-oriented primary care. It is a model that incorporates the elements of the IOM model but adds a population-based approach that identifies and addresses community health needs (Shi and Singh, 1998, p. 225).

    (1) The traditional definition of primary care centered on a biopsychosocial paradigm with medical care rendered to the individual in an encounter-based system.

    (2) The evolving community-oriented primary care (COPC) model has a broader biopsychosocial paradigm, one that emphasizes the health of populations as well as the individual.

 3. In primary care, the relationship of provider and consumer is one of partnership.

  a. Roles played by each will vary over time and circumstances.

  b. The hallmarks of the partnership are mutual trust, respect, and responsibility (Shi and Singh, 1998, p. 223).

 4. Primary care "specialties" are capable of addressing a wide variety of health care needs. They are most commonly designated as:

  a. Adult medicine.

  b. Pediatrics.

  c. Family practice.

  d. Obstetrics and gynecology (OB/GYN)—some practice settings consider OB/GYN a specialty rather than primary care.

 5. Primary care, the conceptual foundation for ambulatory health services, is expected to coordinate access to and use of *secondary care* levels, for example, routine hospitalization and surgery, specialty referrals, advanced diagnostic/therapeutic care and *tertiary care,* (i.e., highly specialized and highly technological care) (Shi and Singh, 1998, p. 224).

B. Ambulatory care settings: ambulatory health care occurs in a wide variety of settings that are generally defined by a community's demographics, health needs, and the resources available (refer to Chapter 2 for a listing of ambulatory care settings).

C. The nature of the modern ambulatory care environment is dynamic—patients initiate scheduled and unscheduled visits, often with the specific nature of their problems initially unknown. Hallmarks of ambulatory care settings include:

 1. High volume, time sensitive encounters, generally based on an appointment schedule.

 2. Patients ordinarily initiate the encounter through the appointment procedure.

 3. However, it is common for patients to present themselves for care (walk in) without appointments.

 4. The true nature of an individual's presenting problem(s) is frequently unknown until he or she accesses the system. Problems have a broad scope, ranging from emergency or urgent situations, through acute illness and minor problems, to a patient's desire for health care at their convenience.

D. Changes in the services available: the single physician as provider is uncommon today; rather the physician now serves as a fulcrum to a diverse managed care system.

   1. From the historical perspective, ambulatory services are as old as the healing arts themselves (Williams, 1993).

      a. The physician was traditionally the central point of care—he or she treated patients in offices and/or during home visits.

      b. Rapidly advancing technology dating from the mid-20th century initiated a shift in the locus of ambulatory treatment, from offices and homes to the community hospital setting.

      c. Physicians gravitated toward hospital-based offices that offered easier access to diagnostic services, pharmacy, etc.

      d. Today, physicians commonly serve as leverage for individual consumers to access comprehensive arrays of health services in a now managed care environment.

E. The managed care environment—the concept and realities of managed care have evolved over the past quarter-century in response to societal concerns about rising health care costs and efforts to contain them.

   1. Definition of managed care—incorporation of controls over the health care utilization behaviors of both providers and consumers (Shi and Singh, 1998, p. 299).

      a. Managed care can be considered in two different contexts.

         (1) As a *mechanism or process* of providing health care services that integrates the key functions of insurance, care delivery, and payment in one organizational setting that exercises control over utilization.

         (2) As a *type of organizational form* (Shi and Singh, 1998, p. 303).

      b. Types of ambulatory care organizational forms include three general types of managed care organizations.

         (1) Health Maintenance Organization (HMO) is characterized by:

            (a) The provision of illness and wellness care with an emphasis on preventive measures (e.g., routine physicals, immunizations, etc.).

            (b) Establishing a fixed fee per member per month that allows access to a range of defined services.

            (c) HMO members must receive care from authorized providers with no choice of providers permitted outside the plan.

            (d) Strong quality assurance and performance improvement programs.

         (2) Preferred Provider Organization (PPO) is a corporate model that contracts with physicians for services at discounted fee-for-service rates.

        (a) Utilizes fee-for-service structure rather then capitation.

        (b) Enrollees can use any provider with a consumer co-pay caveat.

           (i) A co-pay is required for using a non-contract provider.

           (ii) No co-pay is required for using a contractual provider.

    (3) Point of Service (POS) plan is an organizational model that combines the features of the classic HMO with some characteristics of enrollee choice seen in PPOs.

        (a) HMO features include capitation and gatekeeping to restrict inappropriate utilization.

        (b) PPO features include the need for authorization of services with the use of out-of-plan providers permitted at extra cost to the consumer.

  2. Factors contributing to the emergence of today's managed care includes events that resulted from cost containment efforts.

    a. The emergence of hospital insurance before World War II and advances in technology after World War II spurred the fiscal growth and care capabilities of the health care industry.

    b. 1965: the amendments to the Social Security Act created Medicare and Medicaid legislation, made subsidized hospital care available to the aged and poor. This landmark legislation created equal opportunity for health care for the elderly and poverty level populations but also spurred the rise of health care costs.

    c. 1970s: rising costs initiated the first serious cost control efforts including the Health Maintenance Act of 1973 that:

      (1) Allocated federal funds to establish and expand new HMOs.

      (2) Represented the government's first attempt to establish alternatives to fee-for-service reimbursement.

      (3) Required employers with 25+ employees to offer an HMO option as an employee benefit.

    d. 1980s: explosive growth of prepaid, capitated health plans.

    e. 1990s: managed care arrangements dominate health care delivery and utilization (Shi and Singh, 1998, pp. 306-307).

F. Concomitant with the rise of managed care was the emergence of service industry approaches, most notably the notion of placing the "customer" at the center of all plans and activities.

CUSTOMER-FOCUSED HEALTH CARE IN AMBULATORY SETTINGS

Over the decade of the 1990s, marketing approaches evolved in ambulatory care settings in a manner similar to the hospital industry adopting marketing approaches in 1980s. Increasingly, organizations are encouraging service industry strategies in provider-patient encounters as well as for the staff to use in their work relationships. The "customer" is defined differently from different perspectives but, in all cases, is the person, group, or population that is the central focus of the action or interaction.

A. The consumer as customer: in ambulatory settings, the consumer generally initiates the encounter, expecting high levels of care and service from each member of the health care team.

1. Ambulatory health care is largely *self-administered by the individual* in the context of the family, the social, and cultural environments, along with economic and other community factors.

2. The focus of care is on the dignity and worth of the individual and his/her right to participate in:

   a. Making decisions about his/her health care.

   b. Setting goals about his/her health care.

   c. Being informed about and participating in the choice of therapy from among alternative therapies.

3. There are 3 categories of consumer concerns.

   a. Access to health care is conceptually defined "as the fit among personal, sociocultural, economic, and system-related factors that enable individuals, families and communities to have timely, needed, necessary, continuous, and satisfactory health services"(Gulzar, 1999, p. 17). Access addresses the availability of providers to consumers when they need or want an appointment.

      (1) Consumer expectations about waiting for access (or an appointment) vary, depending on the individual's perception of the urgency of the need or want.

      (2) Different providers on the health care team ensure access according to their unique professional expertise.

         (a) Physicians generally care for patients with medical emergencies, severe illness, and those with complex medical problems.

         (b) Advanced nurse practitioners have a variety of roles, depending on the practice setting and the practice styles of others on the team. In general they care for patients with acute minor illness, those who need oversight for the management of chronic disease and/or health education, and those with health and/or wellness concerns.

         (c) In many settings, clinical nurses triage unexpected demand for care, administer appropriate nursing interventions in acute situations, provide health education about disease prevention and health promotion, and serve as the conduit for information between the patient, the physician, and the organization.

         (d) Technicians and unlicensed personnel furnish technical support (e.g., apply casts, screen vital signs, prepare patients for physical examinations, make follow-up appointments, etc.).

   b. Reasonable costs: American consumers generally desire quality health care services with minimal out of pocket costs. Costs of care should be fully disclosed and the payment plan(s) appropriately addressed.

   c. Quality health care: consumers expect high quality care, usually defined from their perspective in terms of:

      (1) Rapid, accurate diagnosis of their health care problem.

      (2) Appropriate therapies and pharmaceuticals that relieve their symptoms and restore them to their normal lifestyle.

      (3) Reassurance that their health concern(s) can be cured, minimized, or managed.

      (4) Receiving information about their condition that is complete, accurate, and understandable.

      (5) Health care team members who are courteous, caring, and treat them and their family members with dignity and respect.

  4. Consumers expect care that is focused on their individual differences and uniqueness.

B. The provider team members as customer: regardless of the particular setting, ambulatory health care delivery usually occurs within the context of a multidisciplinary team of providers in partnership with the patient, their family and significant others.

  1. Service industry approaches include providers approaching each other as a customer.

  2. Ambulatory care staff practice as *members of teams of health care providers* that include a range of professional and allied staff.

    a. Physicians.

    b. Advanced Practice Nurses (APNs) and Physician Assistants (PAs).

    c. Registered Nurses.

    d. Other licensed health care professionals such as physical therapists, occupational therapists, and social workers.

    e. Technicians (staff who are not licensed but are usually certified and/or experienced in a defined specialty [e.g., orthopedic technicians, allergy technicians]).

    f. Unlicensed assistive personnel (UAPs) (e.g., medical assistants, nursing assistants, receptionists, and volunteers).

  3. Modern teams are expected to relate among themselves and with other institutional staff with customer-oriented approaches, that is, placing the other person at the center of the interaction.

    a. Interact with each other with consideration, respect, and dignity.

    b. Work to meet or exceed the other person's expectations.

C. Nursing roles on the ambulatory health care team.

  1. Historically nursing roles focused on technical care (e.g., injections, intravenous therapy, assisting with procedures, etc.).

  2. Increasingly, today's nursing role is collaborative professional practice and includes (Haas and Hackbarth, 1995):

    a. Assisting patients/families to coordinate their health care.

    b. Performing professional nursing interventions.

    c. Communicating nursing interventions and outcomes among team members.

    d. Evaluating nursing performance and outcomes of care.

3. Trends influencing the evolution of nursing roles in ambulatory care.

    a. Consumers are more knowledgeable and service oriented.

    b. Advancing technology allows treatments, traditionally delivered in hospitals, to be delivered on an ambulatory basis.

    c. Regulatory agencies mandate that health care be coordinated across the continuum of care not just within each setting.

    d. Increasing emphasis on disease prevention, health promotion, and wellness.

    e. Growing complexity of health care delivery systems.

4. The sponsoring organization influences the structure and operating style of the multidisciplinary team.

    a. Historical origins of the organization (e.g., hospital based, private practice, HMOs) affect beliefs, strategies, and the way the individual practice environment serves its consumer population.

    b. Roles and functions of team members, including nurses, vary within different organizations and even within different units of the same organization.

        (1) Traditional: physician is leader and chief decision-maker; team members function according to physician directions (commonly seen in, but not exclusive to, private physician offices).

        (2) Care partners: physician and nurse team to assume responsibility for the health care of a designated population (e.g., oncology or oncology patients).

            (a) Follow patients across the continuum of care (hospital, clinic, and home).

            (b) The nurse sometimes referred to as the "primary nurse" (Bedlek, 1996).

        (3) Participatory, multidisciplinary teams: physicians, advanced practitioners, managers, nurses, staff, etc. work collaboratively according to mutually developed and clearly defined roles and functions.

    c. Regardless of the configurations of team roles/functions within an individual setting, societal and regulatory mandates expect designated accountability and responsibility for the health services provided, including outreach, diagnosis, treatment, and follow-up.

    d. Ambulatory care includes the family or significant other in care practices.

        (1) The family is the individual patient's major support system.

        (2) Providing support and information to the patient's caregiver/s is a critical dimension in acute situations, chronic illness, or terminal stages of life.

    e. Customer-focused ambulatory health care services include expectations for cultural competence.

CULTURAL COMPETENCE

Culture is "the totality of socially transmitted behavioral patterns, arts, beliefs, values, customs, lifeways, and all other products of human work and thought characteristics of a population of people that guide their world view and decision making. Becoming culturally competent is a conscious process that is acquired, in a not necessarily linear manner" (Purnell and Paulanka, 1998, p. 2). Developing cultural competence is a professional and social mandate in modern health care. Acquiring cultural expertise can enhance relationships, processes, and outcomes for consumers and providers.

A. Definitions of cultural competence include notions of:
1. Cultural receptivity, that is, knowing, valuing, respecting, and enjoying differences among individuals (Kendall, 1995; Thomas, 1996; Sullivan, 1998, p. 4; DuBrin, 1998, p. 110).
2. Integrating self with the cultural differences of others in a process that usually encompasses (Purnell and Paulanka, 1998, p. 2):
   a. Developing and appreciating an awareness of one's own existence, sensations, thoughts, and surroundings without letting it have an untoward influence on others.
   b. Demonstrating knowledge and understanding of the cultural preferences of others (patients, family, colleagues, etc.).
   c. Accepting and respecting the cultural differences of others.
   d. Adapting professional practice so that it is congruent with the culture of others.
3. Cultural competence addresses differences among the health care team members as well as between providers and patients, families, and the community.
4. Individuals are diverse in multiple dimensions including (DuBrin, 1998, pp. 111-112):
   a. Race.
   b. Gender.
   c. Religion.
   d. Age.
   e. Weight.
   f. Ethnicity (country/geographic area/culture of origin).
   g. Education.
   h. Physical and mental abilities and disabilities.
   i. Job-relevant abilities.
   j. Sexual orientation (heterosexual, homosexual, bisexual, asexual).
   k. Marital status (single, married, divorced, cohabitating, widow/widower).
   l. Family status (children, childless, single parent, two parent, single, grandparent).
   m. Appearance and clothing preferences (casual, formal, professional, business).
   n. Personality traits.
   o. Interest in technology (high-tech, low-tech, technophobe).
   p. Values and motivation.

5. Cultural competence begins with the systematic assessment of key aspects of culturally based behaviors and progresses with the development and application of skills that integrate cultural differences into professional practice activities (Giger and Mood, 1997, pp. 14-18). Key behaviors to address include:

a. Communication styles: communication is the mechanism whereby individuals and groups connect.

   (1) Assessing communication styles and patterns from the cultural perspective can include the following:

      (a) Visit areas where different ethnic communities gather, watching and listening how they interact and conduct business.

      (b) Observe how individuals interact with regard to dialect, volume of speech and silence, the context of speech including emotional tone, and kinesics (gestures, stance, eye behavior).

      (c) Determine from reliable resources the implications of the behaviors you observe in different cultural groups.

   (2) To develop and apply culturally competent communication skills that are central to positive working relationships, nurses and other professionals would:

      (a) Modify communication patterns to adapt to the style of the individual or group addressed.

      (b) Identify and avoid using gestures that individuals or groups find threatening.

      (c) Use clarifying and validating techniques.

      (d) Utilize team members from different cultures as resources in learning about and using culturally sensitive behaviors.

      (e) Employ interpreters as appropriate.

      (f) Explain legal requirements.

b. Use space effectively: *space*, in terms of cultural behavior, is defined as the physical distance occurring in personal interactions and the intimacy techniques utilized when relating to others both verbally and nonverbally.

   (1) Assessing the relevance of space includes acknowledging that space has distinct zones for different interactions.

      (a) Intimate.

      (b) Personal.

      (c) Public.

   (2) Acquire knowledge of the appropriate distances to maintain in different cultures. Comfort with space and distance has different meanings in different cultures.

   (3) Integrating culturally competent space skills includes the ability to:

      (a) Honor space distances according to cultural and personal preference.

(b) Communicate personal space comfort levels appropriately.
c. Social organization as a cultural dimension refers to the values that individuals place on important groups in their life (e.g., family, work group, etc.).
   (1) Assess the importance and value individuals place on the different groups in their lives.
   (2) Value, respect, and integrate individual differences for preferred social organization into professional interactions with individuals and groups.
d. Time as a key element in culture is defined certainly by the clock and the calendar but also includes a person's orientation to the past, present, and future.
   (1) Past-oriented people have a tendency to value tradition and stability.
   (2) Present-oriented people tend to focus on activities that meet current demands.
   (3) Future-oriented people tend to conduct activities in light of their contributions to achieving goals.
   (4) Assessing and integrating cultural competency regarding time includes evaluating an individual's or group's orientation to time (e.g., are they prompt, on time or late for appointments, how are they oriented to the past/present/future).
   (5) Using time in a culturally sensitive manner includes engaging in activities and interactions that utilize time orientation to the individual's and the group's benefit.
e. Environmental control refers to an individual's perceived ability to control external occurrences. These perceptions are a source of the individual's feelings of safety and security.
   (1) Environmental control has two aspects.
      (a) An individual's attachment to a certain terrain, climate, or location (e.g., individual preferences or affinity with a particular country or section of a country, desert living, or locating by water).
      (b) An individual's belief about the degree to which they control events. This belief has two general categories.
         (i) Internal locus of control: a person believe actions can evoke events.
         (ii) External locus of control: a person believes that events occur by chance, luck, or fate.
   (2) Cultural competency regarding environmental control includes:
      (a) Assessing the individual's or group's perception/s about their ability to control external events.
      (b) Framing interventions and programs that meet others' comfort levels.
f. Biological variation, as a dimension in cultural competence, refers to the genetic differences among individuals.

(1) Genetic biological variations among specific ethnic, gender, or cultural groups can be associated with risk factors for specific diseases or responses to therapeutic pharmaceuticals or regimens (Kudzma, 1999).

(2) Cultural competence regarding biological variations includes
   (a) Developing knowledge about cultural differences.
   (b) Assessing for them.
   (c) Adapting interventions to minimize risk from disability and disease.

6. Cultural competence is a social, moral, and professional mandate for all health care professionals and will foster improved health care practices and environments.

7. Cultural competence benefits the individual and the organization in that it:
   a. Fosters mutual trust and respect for differences among individuals and groups.
   b. Acknowledges the contributions of each individual involved.
   c. Values and utilizes cultural variations to the benefit of all.
   d. Maintains a learning environment where cultural behavior is assessed, interpretations are pursued and valued as well as integrated into health care and nursing care delivery (Kendall, 1995; Giger and Mood, 1997, p. 19; Sullivan, 1998).

NURSING CARE DELIVERY MODELS IN AMBULATORY CARE

Nursing models in ambulatory care have developed and evolved as part of the changing concepts about health, advancing technology, the shift of care to outpatient settings, and the practices supportive of a managed care environment. There are a number of diverse models but regardless of which type, professional ambulatory nursing practice is predicated on:

A. Standards that address important professional issues.
   1. Standards.
      a. Ambulatory care nursing administration and practice standards (AAACN, 2000).
      b. Telephone nursing practice standards (AAACN, 1997).
   2. The use of the nursing process in nurse-client interactions.

B. Nursing care delivery models in ambulatory care are presented classified in three major categories: facilitating access to care, direct intervention, and care coordination.
   1. Models that facilitate access: these types of nursing models function to ensure that consumers have access to the health care system.
      a. Nurse-triage services in clinics and offices are an example of an access model that requires expert assessment skills, critical thinking, and problem-solving skills as well as the ability to deal with diverse and often serious, acute health conditions.

    b. Telephone nursing practice is a subspecialty nursing domain that pervades ambulatory nursing practice in all settings.

        (1) The two general categories of telephone nursing practice settings are:

            (a) Centralized call centers are formal settings where nurses ensure consumers have access by telephone to appropriate health care services.

            (b) Decentralized telephone practice: nurses maintain telephone communication with individuals and families regarding their health care inquiries as a part of their daily practice regardless of the practice setting.

        (2) Nursing roles in telephone practice include the ability to:

            (a) Triage responsibilities regarding queries from clients about health problems that may range from emergency or urgent situations to the inconsequential.

            (b) Assist the caller to access the appropriate provider.

            (c) Provide information about diagnostic test results.

            (d) Call pharmacies with prescriptions.

            (e) Health care education: give medical and health care advice according to standardized protocols.

            (f) Conduct follow-up inquiry and evaluation after treatment.

        (3) Standards of telephone nursing practice were developed and published first by the American Academy of Ambulatory Care Nursing in 1997.

    c. Parish nursing is an example of an access model where nurses are available within a religious or faith community.

        (1) Philosophically parish nursing promotes the health of a faith community by working with the clergy and staff to integrate the theological, sociological, and physiological perspectives of health and healing into word, liturgies, and service of the congregation (O'Brien, 1999, p. 200).

        (2) History: parish nursing, as it is evolving in America today, can trace its roots to Europe.

            (a) Groups such as the German Christian deaconesses (Gemeindeschwestern) were active in the 19th century.

            (b) U.S. contemporary parish nursing was instituted during the mid-1980s by Granger Westberg, a Lutheran pastor, as an outgrowth of a holistic health center project funded jointly by the Kellogg Foundation and the University of Illinois College of Medicine (O'Brien, 1999, p. 200).

        (3) Parish nurses serve as volunteers or as paid staff, affiliated with a particular church or with a specific health care institution in partnership with a local church.

        (4) Parish nurses visit individuals and families in homes, churches, hospitals, extended care facilities, and other community sites.

        (5) Parish nurse roles focus on integrating the spiritual and religious

dimension with wellness, illness, and adaptation to chronic disease.

(6) Roles can vary by individual practice but generally include:

(a) *Health counselor*—answers health question, provides grief/bereavement assistance, counseling for marriage and family problems, substance abuse, dysfunctional behaviors, and other personal needs.

(b) *Health educator*—conducts health screenings and wellness activities (e.g., age-specific health programs, maintain a health-related library and pamphlet file, expand understanding about the role of the parish nurse).

(c) *Health facilitator*—trains volunteers to assist in family crises, refers individuals and families to community resources, facilitates small groups (single parents, marriage encounter, loss support), participates in healing services, and coordinates outreach efforts.

(d) *Liaison* to health services and professionals in the local community (e.g., work in partnership with and as a referral source to physicians and public health nurses) (O'Brien, 1999, pp.201-202).

2. Nursing models providing health care directly to consumers. The second general category of nursing models in ambulatory care includes those that provide direct nursing care. These embody the following care delivery systems.

a. Nursing Centers or Nurse-Managed Clinics—are both a concept and a place (Frenn, Lundeen, Martin, Riesch, and Wilson, 1998).

(1) Conceptual definitions of nursing centers require two dimensions:

(a) That the nursing care is directly accessible to the client, family, or community.

(b) That all nursing practice is directly controlled by nurses.

(2) Geographically, nursing centers operate within a specific locale.

(3) Classified in three types (Reisch, 1992).

(a) Community Health and Institutional Outreach models: can be freestanding or institution-sponsored.

(i) Provide primary care services to medically underserved populations.

(ii) Use a multidisciplinary staff.

(iii) Are funded by diverse public and private sources.

(b) Wellness and health promotion models: based on community needs with services developed to focus on promoting health.

(i) Services often delivered where groups gather (work, school, church, shelters).

(ii) Often viewed as alternatives to traditional health care delivery.

(c) Faculty practice, independent practice, and nurse entrepreneurship models: include agencies and services owned and operated by nurses (Frenn, et al, 1999, p. 55).

b. Clinical nurses in medical offices (hospital-based, HMO, community, etc.): function according to the practices of the institution.

(1) Triage patient problems and needs in face-to-face and telephone encounters.

(2) Monitor patient conditions and health status.

(3) Perform nursing therapies for treatment of illness/disease (intravenous therapy for dehydration, medication administration, immunizations, etc.).

(4) Educate patients and families about managing their disease (diabetic teaching, asthma control, etc.).

(5) Communicate health information between physicians and patients (follow-up reports on laboratory/radiology findings, changes in medications or therapies, etc.).

(6) Assist patients and families to access other relevant providers (e.g., specialist referrals, diagnostic studies, other treatments such as physical, occupational, or speech therapy, etc.).

3. Care coordination is the third category of nursing care delivery models found in ambulatory settings.

a. Care coordination emerged from managed care environments as they expended efforts to reduce unnecessary costs. Currently, regulatory agencies are mandating that health care be coordinated across the continuum of care, not just in separate agencies (JCAHO, 1998).

b. Definition: *care coordination* is a process that seeks to achieve the optimal cost-effective use of scarce resources by helping individuals get health, social, and support services that meet their needs at a given point in time or across the life span (Powell, 2000a).

c. The care coordination process includes (Case Management Society of America, 1995; Powell, 2000b):

(1) Outreach efforts, that is selecting, locating, and contacting the appropriate individuals and populations.

(2) Identifying appropriate community health services and funding sources.

(3) Matching the health service and funding resource with the individual's need/s.

(4) Coordinating health care decisions, plans, and activities among the individual and/or family, the clinician, and the provider organization.

(5) Communicating, evaluating, and reporting outcomes.

d. Care coordination historically has been known by the terms care management and/or case management.

e. Types of care coordination models: can be classified in several ways.

(1) Institution-based vs. outpatient settings.

(2) Individual case focus vs. population focus (e.g., geriatrics, special needs, pediatrics).

(3) Disease management models: those that deal with specific

disease (e.g., diabetes, asthma, behavioral and mental health disorders, etc.).

f. Care coordination integrates two major processes (Forbes, 1999).

(1) Case or care management: "a collaborative process which assesses, plans, implements, coordinates, monitors, and evaluates options and services to meet an individual's health needs through communication and available resources to promote quality, cost-effective outcomes" (Case Management Society of America, 1995, p. 8).

(a) Includes screening for and identifying individuals/groups at risk for illness or disease to focus resources for patients and/or families with greatest need.

(b) Ensures timely, appropriate access to and utilization of health care benefits and services.

(c) Communicates appropriate information to consumers and providers that improves the management and mediation of disease symptoms and promotes positive health behaviors.

(d) Measures, monitors, evaluates, and reports outcomes in terms of improvements in patients' health and well-being and reduced costs.

(e) Educates physicians, health professionals, and consumers as to the roles of care managers and the benefits of holistic care coordination.

(2) Utilization management, the second process of care coordination across the continuum of care, is the management and "evaluation of the medical necessity, appropriateness, and efficiency of the use of health care services, procedures, and facilities under the auspices of the applicable health benefit plan" (Carneal, 1998).

(a) Historically conceptualized and operationalized as the review of hospital medical records for appropriate lengths of stay.

(b) Currently expanded from the ambulatory perspective to include evaluating:

(i) The best type of institution to provide the care (hospital, subacute facility, home, etc.).

(ii) The type of provider required to provide appropriate care (physician, advanced practitioner, nurse, pharmacist, nutritionist, etc.).

(c) A tool of utilization management is the review of the clinical situation and/or the medical record. Reviews are conducted in different time frames (Shi and Singh, 1998, pp. 311-312).

(i) *Prospective utilization review* is performed before the care is delivered using guidelines to determine appropriateness.

(ii) *Concurrent utilization review* occurs during the course of health care utilization (e.g., hospitalization) and plans are developed for appropriate, timely discharge from services.

(iii) *Retrospective utilization review* occurs after the service has been consumed in efforts to determine improved utilization, often profiling and comparing practices among different providers.

(d) Evaluation of optimal utilization is dependent on the:
  (i) Severity and acuity of the presenting situation.
  (ii) Skill and competence of the provider/s.
  (iii) Type of therapy or intervention required.
  (iv) Consumer preference.

g. Care coordination model, coordinating the health care of individuals or populations with specific diseases or conditions that put them at risk requires integrating diverse systems, processes, and tools (Figure 3-1, AAACN-ANA, 1997, pp. 44-45).

(1) Specify a clear vision statement that contains expected outcomes, goals, and specific objectives relevant to:
  (a) Managing the disease or presenting situation.
  (b) Improving health outcomes.
  (c) Reducing costs.

(2) Designate the multidisciplinary team of providers (network) with clearly written roles and functions.
  (a) Core providers: those primarily responsible and accountable for coordinating access to and appropriate utilization of health services.
  (b) Resource providers: those used on an ad hoc or referral basis.

(3) Establish written standards for the care coordination process that include:
  (a) Clinical guidelines for care.
  (b) Program management protocols: methods used in program operations (e.g., policies and procedures).

(4) Implement a well-formulated quality assurance and performance improvement program and system.
  (a) Specify indicators that measure success.
  (b) Establish monitoring, tracking, and evaluation systems.
  (c) Disseminate relevant, user-friendly reports that support informed decision making.

(5) Execute a planned, clear system of communication that addresses modes of team member interactions, the reporting of outcomes, and the revisions needed to improve outcomes (Mastal, 1999).
  (a) Establish a written plan of care that addresses the client's health problems, treatment goals, therapeutic interventions, and expected outcomes.

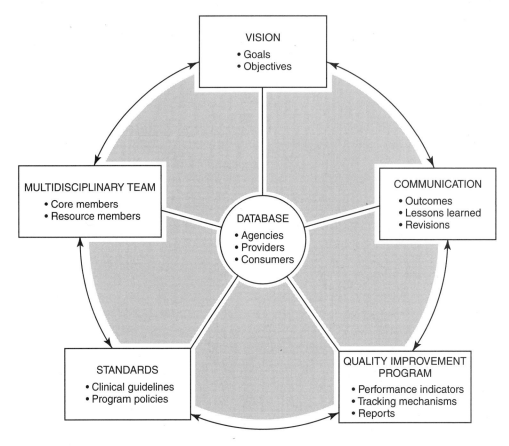

FIGURE 3-1 ■ Conceptual model: health care coordination (Developed by Margaret Mastal. Adapted from AAACN/ANA [1999]: *Conceptual model: managing patient populations.* Washington DC. American Nurses Publishing.)

    (b) Specify how changes in the client's status are communicated among team members (written and verbal).

    (c) Identify systematic evaluation periods and revisions to the plan of care.

    (d) Establish timetables for the collection and reporting of data and information (e.g., client outcomes, costs, etc.).

(6) Establish and maintain an accurate, formal database.

    (a) The database must minimally contain:

        (i) Demographic and credentialing information about agencies and providers.

        (ii) Demographic and clinical information about consumers, both at the individual and population levels.

    (b) The database optimally will be:

        (i) Electronic for ease of data retrieval and reporting.

      (ii) Able to be linked to other databases for use across the consumer's life span.

  C. Evolving concepts of health that expand the notion beyond curing illness to include emphasizing disease prevention and health promotion for both individuals and populations have changed the face of ambulatory care.

    1. These concepts have spurred the emergence of new expectations and practices for providers and consumers across diverse outpatient settings.

    2. Multidisciplinary teams of providers, partnering with consumers, focus on wellness, disease prevention, recovery from acute illness, adaptation to chronic disease, and palliation with dignity at the end of life.

    3. Changes in the health care environment have presented new, expanded, evolving roles for the nurse as an integral member of the provider team and the consumer community.

REFERENCES

American Academy of Ambulatory Care Nursing (2000): *Ambulatory care nursing administration and practice standards.* Pitman, NJ: Author.

American Academy of Ambulatory Care Nursing (1997): *Telephone nursing practice administration and practice standards.* Pitman, NJ: Author.

American Academy of Ambulatory Care Nursing/American Nurses' Association (1997): *Nursing in ambulatory care: the future is here.* Washington, DC: American Nurses Publishing.

American Nurses' Association (1995): *Nursing: a social policy statement.* Kansas City, MO: Author.

Bedlek AK (1996): A new approach to primary nursing. *AAACN Viewpoint,* 18 (1).

Butterfield P (1990): Thinking upstream: Nurturing a conceptual understanding of the societal context of health behavior. *Adv Nurs Sci* 12(2):1-8.

Carneal G (1998): Getting accredited. *Continuing Care,* 17(10):18-24, 42.

Case Management Society of America (1995): *Standards of practice for case management.* Little Rock: Author.

DuBrin A J (1998): *The complete idiot's guide to leadership.* New York: Alpha Books.

Forbes MA (1999): The practice of professional nurse case management. *Nursing Case Management,* 4(1):28-33.

Frenn M, Lundeen S L, Martin KS, Riesch SK, Wilson SA (1998): Symposium of nursing centers: past, present and future. *J Nurs Ed,* 35(2): 4-62.

Giger JN, Mood LH (1997): Culturally competent teamwork. In Dienemann J, editor: *Cultural diversity in nursing: issues, strategies, and outcomes.* Washington, DC: American Academy of Nursing.

Gulzar L (1999): Access to health care. *Image,* 31(1):13-19.

Haas S, Hackbarth D (1995): Dimensions of the staff nurse role in ambulatory care: Part II—comparison of role dimension in four ambulatory settings. *Nurs Econ,* 13 (3):152-165.

Hackbarth D (1995): Institute of Medicine revises definition of primary care. *AAACN Viewpoint,* 17(4).

Institute of Medicine (1978): Primary care in medicine: a definition. *A manpower policy for primary health care: report of a study.* Washington, DC: National Academy Press.

Institute of Medicine (1996): *Primary care: America's health in a new era.* Washington, DC: National Academy Press.

Joint Commission on Accreditation of Healthcare Organizations (JCAHO) (1998): *Comprehensive accreditation manual for health care networks.* Oakbrook Terrace, IL: Author.

Kendall F E (1995): Valuing diversity. In Griggs LB, Louw LL, editors: *Valuing diversity new tools for a new reality.* New York: McGraw-Hill.

Kudzma E C (1999): Culturally competent drug administration. *Am J Nurs* 99(8):46-51.

Mastal M (1999): Coordinating the health care of children with special needs. International Council of Nurses Centennial Conference, London, England.

McDonald G, Bunton R (1992): Health promotion: discipline or disciplines? In R. Bunton R, McDonald G, editors: *Health promotion: disciplines and diversity* (1-9). London: Routledge.

Morgan IS, Marsh GW (1998): Historic and future health promotion contexts for nursing. *Image: J Nurs Scholarship,* 30(4):379-383.

O'Brien ME (1999): *Spirituality in nursing.* Sudbury MA: Jones and Bartlett.

Powell SK (2000a): *Case management a practical guide to success in managed care.* Philadelphia: Lippincott.

Powell SK (2000b): *Advanced case management outcomes and beyond.* Philadelphia: Lippincott.

Purnell LD Paulanka BJ (1998): *Transcultural health care.* Philadelphia: FA Davis.

Riesch SK (1992): Nursing centers. In Fitzpatrick JJ, Jacox A, Taunton RL, editors: *Annual review of nursing research,* vol 10. *Part II: Research on nursing care delivery.* New York: Springer.

Rush K (1997): Health promotion ideology and nursing education. *J Adv Nurs* 25:1292-1298.

Shi L Singh DA (1998): *Delivering health care in America: a systems approach.* Gaithersburg, MD: Aspen.

Sullivan EJ (1998): President's message on differences. *Reflections* 24(2):4.

Thomas RR (1996): *Redefining diversity.* New York: American Management Association.

U.S. Department of Health and Human Services (DHHS) (1991): *Healthy people 2000: national health promotion and disease prevention objectives.* DHHS Publication No. (PHS) 91-50213. Washington, DC: Author.

U.S. Department of Health and Human Services (DHHS) (1999): Website of the Secretary's Council on National Health Promotion and Disease Prevention Objectives for 2010. Available at: http://web.health.gov/healthypeople

U.S. Department of Health and Human Services (DHHS) (2000): *Healthy people 2010: understanding and improving health.* Washington, DC: DHHS Government Printing Office.

Williams SJ (1993): Ambulatory health care services. In Williams SJ, Torrens PR, editors: *Introduction to health services.* New York: Delmar.

World Health Organization (1978): *Primary health care. Report of the international conference on primary health care,* Alma Ata, USSR. Geneva: Author.

World Health Organization (1987): Ottawa charter for health promotion. *Health Promotion* 1(4):iii-iv.

4 Ambulatory Care Team

ROSE BROWNE, MSN, RN-C

OBJECTIVES

Study of the information presented in this chapter will enable the learner to:

1. Understand why the roles of both professionals and nonprofessionals working in ambulatory care are changing.

2. Describe a typical ambulatory care team and the evolving role of the professional nurse on the team.

3. Discuss current strategies being used to improve collaboration and build effective teams.

4. Describe priority management in ambulatory care.

5. Develop an understanding of the extent to which the professional nurse working in ambulatory care must master the skills of both supervision and delegation.

6. Recognize that conflict exists and can often be used for positive change.

The growing emphasis on ambulatory care has created new and innovative roles for the entire health care workforce in the outpatient setting. Most notable is the prominence being placed on primary care—the coordinated, interdisciplinary provision of comprehensive health care and the point at which the patient first seeks assistance from the health care system (Dowling, et al., 1996). Primary care's increased utilization of teams, with their attention on health promotion and disease prevention, positions nurses in the forefront of this health care revolution. The historical role of nurses as patient health educators, as well as their global involvement in the entire spectrum of the patient's care makes them the members of the team most qualified to effectively coordinate that care. In order to accomplish this, professional nurses must be comfortable with the collaborative nature of ambulatory care, understand how to prioritize their nursing interventions, and improve their skills in supervision and delegation. As competition increases, the professional nurse must also be able to recognize and deal with conflict so that the team can work in partnership to fully maximize the benefit to the patient. Physicians, physician assistants (PAs), and nurse practitioners (NPs) still determine the type of care patients receive but they are no longer solely responsible. "Instead it is a team effort and the nurse . . . is the thread that ties it all together" (Browne and Biancolillo, 1997, p. 31).

DIFFERENTIATED PRACTICE IN AMBULATORY CARE

Nursing practice in ambulatory care is differentiated by the qualifications of the nurse and the role the nurse plays in different settings. Increasingly, roles of low complexity are being filled by unlicensed assistive personnel (UAP) and/or licensed practical nurses (LPNs) while the complex roles of nurse-run clinics or case management are being filled by registered nurses (American Academy of Ambulatory Care Nursing [AAACN] and American Nurses' Association [ANA], 1997).

A. Distinguishing the role of the registered nurse (RN) within the ambulatory care setting is problematic for the following reasons:
  1. Nurses in ambulatory care usually work as members of a multidisciplinary team in which the role of the professional nurse is still evolving.
  2. The need for nursing is not universal in ambulatory care settings. Historically, it is the patient who initiates the encounter for the purposes of medical services (AAACN and ANA, 1997).
  3. Several disciplines, both professional and nonprofessional, practice simultaneously, often providing similar or overlapping services.
  4. The need to contain costs will more than likely determine who performs which role.

B. Role definition.
  1. All of the health care workforce in the ambulatory care setting, not just nursing, is grappling with the issue of role definition.
  2. Each discipline is reassessing their roles and their relationship both to the delivery system and to other workers.
  3. More than likely, financing will be a key factor in determining how both health care is delivered and by whom. The result will be increased competition which can be seen by the following:
    a. Nurse practitioners (NPs) and physician assistants (PAs) are increasingly assuming responsibilities originally within the domain of the physician. It costs far less to educate an NP or a PA than to educate a physician.
    b. As the supply of specialty physicians increases, more specialists will attempt to provide primary care.
    c. Increasingly, optometrists are performing procedures originally performed only by ophthalmologists.
    d. LPNs and UAP are increasingly being used to fill many of the low complexity tasks originally done by the professional nurse.

C. Role of nursing.
  1. In spite of the presence of multiple disciplines, nursing has a unique role in ambulatory care.
  2. The professional nurse provides direct care to the patient while at the same time providing care coordination to ensure that:
    a. The patient progresses through the system appropriately.
    b. Referrals for needed services are initiated.
    c. Education on self-care management, health promotion, and disease prevention is provided.
    d. Case management for high-risk patients is planned.

3. Telephone management: RNs provide guidance and care to patients over the phone. RNs are ideal for telephone triage because of their skills in giving advice and directing patients to the appropriate level of care (Richter and Felix, 1999).
4. It is usually the professional nurse, by virtue of his/her training, who possesses the leadership skills necessary to ensure that:
   a. The environment is safe and secure to meet the patient's needs.
   b. The clinic work flows smoothly and efficiently.

AMBULATORY CARE TEAM

An ambulatory care team can be any patient and his/her family partnered with any group of health care workers who provide care in an outpatient setting. As a team, they collaborate to ensure that assessments are multidisciplinary, to develop a treatment plan to assure that care is continuous and that scarce resources are not wasted doing discipline-specific variations on the same task. They negotiate where responsibilities lie when more than one provider can provide services to meet patient needs (AAACN and ANA, 1997). The team recognizes that control over the encounter remains primarily with the patient and/or family and that acceptance and compliance with treatment plans are determined by the patient (AAACN and ANA).

A. Ambulatory care is personal health care provided to individuals or a population of individuals who are not occupying a bed in a health care institution or at home (Mezey, 1999).
B. Ambulatory care can be practiced in a variety of settings (see Chapter 2).
C. Most significant is the emphasis being placed on primary care. Primary care is "the provision of integrated, accessible care services by clinicians who are accountable for addressing a large majority of the personal health care needs of their patients over a period of time, with the understanding that the patient may sometimes need others to care for those health needs (e.g., physician subspecialists, physical therapists, social workers). It is also implicit in this definition that the primary care provider must act as a coordinator for those health needs" (Mezey, 1999, p. 188).
D. Primary care teams.
   1. As an increased number of health care organizations move toward a primary care delivery system, it is likely that the primary care provider will be a *primary care team.*
      a. A primary care provider can be a physician, a nurse practitioner, or a physician assistant.
      b. A primary care team is usually a primary care provider aligned with a group of other health care providers consisting of but not limited to physicians, nurses, social workers, dietitians, pharmacists, and clerical support staff. This team is responsible for:
         (1) Providing comprehensive health care to a patient and/or to a panel of patients on their team.
         (2) Serving as the point of access to the system.

(3) Ensuring that the highest quality care is provided in the most cost-effective manner possible.

(4) Focusing their treatment and their education on self-care management, health promotion, and disease prevention.

E. Roles of team members in primary care—the disciplines most commonly included as core members of the primary care team (PCT) include:

1. *Physicians/NPs/PAs*—responsible to deliver comprehensive general health care to a panel of patients ensuring that the patient's care is consolidated within the hands of the primary care team.

2. *Social workers*—provide psychosocial assessments, ongoing counseling and treatment, and serve as consultants on psychosocial issues to other team members.

3. *Dietitians*—perform nutritional screening and/or assessment and develop, implement, and educate the patient and family members in an appropriate nutrition therapy plan.

4. *Pharmacists*—educate patients about medication regime including side effects.

5. *Clerks*—enroll new patients, set up clinics, schedule appointments, and retrieve charts to ensure the providers are able to deliver care.

6. *Psychologists*—more recently, many teams have incorporated a psychologist as a member in order to identify and treat the growing number of mental health patients requiring more intense treatment than that able to be provided by the core members.

7. Nurses.

F. Nurses in primary care.

1. Nursing plays an integral role as a member of the primary care team.

2. As the member of the team who is most likely to be present at all times, the professional staff nurse provides direct care as well as coordination of care for the patients on their team, ensuring continuity.

3. A significant contribution of nursing is the ability to carry out many of the roles of other members of the team often adding such responsibilities as dietary education, psychosocial support, and clerical duties in the event that these team members are not available.

4. Specific role dimensions that routinely fall to the RN on the team include:

a. Triage to determine an appropriate course of action.

(1) Immediate intervention, either to the emergency department or to an urgent care center to divert patients from the expense of an emergency room visit.

(2) Intervention within 24 hours.

(3) A routine appointment.

b. Referrals to other members of the team or to community services such as home care, assisted living facilities, or nursing homes.

c. Case management.

(1) According to Bower (1992) case management (as cited in Richter and Felix, 1999, p. 227) is a "collaborative process that assesses,

plans, implements, coordinates, monitors, and evaluates options and services for meeting an individual's health needs and promoting quality cost-effective outcomes."

(2) Although case management programs are not exclusively run by RNs, it is the RN who has the appropriate skills to coordinate the care of the patient across the continuum of care. Thus the professional nurse on the primary care team is positioned in such a manner that encourages and supports a case manager role.

d. LPN/UAP supervision: as roles evolve the ability to supervise and delegate responsibilities to LPNs and UAP will be essential.

e. Telephone advice/screening.

(1) Call centers with formalized triage protocols for specific complaints are usually used.

(2) However, a study done by Mayo (1998) suggests that using protocols for every patient is not always possible because protocols do not always cover all the patient symptoms encountered. This study found that, in many cases, nurses felt that connecting with the patient was just as important and more beneficial to the patient. Thus the advantage of using the team nurse in this role should be considered.

f. Patient advocacy.

(1) In this dimension, the nurse must balance the needs of the patient with the needs of the organization.

(2) Recent efforts to manage health care have involved a supply approach that typically uses techniques that in some way restrict consumer access to health care services and/or steer them to lower cost services.

(3) Increasing evidence shows that although the supply side approach has decreased costs, it has performed poorly in the areas of patient satisfaction and quality of care (Veterans Administration [VA] Office of Primary and Ambulatory Care, 1998).

(4) Demand management, a shared patient-provider decision-making strategy, "leads to a reduction in both the actual and perceived need for healthcare services such as hospitalization, office visits, and emergency room visits. The decrease in the demand for services lowers patterns of utilization and reduces healthcare costs while maintaining quality and improving customer satisfaction" (VA Office of Primary Care, p. 1). It accomplishes this by:

(a) Focusing on providing the right care at the right time in the right place.

(b) Using alternative care such as telephone advice.

(c) Educating patients on chronic disease management, self-care and wise consumerism by informing patients on how and when to use the health care system.

(d) Encouraging the use of complementary services such as health promotion and screening programs.

g. Patient health education: Although the entire team is responsible for patient health education, a major portion usually falls to the RN because he/she often spends substantially more time with the patient than other professionals on the team. Additionally, nurses have historically been patient health educators by virtue of their education and their skills. This education:

(1) Should include an assessment of the patient's readiness to learn, the goal of the teaching, the content taught, who was taught, the method used, any barriers to learning the patient may have, and the patient's response.

(2) Includes information on disease, medication, self-care management, and lifestyle risk factors.

(3) Focuses on health promotion and disease prevention to both individuals and groups.

(4) Should be consistent with the *Healthy People 2010 Objectives* being proposed by the U.S. Department of Health and Human Services, which mandates a heightened awareness of prevention (U.S. Department of Health and Human Services, 1999).

(5) Should be congruent with nursing theory, such as Dorothea E. Orem's (1995) theory of self-care in which the nurse designs an effective supportive-educative nursing system that is holistic in approach. The goal of a supportive-educative system is for the patient to become an effective self-care agent, which is the ability to perform self-care activities. This premise is contemporary with today's concepts of health promotion and health maintenance and promotes the individuals' and families' responsibility for health care, which is essential when considering today's emphasis on outpatient services and home care.

(6) Encourages the participation of family members and significant others whenever possible.

(7) Takes into consideration the increase in the number of elderly patients as well as those with chronic diseases.

(a) The number of people over age 65 will double in the next 25 years, driving up the demand for health services that focus on chronic illness and supportive services (Knickman, 1999).

(b) Nurses will need to increase their awareness of the complex health care needs of the elderly, encourage and solicit family involvement, and concentrate their education on health-promoting behaviors that foster independence for as long as possible.

(c) Additionally, this education should include information about available options when independence becomes more difficult. Nursing homes are no longer the only choice. Other sources of care becoming increasingly popular are home care and assisted living facilities (Knickman, 1999).

(8) Evaluates when end-of-life planning should be initiated so that patients can be educated about their rights to plan their medical care and to have information regarding advance directives (i.e., living wills, health care proxies, and treatment preferences).

(9) Recognizes the importance of confidentiality.

   h. Quality improvement activities.

(1) In spite of the interdisciplinary approach in primary care, nurses often lead the way in identifying quality improvement activities for the entire team.

(2) Because nurses are heavily involved in so many aspects of delivering health care they are the ones most likely to be able to identify the problems or topics to be evaluated while ensuring that professional assessment and judgment are incorporated into the quality improvement process.

(3) As the amount of care provided in the outpatient setting increases so too will the amount of quality improvement activities increase to include, but not be limited to, the following:

(a) Accessibility and timeliness of care.

(b) Telephone access to care.

(c) Access to specialists for complex health-related issues.

(d) Availability of preventive services.

(e) Outcomes of clinical interventions, including patient education.

(f) Patient satisfaction.

5. The professional nurse must recognize that his/her knowledge and understanding of all aspects of a patient's care does not mandate that the nurse perform everyone's role. Instead, this knowledge makes him/her the person most qualified to:

   a. Coordinate the care of the patient.

   b. Delegate appropriate tasks to the appropriate member of the team.

   c. Fully utilize leadership and delegation skills to ensure a collaborative team effort and a smooth flow of clinic activities.

COLLABORATION

Collaboration is to work together toward a common goal. "In a collaborative relationship, there is an agreement to pursue a common purpose and a sharing of knowledge to resolve problems, decide issues, and set goals within a structure of collegiality" (Rowland and Rowland, 1997, p. 50).

   A. The egalitarian nature of ambulatory care requires that collaboration occur within and across disciplinary lines.

1. Physicians still determine what type of medical care is provided, and they share the responsibility with other professionals on the health care team for the delivery of all health care services.
2. As a result, greater collaboration and cooperation is essential.
3. All disciplines must concur and agree on who will provide what for the patient.
4. The common goal is the provision of cost-effective quality care. It is paramount to the success of the ambulatory care team.

B. Critical attributes for collaborative practice (Hertz, 1996; Liedtka and Whitten, 1997; Stapleton, 1998).
  1. Characteristics of a collaborative team.
    a. Goals, values, and vision are developed and agreed upon.
    b. Roles and responsibilities have been defined.
    c. Specific tasks and relevant time frames have been identified.
    d. Monitors are in place to evaluate team performance.
    e. Team norms or practice/process parameters have been established (e.g., conflict resolution, decision-making).
    f. Open, honest communication is practiced and team members are willing to discuss differences.
    g. The team deals with problems, concerns, issues, etc.
    h. A unified front: mutual trust, respect, and support.
    i. Diversity in style and scope of practice is acknowledged and valued.
    j. Responsibility and accountability are shared.
    k. Financial issues, which affect the team, are discussed with the group.
    l. Data measures, reports, and analytical processes are familiar to all team members.
  2. Individual team member characteristics (Leidtka and Whitten, 1997; Stapleton, 1998).
    a. Has expertise that contributes to the overall functioning of the team.
    b. Is willing to devote time and energy to the relationship.
    c. Is professionally competent.
    d. Understands the value and contribution of each of the other team members.
    e. Recognizes individual strengths, abilities, and personal power.
    f. Recognizes collaboration as an opportunity for improvement.
    g. Accepts their role within the context of a larger system.

C. Outcomes of collaboration (Dunevitz, 1997; McCloskey and Maas, 1998).
  1. Health care accessibility is enhanced.
  2. Choices and options for patient and providers are improved.
  3. Quality care is maintained.
  4. Patient and provider satisfaction is improved.
  5. Resources are optimized.
  6. Rework is minimized and assignment turnover is improved.

D. Barriers to collaboration (Stapleton, 1998).
  1. Practice styles or thought processes are not well understood as a result of separate training for each health care provider.

2. A hierarchical culture of health care delivery does not involve equality and autonomy for all professionals within their scope of practice and may not be conducive to providers practicing collaboratively.
3. Gender oriented ways of thinking and communicating.
4. Dominance of the medical profession in the health care system with a potential lack of understanding and appreciation for the value and contributions of other professions.
5. The traditionally independent nature of medical practice.
6. The impact of social status on professional interactions and on the parity and equality implied in a collaborative relationship.
E. Administrative and organizational support required for a collaborative team (Liedtka, 1997).
   1. In order to create environments that support successful collaboration, the organization and administrators should:
      a. Acknowledge collaborative teams as a valued model of practice and part of the organizational culture.
      b. Provide encouragement and incentives.
      c. Model collaboration and open communication.
      d. Assure measurement systems are in place to link practice behaviors with financial outcomes.
      e. Lead by supporting and facilitating versus managing through authority.
      f. Take responsibility for proper functioning of the team and for resolution of issues.
      g. Monitor development of protocols for team improvement and evaluation, standardization of practice, and outcomes information.
      h. Commit time and resources for team development.
F. Skills required for collaborative team members (Hertz, 1996; Schraeder, Dworak, and Shelton, 1997).
   1. Know how to collaborate as a team member and foster collaboration as a team leader.
   2. Be able to facilitate and lead high performance teams to demonstrate excellent team efficiency, dynamics, and group thinking.
   3. Develop an excellent personal interaction style fostered by specific actions on which people can easily focus.
   4. Use group dynamic skills effectively.
   5. Use methods to engage a team in problem-solving.
   6. Use conflict management skills.
   7. Know how to give and receive constructive feedback.
   8. Know how to honor and work with culturally diverse organizations, teams, and individuals.

PRIORITY MANAGEMENT

In ambulatory care, priority management refers to the ability to direct the flow of patients so that the clinic runs smoothly and efficiently.

A. This means that patients:
1. With acute problems are triaged and treated quickly and efficiently.
2. Are seen in a timely manner and as close to their appointment time as possible.
3. Are provided with the appropriate care at the appropriate level.
B. Obstacles: although patients have scheduled appointments, it is often difficult to predict the flow of the clinic because changes in volume, which occur frequently as a result of:
1. A high number of walk-ins.
2. A high number of no-shows.
3. A high number of overbooks/add-ons.
4. Sicker patients.
5. Emergencies.
C. Strategies to maintain an optimum flow.
1. Allow the routine flow to be accomplished by assistive personnel.
2. Identify the nature of the patient visit and assign the patient to the appropriate caregiver or member of the team.
3. Focus nursing interventions on those patients or groups of patients with complex nursing needs.
4. Delegate tasks with low complexity to assistive personnel.

SUPERVISION AND DELEGATION

The central meaning of supervision is to have the direction and oversight of the performance of others whereas delegation is to commit or entrust to another, to delegate a task (*American Heritage Dictionary*, 1992).

A. Supervision.
1. The professional nurse working in the ambulatory care setting has a great deal of autonomy as a result of the following:
a. In many instances, the nurse reports to a physician or a clinic manager who may not be a nurse.
b. The nurse may be the only RN on a team functioning in one of the many off-site or freestanding facilities being erected in multiple locations in an effort to bring care closer to the community.
c. In instances where an identified nurse-manager does exist, this manager is often responsible for several areas and is not always readily available.
2. The autonomous role will require that the staff nurse in ambulatory care develop the skills necessary to:
a. Direct and guide other professional members on their team.
b. Direct and guide the outcomes of the performance of LPNs and UAP on their team.
c. Provide the direction necessary to ensure completion of the task.
d. Develop a broad understanding of primary care practice.
3. Supervision of unlicensed assistive personnel (UAP).

a. Rising health care costs, downsizing, and the implementation of new care models has resulted in an increase in the use of UAP.

b. UAP function in an assistive capacity to the RN in the delivery of patient care (Badovinac, Wilson, and Woodhouse, 1999).

c. Because of the increase in the number of UAP, staff nurses are increasingly finding themselves in supervisory roles for which they are ill prepared. Their concerns include (Haas and Gold, 1997):

  (1) Resentment over the amount of time it takes to supervise UAP.

  (2) Discomfort in giving feedback, both negative and positive.

  (3) False ideas about legal responsibilities related to supervision.

d. Strategies that staff nurses should develop for effective supervision (Haas and Gold, 1997).

  (1) Know your assistive workers, their role expectations, and their levels of competence. The best way to accomplish this is to consistently assign the assistive worker to the same nurse and the same team(s) and/or clinic(s).

  (2) Allocate time for supervision and for evaluating the progress of care delivery. Time for oversight of the work of UAP must be built into the care model so that work performance can be observed and timely performance feedback given.

  (3) Allow for open lines of communication.

    (a) The staff nurse supervising UAP must be willing to recognize the importance of open, respectful, constructive communication.

    (b) When conflict occurs, communication should be nonconfrontational and should focus on actual occurrences, behaviors, and job expectations.

  (4) Adhere to patient care and work performance standards. The staff nurse in a supervisory role must serve as a role model and adhere closely to the standards of care and the mission of the institution in which he/she works.

  (5) Give timely feedback, both positive and negative.

    (a) Personnel, especially those in new positions, should be made aware of how they are progressing.

    (b) Just as patterns of behavior that compromise patients should be addressed immediately, so, too, should a job well done be complimented.

    (c) UAPs should also be encouraged to offer their own feedback and suggestions on how work should be done.

e. Staff nurses should be aware of the following:

  (1) Supervision is a role expectation for all nurses.

  (2) The professional nurse who delegates to a UAP is accountable to supervise the UAP and is not held liable if the UAP is negligent as long as the UAP has been trained and deemed competent.

(3) However, the nurse can be held liable for his/her lack of competence in performing the duties of supervision (Douglas, 1996).

(4) The nurse practice act in their state.

f. Staff nurses should expect the following from their nurse executives and managers (Haas and Gold, 1997).

(1) The opportunity and support needed to learn and perform the act of supervision.

(2) The allocation of enough time so they can supervise appropriately.

(3) Assistance in finding rewards and satisfaction for the role of supervisor.

B. Delegation.

1. "Delegation knowledge is crucial to the successful direction of the health care team in the managed care environment" (Parsons, 1998, p. 26).

2. The professional nurse working on the ambulatory care team must be able to recognize that:

a. One person will be unable to care for the multiple, myriad needs of the patient especially in the current health care environment, which expects a more holistic approach to care.

b. In order to fully utilize and expand his/her professional skills, delegation of certain responsibilities and/or tasks to LPNs and UAP will be an absolute necessity.

c. At times, this delegation may extend to other members of the health care team including clerical support staff, dietitians, social workers, and sometimes the primary provider.

d. The current economic climate will necessitate that decisions be made as to who can best meet the needs of the patient so that everyone is not performing a variation of the same task, but rather complementing one another so that quality care can be provided in the most cost-effective manner possible.

3. In delegating tasks the following should be considered:

a. That the delegation adheres to state laws governing nursing practice.

b. That the right task is assigned to the right person.

c. That a clear, concise description is given of the task to be performed.

d. That the appropriate direction, monitoring, and evaluation are provided as needed depending on to whom the task is assigned.

e. That in ambulatory care, it is not always clear who should perform which task, and team collaboration will be necessary.

f. The need to develop mechanisms for clarification of roles.

4. Barriers to delegation.

a. Confusion in responsibilities and delegation.

b. Preference for doing everything yourself.

c. Lack of experience in the job or in delegating.

d. Lack of confidence in others' abilities to complete the job.

e. Uncertainty over tasks.

    f. Failure to establish effective communication and to follow up.

    g. Blurring of roles.

  5. Effective delegation will require that the professional nurse:

    a. Be familiar with his/her scope of practice within his/her individual institution.

    b. Have knowledge of the state nurse practice act.

    c. Have a good understanding of professional practice standards.

    d. Assign only those activities that are not in the legally protected scope of nursing practice.

    e. Be aware that patient assessment and coordination of care are professional activities that cannot be delegated.

CONFLICT RESOLUTION

Conflict resolution is the use of effective techniques to achieve the desired level of conflict.

A. Conflict can be defined as a process that begins when one party perceives that another party has negatively affected, or is about to negatively affect, something that the first party cares about (Robbins, 1993).

B. In viewing conflict it is important to remember that:

  1. Not all conflict is negative, and, at times, conflict may actually increase creativity, satisfaction, performance, and team effectiveness.

  2. It is inevitable and exists in most healthy organizations.

  3. It can be either internal or external.

  4. It can be overt or covert.

  5. It must be acknowledged before it can be dealt with so that the solution is one that benefits the team.

C. Sources of conflict.

  1. Incompatibility of goals.

  2. Differences and/or perceptions in interpretation of facts.

  3. Disagreements based on behavioral expectations.

  4. Competition for status.

  5. Lack of resources.

  6. Varying beliefs on how things should be done, especially when working in different functional departments.

  7. Difference of position in the hierarchy.

  8. Differences in styles of communication.

D. Sources of conflict within the ambulatory care team.

  1. Rapid, fundamental changes within the ambulatory care arena.

  2. Increased emphasis on teams and the need to work together in an egalitarian environment.

  3. Growing competition among professionals.

  4. Growing competition between professionals and assistive personnel.

  5. Increased pressure to control costs.

  6. Lack of adequate resources within this new competitive market.

  7. Misunderstanding about roles.

8. Lack of communication between disciplines.
9. Interpersonal differences within the team.
10. Disagreements over allocation of space.

E. Managing conflict effectively can contribute to effective changes within the team and improve its performance. Thomas (1976) describes five behavioral approaches used to manage conflict (as cited in Baker, 1995).
   1. Avoiding involves behavior that is unassertive and uncooperative and is characterized by simply not addressing the issues.
   2. Competing is an assertive but uncooperative method of dealing with conflict. With this method individuals pursue their own personal goals without regard for team goals.
   3. Accommodating is a cooperative but unassertive method in which harmony is maintained but issues are not addressed.
   4. Compromise is a cooperative and assertive method in which a workable solution is sought. It is based on give and take involving a series of negotiations and concessions. In comparison to collaboration compromise does not maximize joint satisfaction.
   5. Collaboration, the most desired, is a highly cooperative and assertive method. It represents a desire to maximize joint outcomes. True collaboration is a joint effort of problem solving (Littlefield, 1995). The five steps in problem solving include:
      a. Recognize that conflict exists and that everyone has legitimate concerns.
      b. Analyze the cause or causes of the conflict.
      c. Propose solutions based on everyone's thoughts and feelings on the issue with a clear understanding of the goals.
      d. Select the solution that maximizes the goals and improves patient care.
      e. Implement the solution.
      f. Evaluate and refine the solution—this is an ongoing process and necessary to ensure team maintenance.

F. As health care organizations restructure their organizations based on team-managed philosophy, staff nurses will need improved conflict resolution skills (Baker, 1995). They will need to:
   1. Learn to deal with conflict openly.
   2. Understand the various types of behavioral approaches used to manage conflict.
   3. Recognize that an individual's use of certain conflict resolution behaviors is not only influenced by the culture of the organization but by personal values and beliefs.
   4. Understand that conflict resolution is an ongoing process and that the solution to the conflict needs to be tailored to the individual event.
   5. Develop skills that foster collaborative conflict resolution methods (refer to the Collaboration section earlier in this chapter).

G. Whatever strategy is chosen to reduce conflict nurses will need to learn to "work as team members and many times as team leaders. This means knowing how to delegate . . . and [how] to lead other workers who are highly skilled, but whose specialty skill is outside the traditional role of nursing" (Myers, 1998, p.187). Developing effective conflict resolution skills will be a necessity in order for nurses to be successful in this environment.

REFERENCES

American Academy of Ambulatory Care Nursing (AAACN) & American Nurses' Association (ANA) (1997): *Nursing in ambulatory care: the future is here.* Washington, DC: American Nurses Publishing.

American Heritage Dictionary, ed 3 (1992): Boston: Houghton Mifflin.

Badovinac C, Wilson S, Woodhouse D (1999): The use of unlicensed assistive personnel and selected outcome indicators. *Nurs Econ* 17(4):194-200.

Baker KM (1995): Improving staff nurse conflict resolution skills. *Nurs Econ* 13(5):295-298.

Browne R, Biancolillo K (1997): Fusing roles: the ambulatory care nurse as case manager. *Nurs Management* 28(9):30-31.

Douglass L (1996): *The effective nurse leader and manager,* ed 3. St Louis: Mosby.

Dowling M, Biancolillo K, Blumenthal D, Craig T, Dennis A, Eng J, Evans E, Gozenbach S, Leung J (1996): *VISN 3 primary care product line team final report.* Unpublished manuscript.

Dunevitz B (1997): Collaboration, in a variety of ways, creates health care value. *Nurs Econ* 15(4):218-219.

Haas S, Gold C (1997): Supervision of unlicensed assistive workers in ambulatory settings. *Nurs Econ* 15(1):57-59.

Hertz P (1996): The leader's role in building collaborative teams. *Seminars for Nurse Managers* 4(4):205-206.

Knickman JR (1999): Futures. In Kovner AR, Jones S, editors: *Health care delivery in the United States.* New York: Springer, pp. 505-526.

Liedtka J, Whitten EL (1997): Building better patient care services: a collaborative approach. *Health Care Management Review* 22(3):16-24.

McCloskey JC, Maas M (1998): Interdisciplinary team: the nursing perspective is essential. *Nursing Outlook* 46(4):157-163.

Mayo AM (1998): The role of the telephone advice/triage nurse. *AAACN Viewpoint* 20(6):9-10.

Mezey AP (1999): Ambulatory care. In Kovner AR, Jonas S, editors: *Health care delivery in the United States.* New York: Springer, pp. 183-205).

Myers SM (1998): Patient-focused care: what managers should know. *Nurs Econ* 16(1):180-188.

Orem DE (1995): *Nursing concepts of practice,* ed 5. St. Louis: Mosby.

Parsons LC (1998): Delegation skills and nurse job satisfaction. *Nurs Econ* 16(1):18-26.

Richter P, Felix K (1999): Adding value by expanding RN roles in ambulatory care. *Nurs Econ* 17(4):225-228.

Robbins SP (1993): *Organizational behavior: concepts, controversies, and applications,* ed 6. New Jersey: Simon & Schuster.

Rowland HS, Rowland BL (1997): *Nursing administration handbook,* ed 4. Gaithersburg, MD: Aspen.

Schraeder C, Britt T, Dworak D, Shelton P (1997): Management of nursing within a collaborative physician group practice. *Seminars for Nurse Managers* 5(3):133-138.

Stapleton SR (1998): Team-building: making collaborative practice work. *J Nurse-Midwifery* 43(1):12-18.

U.S. Department of Health and Human Services (1999): *Healthy people 2010 objectives.* Available: http://www.health.gov

Veterans Administration Office of Primary and Ambulatory Care (1998): *Demand Management Fact Sheet.* Unpublished fact sheet.

5 Practice/Office Support

CINDY ANGIULO, MSN, RN, Cm
ELIZABETH DICKEY, MPH, RN, FNP

OBJECTIVES

Study of the information presented in this chapter will enable the learner to:

1. Schedule patients more efficiently.

2. Design more productive workspaces.

3. Maintain safe patient care environments.

4. Control environmental hazards and risks in work settings.

■■ The quality of patient care provided in any ambulatory setting is as dependent on the soundness of the delivery systems and environmental supports as it is the skills and abilities of providers. Nurses play a key role in assuring quality, and therefore this chapter outlines important aspects of patient scheduling, facility design, and environmental management, the latter now largely a matter of regulatory compliance.

SCHEDULING

Scheduling is the prearranged timing of patient visits intended to reduce waiting time for patients and providers. Efficient scheduling will enhance utilization of support staff, space, and ancillary services, such as lab and radiology; and will improve visit planning with regard to financial matters, prior tests and reports, and specific patient preparation. Nurses working in ambulatory care, whether as providers or supporters of that care, must fully comprehend the intricacies of the scheduling system, because the degree to which that system functions effectively has profound effects on work volume and work flow.

    A. Scheduling types (Barnett and Mayer, 1992).

        1. Type of visit.

            a. New patient vs. established patient.

            b. Advance vs. same-day.

            c. Primary care vs. specialty care.

            d. Type of specialty and/or requirement for procedures.

    2. Type of scheduling.

       a. Set time (e.g., 4 patients: 9:00, 9:15, 9:30, 9:45) vs. block time (e.g., 4 patients: all at 9:00).

       b. Fixed time increments (e.g., 1:00, 1:15, 1:30, 1:45) vs. varied time increments (e.g., 1:00, 1:05, 1:10, 1:20, 1:40).

       c. Individual (e.g., one patient per time slot) vs. group (e.g., several patients per time slot).

       d. Provider-specific (e.g., appointment with Dr. Smith) vs. clinic-specific (e.g., appointment with pediatric clinic).

B. Provider variables.

    1. Type of provider (e.g., internist vs. general surgeon; nurse practitioner vs. nurse educator).

    2. Personal traits.

       a. Fast vs. slow worker.

       b. Early, on-time, late starter.

       c. No lunch, short lunch, long lunch.

       d. Needs no support, some support, a lot of support.

    3. Provider-specific show rate (i.e., do not double-book procedures with 90% to 100% show rates).

    4. Specialist-specific issues.

       a. Appropriateness of referral vis-à-vis lack of referral.

       b. Completeness of prior workup.

       c. Previsit planning requirements.

    5. Providers' overall schedule and availability.

       a. On-call requirements.

       b. Meeting requirements.

       c. Teaching schedules.

       d. Planned leaves of absence (e.g., vacation, continuing education).

C. Patient variables.

    1. Urgency of problem and/or follow-up.

       a. Medically urgent.

       b. Medically non-urgent.

       c. Follow-up is time-sensitive.

       d. Follow-up is not time-sensitive.

    2. Newness of the problem.

       a. New patient/new problem.

       b. New patient/existing problem.

       c. Established patient/new problem.

       d. Established patient/existing problem.

    3. Database requirements.

       a. Complete history and physical vs. focused history and physical.

       b. Existence/availability of prior databases/test results.

       c. Need for pre-visit triage and/or assessment.

    4. Special needs.

       a. Foreign language and/or American Sign Language (ASL) interpreters.

      b. Physical limitations including wheelchair users and blind patients.

      c. Acutely ill or debilitated patients using stretchers.

D. Support variables.

   1. Staff.

      a. Number available (ratio of supporters/providers).

      b. Teamed or unteamed.

      c. Type and mix of staff (RN, LPN, NA/MA/technician).

   2. Space.

      a. Number of exam rooms available (ratio of rooms:provider).

      b. Exam room configuration vis-à-vis visit type (room is properly sized and equipped for the type of visit conducted).

   3. Support variables.

      a. Insurance verification/authorization.

      b. Closed vs. open practice (e.g. accepting new patients or restricted to established patients).

   4. Other.

      a. Special equipment availability.

      b. Test results, consult reports availability.

E. Scheduling system features and qualities (Ross, 1998).

   1. Computerized systems should include:

      a. Search capability by:

         (1) Provider.

         (2) Patient.

         (3) Clinic.

         (4) Day/date/time.

      b. Interface with patient registration and financial eligibility.

      c. Coordinate and link two or more visit types or services.

      d. 24-hour interdepartmental access and scheduling capacity.

      e. Trigger for medical record pull and printing of health summary (when available).

   2. All systems should be:

      a. Flexible in response to:

         (1) Varying demand.

         (2) Special needs/requests.

      b. Realistic (i.e., based on actual experience as well as targeted goals).

F. No-shows, cancellations, and late arrivals.

   1. Preventive strategies.

      a. Pre-visit calls to new patients.

      b. Reminder calls to all patients.

      c. Policies for handling chronic failures to appear for appointment.

      d. Tailor appointment time to patient's schedule.

   2. Management strategies that enhance scheduling.

      a. Medical records reviews.

      b. Follow-up calls.

      c. Re-appointing processes/policies.

      d. Outreach to high-risk patients.

   e. Late arrival process/policy.
   f. Statistical monitoring.

FACILITY PLANNING AND SPACE UTILIZATION

The location and design of an ambulatory care facility can make or break a practice. The overall facility must be accessible to patients and staff (parking is a big issue); convenient to home, work, and hospitals; project a positive, healthy image; be capable of expansion and functional change; and support good flow and productivity. Nurses in management positions play a major role in facility planning, design, and oversight, and those in provider roles need an awareness of how space affects productivity and quality of care.

   A. Location issues (Barnett and Mayer, 1992).
      1. Accessibility.
         a. Traffic and congestion patterns.
         b. Adequate, close-in parking (5 to 6 spaces per 1000 sq. ft. of office space).
         c. On bus or metro transit route with convenient stop.
         d. Near home, office, shopping district, or community center.
         e. In compliance with Americans with Disabilities Act (ADA-P.L.#101-336, 1990).
      2. Visibility.
         a. Adequate signage.
         b. Easy entry and egress.
      3. Area safety.
         a. Safe neighborhood.
         b. Adequate police/security protection.
         c. Well-lighted area.
         d. Secure entryways and limited access.
      4. Image.
         a. Not in proximity to noisy, dangerous, odorous, or otherwise offensive business or industry.
         b. Clean.
         c. Low clutter.
      5. Expandability.
         a. For building expansion.
         b. For parking expansion.
   B. Layout and design issues (Barnett and Mayer, 1992).
      1. ADA compliance, especially new and renovated space, and compliance with state and local regulations.
      2. Reception/main waiting.
         a. Patient entryway separate from staff entry.
         b. Sufficient number of public restrooms, telephones.
         c. Main waiting/reception areas sized to accommodate patients, family, and/or friends. Separate adults from children and sick children from well.

    d. Warm, welcoming space with easy access to reception and information.

    e. Private and secure areas for patient registration, insurance authorization, billing discussions, and payment transactions.

3. Exam/direct care space.

    a. Triage/consult space.

        (1) Confidential (i.e., soundproof, doors close).

        (2) For triage locate between waiting area and exam area.

        (3) To accommodate patient plus one adult or two children, interpreter.

        (4) Limit clutter and equipment to reduce distraction.

        (5) Separate telephone triage space from on-site triage space.

        (6) Consult rooms regularly used for patient education, discharge, teaching. Need storage for brochures and educational materials, and may need space for TV monitor, VCR, and computer.

        (7) Triage areas should accommodate computer hook-ups.

    b. Vital sign and measurement areas: These functions may be performed in the triage/interview room, in the exam room, or in an area specially designed for this purpose. The following apply regardless of location.

        (1) Area should accommodate use of automatic BP monitors, pulse oximeters, wide platform digital scales (pediatric digital scales when appropriate).

        (2) Attention to ergonomics needed to support productivity in this area.

        (3) Need hooks and/or counters for patient clothing, purses, etc. and place to sit if taking off shoes prior to weighing.

    c. Exam rooms.

        (1) Minimum of two per provider, higher for certain specialties (e.g., obstetrics, orthopedics, dermatology).

        (2) Minimum of 80 to 120 sq. ft. with appropriate configuration for stretcher accommodations. Check state health code for local standards (American Institute of Architects, 1996).

        (3) In general, multipurpose exam rooms (serves different provider/different functions) preferred over single purpose (specific provider/specific function).

        (4) Designed for visual privacy during disrobing and exam, soundproof for communication (see Environmental Management section starting on p. 77).

        (5) Clustered in twos, threes, or fours, depending on minimum number per provider. Consider proximity to nursing area and consultation rooms.

        (6) Infection control and safety issues.

        (7) Able to lighten or darken as needed.

        (8) Flag or light system to facilitate internal communication (e.g., clean/dirty, occupied by patient only, patient and provider, or patient and assistive staff, and assistance needed).

     (9) Adequate seating for provider, patient, and parent or companion, interpreter.

    (10) Adequate storage/counter space for essential supplies and equipment.

    (11) Appropriate and limited art, signage, or instructional material on walls.

    (12) Adequate waiting and/or computer space.

    (13) Attention paid to ergonomic requirements of various exams.

    (14) Isolation rooms may be required, especially in pediatric practice.

  d. Treatment/procedure rooms.

    (1) Number of procedure/treatment rooms dependent on specialty.

    (2) Approximately 120 to 200 sq. ft. minimum (American Institute of Architects, 1996).

    (3) Designed for proximity to key equipment and supplies, ease of circulation of two or more staff members, and generally equipped with oxygen, monitoring equipment, and crash cart.

    (4) Spot lighting essential/consider dimmer capabilities.

    (5) Often doubles as observation area so is best located in close proximity to nursing stations.

  e. Nursing/support staff stations.

    (1) Close proximity to exam room clusters.

    (2) Designed *not* to be magnet area for all staff. Often best to decentralize.

    (3) Sufficient counter space for computers and writing, computer screen privacy, paper and forms storage.

    (4) Easy access to medications, biologicals, supplies, and frequently used equipment.

    (5) Private area for reviewing medical records, test results, entering data into patient registers/logs, and phoning patients.

  f. Special work/storage areas.

    (1) Medication room/storage area with refrigeration, locks, preparation counters.

    (2) Clean utility.

    (3) Soiled utility.

    (4) Lab room/work area for in-office lab procedures, microscopic exam of specimens with appropriate disposal facilities.

    (5) Storage rooms for supplies and equipment. Size and design varies according to specialty.

  g. Paperwork areas.

    (1) Charting, dictation, telephone and computer access, space that is private, soundproof, and close to exam rooms.

    (2) Fax and copy room that is private and soundproof.

    (3) Provider office space (solo or communal) is usually located in the rear of the clinic with restricted access, soundproofing for telephone calls, and computer hook-ups.

(4) Nurses involved in visit/care planning, patient education, and chart reviewing need office space similar to that of providers.

h. Interior patient sub-waiting areas are essential for clinics where waits are common between triage/intake, exam, lab/x-ray, or procedures.

4. In-house lab/x-ray.*
   a. Short distance from clinic area to clinic-based phlebotomy.
   b. Need processes to transfer results and radiographs to the clinic.
   c. Sub-waiting area(s) and separate restroom(s).

5. In-house pharmacy.*
   a. Adjacent to medical records area if pharmacist fills Rx directly from the record.
   b. Separate windows for drop-off, pick-up.
   c. Private consult rooms to educate patients about proper drug/device use.
   d. Restricted access to pharmacy staff.

6. Medical records.*
   a. Adjacent to clinic area or designed for quick movement of records to and from the clinic.
   b. Work space for providers and nurses to review records and do charting.
   c. Restricted access to all except records staff.
   d. Expandable space is crucial (or remote storage plan) so long as paper records are maintained.

7. Business office.
   a. Close physical proximity to medical records highly desirable because billing clerks often need to review patient records.

8. Administrative office.
   a. Can be located away from clinic area but be on-site so administrative personnel are available to staff and patients.

9. Staff lounges.
   a. Close proximity to the clinic enhances productivity.
   b. However, lounges should not be visible to or accessible to patients.

10. Maintenance/cleaning/refuse areas.
   a. Clinic staff should know how to access these areas or contact area-specific personnel to perform these functions.
   b. Medical waste has specific handling, disposable, recycling issues (see Environmental Management section that follows).

11. Other design/layout considerations.
   a. Space planning and scheduling should be linked to staff hiring and scheduling.
   b. Support staff can better manage a group of exam rooms when they have direct visual control of those rooms.
   c. Providers and support staff need proximity or devices that ease communication between them.

---

*Items 4 to 6 include only the design features of significant relevance to ambulatory care nurses.

    d. Separate clinic entrance and egress improves flow. Locate discharge planning/exit discharge consult rooms near point of egress.

    e. Use of computers in the clinical areas will increase many-fold in the coming years. New construction and renovation should anticipate the space, wiring and related needs of computerization.

    f. Proximity and speed of elevators in multi-story facilities affects how quickly patients can move from area to area.

ENVIRONMENTAL MANAGEMENT

The assurance of appropriate management plans to provide a safe, accessible, effective, and functional environment of care. Nurses in ambulatory settings have accountability for proactive evaluation of patient care environments and need to develop safety and infection control plans, ongoing monitoring, and staff education (Joint Commission on Accreditation of Healthcare Organizations, 1997).

  A. Safety.

    1. Recognize factors that affect patient safety.

      a. Physical disability.

      b. Mental status and judgement.

      c. Medication effects.

    2. Assess need for furnishings and equipment suitable for population served.

      a. Age/size appropriate.

        (1) Child safety (i.e., electrical outlet covers).

        (2) Elder safety (i.e., heavy, nonmoveable chairs).

        (3) Safety for large/obese patients (i.e., oversized chairs, scales, and wheelchairs).

      b. Specialty specific.

        (1) Rehabilitation patients (i.e., wheel chair accessible).

        (2) Orthopaedic patients (i.e., higher seating).

    3. Develop plans to monitor/control recalled products and medical devices.

    4. Equip environment to promote staff/provider safety.

      a. Patient transfer devices.

      b. Powered examination/procedure tables.

      c. Wheelchair accessible scales.

      d. Hallway safety rails.

    5. Develop hazardous materials and waste management plans.

      a. Identify types of hazardous materials and waste (i.e., chemicals, air pollutants/gases/vapors, blood-soiled items, and energy sources/lasers/x-ray equipment).

      b. Identify handling, storage, using, and disposing procedures consistent with applicable law and regulation (i.e., Material Safety Data Sheets).

      c. Provide staff orientation and education for maintenance/management of hazardous materials and waste.

      d. Use appropriate precautions when working with potentially harmful chemicals.

      e. Implement emergency procedures for exposures to spills.

      f. Develop performance improvement/preventive actions for subsequent hazardous materials and waste incidents.

  6. Assure reporting and investigation of all incidents of injury, property damage, exposure, and occupational illness.

B. Security.

  1. Establish systems to control access.

      a. Monitor facility entrances and parking facilities.

      b. Provide vehicular access to emergency/urgent care areas.

      c. Secure surgical/procedure areas including specialized equipment (i.e., laser equipment).

      d. Secure prescription pads and all medications including sample medications and controlled substances.

  2. Patient and staff/provider identification.

      a. Patient identification at point of service.

      b. Patient identification (banding) at times of reduced consciousness, blood transfusions, chemotherapy.

      c. Photo identification and appropriate attire/presentation for staff/providers.

  3. Recognize security emergencies and implement emergency plan response.

      a. Escalating/aggressive patient behavior/suicide risk patients.

      b. Patients with possession of weapons (i.e., guns, knives, pepper spray).

      c. Bomb threats (i.e., knowledge of questions to obtain information that may help identification of caller).

C. Medical emergencies.

  1. Ensure staff competence in recognizing acute changes in the patient's condition.

  2. Ensure appropriate placement of age-specific medical equipment to institute emergent patient care (i.e., crash cart, resuscitation equipment, transport gurney).

  3. Provide staff orientation and education.

      a. Role and responsibilities during emergencies.

      b. Skills required.

      c. Competency assessment.

      d. Ongoing performance evaluation/scheduled drills.

  4. Initiate emergent treatment/cardiac/respiratory/resuscitation.

  5. Complete documentation for:

      a. Patient's medical record.

      b. Risk management/incident reporting.

  6. Inspection/oversight of medical equipment (refer to the Management of Equipment and Supplies section later in the chapter).

D. Infection control.

  1. Recognize health exposure risks and presence of infection.

    a. Symptoms of infection (i.e., wound drainage, jaundice, diarrhea).

    b. Airborne diseases (i.e., chicken pox, measles, meningitis, mumps, tuberculosis).

    c. High-risk body fluids (i.e., needle sticks, splash to mucous membranes—eyes, nose, mouth).

2. Provide staff orientation/ongoing education.

    a. General infection control principles and clinic-specific procedures (Barnett and Mayer, 1992).

        (1) Disease transmission.

        (2) Standard Precautions.

        (3) Isolation.

        (4) Employee safety.

    b. Competency assessment.

    c. Ongoing education to update on changing infection control requirements.

3. Clinic-specific environmental infection control policies and procedures (University of Washington Medical Center, 1998).

    a. Patient waiting areas.

        (1) Encourage patients with communicable diseases to stay at home if they can be managed safely by telephone communication.

        (2) Signage to encourage reporting of symptoms to receptionist/nurse upon check-in.

        (3) Immediately remove patients and family members with obvious symptoms/diagnosed infection/immunosuppression to exam area.

        (4) Schedule patients with communicable diseases at end of the day.

        (5) Bring services/equipment to patient in exam area to prevent spread of disease to other facilities (i.e., restroom, lab, pharmacy).

        (6) Explain purposes of isolation/procedures to patient and/or family member.

    b. Exam rooms.

        (1) Cleaning between patients such as changing table paper, removing soiled equipment/linen, and disinfecting soiled surfaces.

        (2) Daily cleaning such as exam tables, counter tops, treatment carts, floors.

        (3) Close room occupied by patient with airborne infection and disinfect before placing another patient in the room.

    c. Equipment and supplies.

        (1) Separate all clean and soiled supplies/linen.

        (2) Disinfect/resterilize soiled and/or outdated equipment according to clinic-specific policies and procedures.

        (3) Discard disposable equipment after each use into designated waste receptacles.

        (4) Discard needles and sharps into appropriate sharps containers.

        (5) Clean the handpiece of electronic thermometers after each use.

(6) Use disposable thermometers on infection/isolation patients.

(7) Discard sterile solutions for irrigation 24 hours after opening or sooner.

(8) Follow prescribed reprocessing/high-level disinfection procedures for fiberoptic endoscopes and accessories.

d. Refrigerators.

(1) Separate medication, food, and specimen storage.

(2) Maintain temperature within safe range (36 to 40° F).

(3) Monitor temperature daily and record on a log.

(4) Clean and defrost at regular intervals.

4. Prevention.

a. Assure good hand washing techniques.

b. Avoid direct contact with blood, respiratory or excretory secretions, wound drainage, aerosols, or contaminated articles/patient belongings.

c. Practice body substance isolation for all patients.

d. Provide equipment and protective apparel appropriate in type and size to clinic-specific activity (Joint Commission on Accreditation of Healthcare Organizations, 1997).

(1) Disposable masks, gowns, gloves.

(2) Protective eyewear, face shields.

(3) Isolation sign.

(4) Exam room with sink (splashguards when appropriate) and door.

(5) High filtration mask for patient with newly diagnosed airborne communicable disease at time of transport.

e. Use appropriate containers to hold contaminated items for transport, disposal, reprocessing (i.e., covered metal containers for speculums, endoscope containers).

5. Postexposure treatment.

a. Implement emergency procedures/administer first aid for exposures.

b. Develop post-exposure prophylaxis procedure (i.e., Centers for Disease Control and Prevention [CDC] recommendations).

6. Reportable diseases.

a. Obtain current list of reportable diseases as regulated by state and federal laws (i.e., Centers for Disease and Prevention [CDC] local public health authorities).

b. Ensure mechanism for timely reporting.

c. Document in-patient/employee medical record.

7. Surveillance monitoring (Barnett and Mayer, 1992).

a. Identify and track infections associated with clinic-specific patient care/treatment (i.e., urinary tract infections after instrumentation, gastroenteritis after endoscopy, surgical wound infections).

b. Ensure patient follow-up on signs of infection and laboratory results reporting (i.e., urine, throat, wound cultures).

c. Develop ongoing quality monitoring program, using results to educate staff and develop/modify policies and procedures.

E. Emergency preparedness.
   1. Identify specific procedures in response to internal and external disasters (i.e., fire, explosion, earthquake, hurricane).
   2. Define facility's role in community-wide disaster.
   3. Provide staff orientation and education.
      a. Role and responsibilities during emergencies.
      b. Skills required.
      c. Competency assessment.
      d. Ongoing performance evaluations/scheduled drills.
   4. Establish communication systems and backup plans during disasters/emergencies.
   5. Develop plans to obtain disaster supplies and equipment.
   6. Develop primary and alternative evacuation plans including access to transport equipment.
   7. Establish plans for utilities disruption/failure.
      a. Alternative sources of essential utilities (i.e., emergency power, water, steam).
      b. Emergency procedures for system failures.
      c. Location of emergency shut-off controls.
      d. Process for repair services.

MANAGEMENT OF EQUIPMENT AND SUPPLIES

This is the process to establish and maintain medical equipment and supplies including a plan to promote safe and effective use of equipment, staff competency assessment and education, and cost-effective purchasing. Nurses in ambulatory care are accountable to assure safe handling, inventory control, and appropriate charging of patient care equipment and supplies.

A. Selecting medical equipment and supplies.
   1. Equipment and supply function(s).
   2. Risks associated with use.
   3. Maintenance requirements.
B. Ordering/purchasing of equipment and supplies.
   1. Identify purchasing specifications and sole source requirements.
   2. Utilize shared purchasing contracts ("group buying") to ensure the best possible cost.
   3. Evaluate service/maintenance contracts and warranties.
   4. Plan for expedited delivery of urgently needed equipment/supplies.
C. Inventory control.
   1. System to monitor current supply "stock on hand" such as:
      a. Description.
      b. Quantity.
      c. Lot number.
      d. Expiration date.
   2. Ability to limit inventory to preserve financial investment.
      a. Increase frequency of purchasing.
      b. Implement agreements for standardization.

      c. Expedite delivery processes.
    3. Accessible vendor information.
    4. Identify storage areas that are in close proximity to point of care.
D. Staff orientation/ongoing education.
    1. Identify learning requirements and competency assessment process for use of equipment.
    2. Evaluate training, technical skills, and current competency as part of the privileging/credentialing process.
    3. Ensure initial and recurring staff training on equipment/supply changes.
    4. Develop training on emergency procedures in an event of failure/user error.
E. Ongoing assessment and monitoring for safe and functional equipment (University of Washington Medical Center, 1998).
    1. Identify responsibility and oversight of medical equipment including:
        a. Policy and procedures.
        b. Equipment maintenance/management plan.
        c. Required inspection labeling.
    2. Provide initial inspection of all powered medical equipment for compliance with appropriate specifications prior to initial use.
    3. Routine preventive maintenance through:
        a. Scheduled inspections.
        b. Ongoing repair/replacement of existing equipment.
    4. Systems for monitoring equipment.
        a. Staff checking equipment before use to ensure good operating condition (i.e., no frayed electrical cords, no evidence of physical damage).
        b. Action plans for hazard alerts and recall notification.
    5. Report equipment problems, failures, and user errors as required by the Safe Medical Device Act of 1990.
    6. Availability of back-up equipment.
F. Charging for supplies.
    1. Determine costs of individual medical/surgical supplies.
    2. Establish price and integrate basic supplies into procedure (i.e., bundled) charges.
    3. Develop charge schedule based on applicable reimbursement coding/ standardize charges across facility.
    4. Determine review schedule for supply charges.
G. Storage.
    1. Ensure appropriately sized storage located in close proximity to point of care (refer to Facility Planning and Space Utilization section starting on p. 73).
    2. Control access to sterilized equipment/storage of expensive equipment.
    3. Use exchange carts to reduce restocking labor costs.
    4. Enclose/cover areas for linen storage.
    5. Preassemble surgical trays/case carts for specialty-specific procedures and locate near point of care.

H. Recycling.
   1. Identify what can safely be recycled.
   2. Provide staff education.
   3. Provide appropriate, labeled containers.
   4. Ensure shredding of confidential papers.
   5. Arrange for regular pick-ups and disposal.

REFERENCES

American Institute of Architects, (1996): *Guidelines for design and construction of hospitals and health care facilities.* Washington, DC: Author.

Barnett AE, Meyer GG (1992): *Ambulatory care management and practice.* Gaithersburg, MD: Aspen.

Joint Commission on Accreditation of Healthcare Organizations (1997): *Comprehensive accreditation manual: for hospitals.* Oakbrook Terrace, IL: Author.

Ross A, Williams SJ, Pavlock EJ (1998): *Ambulatory care organization and management,* ed 3. Albany, NY: Delmar.

U.S. Congress (1990): *Americans with disabilities act of 1990,* 42 U.S.C.A. § 12101 *et seq.* (West 1993).

University of Washington Medical Center (1998): *Administrative policies and operating procedures.* Seattle, WA: Author.

6 Health Care Fiscal Management

CINDY NOA, MS, RN, CNAA
LINDA D'ANGELO, MSN, MBA, RN

OBJECTIVES

Study of the information presented in this chapter will enable the learner to:

1. Explain the financial environment of health care.

2. Acquire knowledge of common revenue sources.

3. Apply knowledge of managed care financial principles in daily practice and mechanisms to ensure quality and appropriate care.

4. Acquire knowledge of common coding systems.

5. Use resource management in daily practice.

6. Gain an understanding of the business of health care and its relationship to the budgeting process.

■■■ In today's health care economic environment, ambulatory care nurses must understand the economics of health care and appreciate their role in controlling costs. The magnitude of public expenditures for health care has resulted in a significant growth in government's role in the financing and regulation of health care. Decisions made by nurses not only affect the financial viability of the organizations for which they work but may directly affect the financial well being of their patients. Ambulatory care nurses must make point-of-care changes quickly to foster cost-effective care delivery. This chapter will provide ambulatory nurses with a basic knowledge of health care finance and will allow them to knowledgeably and actively participate in providing cost-effective patient care services. In this chapter, the ambulatory care nurse will acquire knowledge of commonly used financial terms and acronyms and be able to apply them in the work setting. The nurse will gain understanding of basic financial concepts such as revenue stream, cost accounting, cost benefit analysis, coding and reimbursement mechanisms, and managed care concepts. The nurse will also gain insight into how personal performance affects business viability and acquire additional knowledge of resource management principles. The nurses' awareness of clinical behavior's impact on the cost of health care services is essential in the ambulatory care environment. Failure to understand and apply clinical guidelines and decision pathways may result in avoidable emergency department visits, hospitalizations, and other costly interventions. The ambulatory care nurses' specific role dimension in the continuum of care focuses on the integration of the plan of care, measurement of results (outcomes), education of patients, and ensures access to care. These activities result in lower costs, higher quality, and continuous improvements.

FINANCIAL ENVIRONMENT OF HEALTH CARE ORGANIZATIONS

Cleverley (1997) explains that a health care organization as a provider of health services will be financially viable if it receives revenues from services provided in an amount equal to or greater than the dollars expended to provide the service. Patient service revenue represents the amount that results from the provision of patient care services. Other sources of revenue may include government payments at the local, state, or federal level for such services as educational programs and research or foundation grants.

    A. Fee setting or costing allows organizations or providers the opportunity to recover the cost of rendering a service. Direct and indirect costs must be identified prior to establishing fees.

        1. Direct costs can be traced to a specific service provided. Examples of direct costs are nursing salaries, supplies, and medications.

        2. Indirect costs are usually not attributable to a single service or item. The cost of employee salaries in the business office, rent, and parking expenses are examples of indirect costs.

        3. Desired net income must be determined prior to setting fees.

            a. Net income equals the amount of income, allowing for noncollectible amounts or bad debt, before expenses are paid.

            b. The sum of net income for all goods and services provided equals the net income for the overall business.

            c. Net income is used to develop new programs, fund capital expenses such as information technology systems or building projects, contribute to retained earnings for operations in future years, or is paid out as profits or dividends to shareholders in the for-profit health care entity.

    B. Revenue is the total return or income produced from a given source. The rapidly changing health care environment and a payer (health plan) focus on controlling costs can directly affect an organization's revenue stream or sources and amounts of revenue. Medicare, Medicaid, and other insurance coverage limits and payments change frequently and can significantly affect the revenue stream.

        1. A charge or fee for a service often does not reflect the actual amount collected. The actual amount received is commonly referred to as the collectible.

            a. Bad debt occurs when an insurer, employer, or a patient does not pay a bill.

     b. Usual and customary (U&C) amount is a method used to determine if a fee is usual, customary, and reasonable.

       (1) Usual refers to fees normally charged by a doctor or health care provider for a service.

       (2) Customary according to Kongstvedt (1995) is the normal fee charged in the geographic area for the same service. When a health insurance plan pays 80% of an organization's fee based on U&C the unpaid amount is often not collectible.

     c. Discounts are often negotiated by health care organizations to secure a contract with another organization. This provides some assurance of business volume. An example is physicals performed by a nurse practitioner for a particular company according to a sole provider agreement.

REVENUE SOURCES

The major payers of ambulatory health care services are the primary revenue sources for most organizations.

    A. Government—federal, state, and local governments—funds or provides health plans.

      1. Medicare: government plan that provides some type of coverage for hospital expenses (part A) and physician services (part B) for individuals over 65 and other qualifying individuals.

      2. Medicaid: a plan jointly funded by federal and state governments, introduced in 1966 to cover poor individuals and managed independently by each state.

      3. Civilian Health and Medical Program of the United States (CHAMPUS) is a federal program providing coverage to families of active duty military personnel, military retirees, spouses, and dependents.

      4. Other: some states and local governments provide additional limited coverage of health services based on need or qualification.

    B. Private insurance. Private insurance covers both commercial indemnity plans and managed care plans. Individual chooses type of insurance (e.g., Blue Cross/Blue Shield, Prudential). There are a variety of private insurance plans.

      1. Commercial indemnity plans are a type of insurance contract in which the insurer pays for care received up to a fixed amount per encounter or episode of illness. For example in an 80/20-indemnity plan the insurer would pay 80% of U&C. The insured individual would be responsible for 20% or remainder of the fee.

      2. Managed care plans: for example the insurer may offer health maintenance plans (HMOs), preferred provider plans (PPOs), point of service plans (POS). These will be described under Managed Care Concepts.

    C. Fee for service: reimbursement method in which payment is made for each service or item. May drive up costs because it encourages a doctor or an organization to provide more medical care by paying for each service provided. Examples include preoperative chest x-rays and annual choles-terol screening, which may not be indicated by history and clinical findings.

D. Employer-provided insurance: may elect to offer health plan choices or provide an employer-funded plan where the company bears the risk. Often contract with outside organization to manage the plan, a third party administrator.

E. Private pay: individual pays for health care services he/she receives.

F. Out of pocket expense refers to the portion of health care cost for which the individual is responsible. Could be 100% if an uncovered service such as cosmetic or plastic surgery, 100% if individual has no insurance, or the portion that is not paid by the insurance plan under which an individual is covered.

G. Copayment: out of pocket expense paid by an individual for a specific service defined in the insurance plan. Could be for example, 20% of charges for care or $10 per visit.

MANAGED CARE CONCEPTS

Kongstvedt (1995) describes managed care as a system of care delivery that influences and measures service utilization, cost, and performance. The goals of managed care are quality, cost-effective, and accessible health care. It is a coordinated system of health care, which achieves outcomes (reduced utilization and improved population health) through preventive care, case management, and the provision of medically necessary appropriate care.

A. Prepaid health insurance: a fixed amount is paid to the contracted provider of care each month for each enrollee for specific services defined by the health plan. For example, radiology services may be contracted at specific rates for enrollees in a plan.

B. Capitation: a method for funding expenses of enrollees in prepaid health plans pays providers a fixed fee per member regardless of service provided.
   1. The provider is responsible for delivering or arranging the delivery of all services required under the conditions of the provider contract.
   2. For example a plan which pays a per member per month amount to a physician group to provide primary care services for each enrollee in the plan.
   3. Efforts to reduce duplication and control costs create new professional demands on ambulatory nurses, emphasizing efficient resource alloca-tion, coordinated care planning, and outcomes assessment.

C. Managed careplans: different types of managed care plans define where patients may receive the most cost effective care, which providers are included, and how expenses will be paid.
   1. Preferred provider organization (PPO): a program in which contracts exist between the health plan and care providers, at a discount for services. Typically the plan provides incentives for patients to utilize in-network providers as opposed to nonparticipating providers (inde-pendent/noncontracted) through decreased copayments. Kongstvedt

(1995) describes network providers as providers who are contracted through a health plan to deliver health care to members.

2. Point of service (POS): a plan that defines service providers in the service area outside of usual preferred provider network. According to Hartley (1998), an insured patient pays an increased premium with more out-of-pocket expenses. Service providers are providers outside the network contracted to provide specialty services such as invasive cardiology.

3. Health maintenance organization (HMO): there are two possibilities.
   a. A health plan may place risk on the providers for medical expenses. In this instance, providers are encouraged to provide appropriate medical services but not medically unnecessary services in exchange for larger premiums. The risk lies in the fact that the provider may deliver services for which he may not be paid. They may not be fully paid if they do not achieve certain predefined quality outcomes such as immunization or mammography screening targets.
   b. A health plan that uses physicians as gatekeepers. In this model the patient chooses a primary care provider (PCP) who is responsible for all aspects of care management and must authorize (gatekeeper) or give permission for referral to other providers.
      (1) PCPs are often paid a panel management fee and incented financially for providing more comprehensive services within the provider's own practice. Physicians may receive a standard amount, $2 to $10 per member per month, to actively manage the care for the panel population by offering special programs or services based on the panels' clinical conditions or demographics (e.g., cholesterol screening for hypertensives, retinal screening for diabetics).
   c. Many HMOs have open access, now allowing patients to see specialists within network without the primary care physician's approval.

4. Independent practice association (IPA): Kongstvedt (1995) defines an IPA as a legal entity whose members are independent physicians who contract with the IPA for the purpose of having the IPA contract with one or more HMOs. The health plan contracts with an IPA for provision of services for a negotiated fee.

5. Physician hospital organization (PHO): legal organizations often developed for purposes of contracting with managed care plans. Link physicians to specific hospitals for hospitalization care.

6. Medicare managed care: instead of the traditional fee for service payments, reimbursement is paid on a capitated, per enrollee basis each month.
   a. A fee scale is set based on the average adjusted per capita cost (AAPCC) that has been historically paid in a given region or county for Medicare-eligible enrollees (Kongstvedt, 1995).
   b. As of September 1998, 6.5 million beneficiaries (17.2% of Medicare population) were in managed care plans (Grimaldi, 1999).

7. Medicaid managed care. Managed care plan for Medicaid enrollees. They are relatively new and are experiencing significant difficulty with patient care coordination.

D. Mechanisms to ensure quality/appropriateness.

1. Health Plan Employer Data and Information Set (HEDIS).

   a. Measures plan performance against plan predictions and performance targets such as cervical cancer screening rates or mammogram rates.

   b. Employers may choose not to enter into contracts with health plans if performance goals are not met.

2. Precertification: the process of obtaining authorization or certification from a health plan for routine hospital admissions, referrals, procedures, or tests. Ambulatory nurses are commonly involved in obtaining precertification or authorization from health plans to obtain coverage approval for costly procedures such as surgery and MRIs or for out-of-network referrals.

   a. Enables review for clinical appropriateness for the procedure against standards, and ensures the service is provided in the most cost-effective, appropriate setting (e.g., ambulatory surgery center vs. inpatient admission and main operating room).

3. Concurrent review. Case management of costly cases is often performed by nurses to ensure hospitalized patients are being managed most efficiently relative to length of stay and discharge planning needs. Case management is a method for managing the provision of health care to members/patients with catastrophic or high cost medical conditions. According to Kongstvedt (1995) the focus is on coordinating the care to improve the continuity and quality of care as well as lower costs.

4. Care delivery: nurses providing care—right patient, right setting, right care, right provider at the right time.

   a. Care delivery systems are financially stronger when efficiencies are maximized.

   b. Disease management: method that utilizes standardized care plans based on evidence and best practices to manage patients with chronic diseases.

   (1) Provide uniform care and ensure patients are being properly managed.

   (2) Diabetes care, hypertension management, and anticoagulation clinics are examples in which better care can be provided at less cost through programs, guidelines, or case management.

   c. Health promotion/wellness education key to promoting healthier patients. Self-care promotion provides opportunities for nurses.

   d. Case management for specific populations and care management over time provide enhanced opportunities for nurses to affect (decrease) total cost of care for an episode or condition by early detection of impending health crisis and early intervention. Examples such as congestive heart failure monitoring via home care or telephone will decrease hospital admissions or emergency department visits.

CODING

A standard method used to report patient care services provided to private or government health plans in order to receive payment.

  A. The Health Care Financing Administration (HCFA) is within the U.S. Department of Health and Human Services. Determines the standard rules and reporting mechanisms for health care services.

    1. This oversight group initially introduced a view that payment for inpatient Medicare enrollees should be derived from a cost-based reimbursement system.

    2. Because of escalating costs driven by fee-for-service payment methodology, without quality, appropriateness, or utilization controls, HCFA switched to diagnostic related groups (DRGs) in 1983, paying a fixed amount for defined hospital services based on diagnostic related levels of service provided, length of stay, or cost of care.

    3. It was expected that hospitals would improve operational efficiencies, provide quality care, and maintain financial viability.

  B. Diagnostic related group (DRG) is a system for classifying hospital inpatients into groups using similar quantities of resources according to characteristics such as diagnosis, age, procedure, complications, and comorbidities.

    1. The care costs of DRGs are estimated.

    2. Advances in technology and reduced payments from HCFA have had significant effects on hospital lengths of stay resulting in lesser costs assigned to DRGs.

    3. This cycle has produced system-wide ramifications including a marked shift in care setting from inpatient to ambulatory environments.

    4. Ambulatory care nurses have a significant opportunity to affect the cost of an inpatient admission, a case, an encounter, or a service.

      a. Preadmission and preprocedure patient education and discharge planning begin with the ambulatory nurse.

      b. Proactive planning with the patient and family ensure more efficient processes and allow shorter lengths of stay and faster recovery periods for patients.

  C. Resource based relative value system (RBRVS) is a classification system that attempts to assign within a defined setting the resource requirements based on weights according to relative cost of each service.

    1. RBRVS has been used by HCFA since 1992 for determining payment to physicians for services provided to Medicare enrollees.

    2. RVU, relative value unit, was established by HCFA to approximate the work, practice expense, and malpractice expense for delivery of physician services.

      a. For every procedure the three components reflect the value of a particular service, which make up a classification unit in the RBRVS.

      b. Each RVU according to Cleverley (1997) is multiplied by a regional specific price index to reach the reimbursement rate for that particular service that is paid by HCFA.

  D. HCPCS is the abbreviation for the Health Care Financing Administration (HCFA) Common Procedure Coding System.

1. A uniform method for health care providers and medical suppliers to report professional services, procedures, and supplies to health care plans.
2. Allow for consistent communication of services provided.
3. Ensures validity of profiles for the classification system and fee schedules through standardized coding and enhances education and research by providing local, regional, and national data comparisons.
4. The *Physicians' Current Procedural Terminology* (CPT), CPT 2000 (1999), is published by American Medical Association and is the internationally recognized coding system for reporting medical services and procedures. Nurses use CPT coding guidelines for reporting services provided by nurses. The insurance carrier determines if nurses are an eligible billing provider. There are three levels of HCPCS CPT codes.
   a. CPT Level I.
      (1) Evaluation and Management (E&M): category of CPT codes that represent nonprocedural provider encounters such as an office visit for an earache or a blood pressure monitoring.
      (2) 99211: minimal office visit, CPT 2000 (1999), is the only code that a nurse can bill that is independent of a physician encounter. An example is an office visit for a 20 year-old female who receives an allergy vaccine injection and is observed by a nurse. The assessment and plan of care must be documented to bill, utilizing this code.
   b. CPT Level II represents alphanumeric codes established for services and items not listed in CPT I such as supplies and drugs. An example is 90746 Hepatitis B vaccine, adult dose.
   c. CPT III represents alphanumeric codes established by individual state Medicaid carriers to cover services not listed in Level I or II.
5. ICD 9: *International Classification of Diseases*, 9th revision, clinical modification published by U.S. National Center for Health Statistics is the internationally recognized system for the purposes of international morbidity and mortality and in the United States is used for coding and billing purposes (Schmidt, Hart, and Aaron, 1999).
   a. HCFA requires the use of ICD 9 codes on claims submitted by health care providers.
   b. The numerical code must represent an accurate translation of the diagnostic statement or terminology documented by the provider, and may be a sign, symptom, or condition.
   c. Coders are individuals who are used by many health care organizations.
      (1) Responsible for painting an accurate picture of the patient's condition using numerical codes to translate the physician's documentation into billable services.
      (2) May only apply standardized codes to information that is documented.
   d. Electronic coding systems: though early in development, electronic

systems (computers) translate physician online documentation in clinical information systems into billable service codes.

6. Documentation: medical terminology describing the reason for a patient's encounter must appear on a source document.
   a. Source documents refer to any documentation of a patient encounter.
   b. Encounter forms, emergency reports, billing forms, and patient records are examples of source documents that may vary from facility to facility.
7. Compliance: the provider of health care services must follow standard coding guidelines and be prepared to provide documentation of the service provided. Failure to do so could result in allegations of fraud and significant monetary fines or loss of licenses by hospitals.

E. Ambulatory encounter systems (AES): according to Goldfield (1993), AES measures the ambulatory encounter or visit. Attempt by government to control cost and quality by fixed pricing. Not yet fully implemented. Being tested in some military settings.
   1. AVGs (ambulatory visit groups): single payment for all services provided during an ambulatory visit. Goal to reach prospective payment in ambulatory care groups requiring similar resources based on age, sex, diagnosis, and procedure (severity adjusted).
   2. APGs (ambulatory patient groups): patient classification system designed to explain amount and type of resource used in ambulatory care visit.

RESOURCE MANAGEMENT

Resource management is an organization's ability to effectively manage its resources, people, capital, equipment, and supplies. West, Hicks, Balas, and West (1996) found nurses must participate actively and knowledgeably in the identification of actual costs associated with patient care (costing process).

A. Nonlabor resource management. Management of clerical and surgical supplies, linen, pharmaceuticals, durable medical equipment, etc. Caroselli (1996) demonstrated that nurses can have great opportunity to affect the costs of daily operations when they take an active role and interest in understanding how supply or linen usage or staffing patterns affect costs. Overordering and overstocking leads to waste when supplies sit unused on shelves or expire before use.
   1. Inventory management: par levels: minimum supply levels are determined and maintained to ensure a short shelf life while meeting user demand.
   2. Product evaluation: a standard methodology adopted by organizations to ensure cost-effective purchasing decisions of supplies and other equipment.
      a. Choosing the least expensive alternative that achieves desired results (outcomes) vs. personal preferences.
      b. Product evaluation may be accomplished by committee using studies (product trials within the institution), literature review, etc.

3. Trending and tracking.
   a. Tracking sheets to monitor volume and frequency of use of specific items or supplies.
   b. Invoices are provided by supplier when supplies are received and should be matched against those items ordered or requested.
   c. Budget variance reports identify variances in dollars over or under projected amounts.
B. Labor resource management.
   1. Practice efficiency: staffing for the right level of care and volume.
      a. Length of encounter, waiting times, delay in process, downtime (no-shows, vacant appointments, hold times) can increase the need for support staff.
      b. Efficient management of phone calls, scheduling of procedures, and organizing workflow to meet customers' needs will lead to more cost effective staffing.
   2. Appropriate staffing: the right person, based on educational preparation and licensure, assigned to do the work that must be performed at the right time.

BUDGET

Budgeting is a logical way for a health care organization to plan for and manage its processes. Strategic, longer-term plans drive operational or shorter-term budget cycles.

A. Planning.
   1. A process used to develop specific courses of action to attain organization's goals and objectives.
   2. Can be defined as the process by which organizational plans are expressed in dollars and cents.
   3. Formalized processes in most organizations and key to health care organizations' financial viability.
   4. Built on historical performance (projected numbers of visits, number of encounters, or number of patients in a physician's panel for which she/he will receive capitated fees may be used in planning revenues and expenses).
   5. Requires goals, which are broad statements indicating what is to be achieved, and objectives, which are more specific statements of what is to be achieved within a specific time period.
   6. Forecasts anticipated revenues associated with anticipated expenses.
   7. Benefits of planning a budget.
      a. Promotes effective decision-making.
      b. Allows one to consider alternatives.
      c. Specifies major assumptions, for example, rate of inflation, and fee increase estimates.
      d. Uses financial and statistical indicators that allow both operations and productivity to be monitored.

B. Financial reports.

1. Expenses budgeted (planned) and actual (incurred) are reported and the volume of activity measured (visits or procedures).
2. Productivity indicators, for example paid man-hours per visits.
3. Hospital referral report. Tracks hospital admission days and charges to reconcile with practice.
4. There are many other types of financial reports.

C. Programming: determines the programs an organization will offer to reach its stated goals and objectives.

1. Feasibility study is completed to determine how feasible it is to offer or continue offering a program or service. This might include market studies, patient interest, facility requirements, and identification of similar programs in the area.
2. Cost benefit analysis. A formal financial analysis completed by organizations to determine the cost of a program, projected revenues, and to identify and quantify program benefits. Includes assumptions about specific expenses and potential revenue based on projected volumes (Cleverly, 1997). Usually completed before starting a new program or service. Included in the feasibility study.

D. Types of budgets: the most common ones are capital and operating budgets.

1. Capital budget: departments usually forecast or estimate capital needs for the coming year translated into dollars; includes such items as new and replacement equipment, facility renovation, new technology, and other items that may be paid over several years.
2. Operating budget: includes statistical, revenue, and expense budgets (Cleverly 1997).
   a. Statistical budget provides measures of workload or activity for each responsibility center or service provided.
   b. Expense budget is a projection of expected costs allocated to a specific program or service based on anticipated volume of activities (e.g., payroll and supplies expense). Includes allocation (assignment) of indirect costs such as building and equipment, depreciation and bad debt and allocation of direct identifiable costs related to a specific program budget.
   c. Revenue budget is a projection of expected revenues associated with a specific program or service based on volumes projected in the statistical budget.

E. Accounting: the financial services or accounting department collects and reports information on revenues and expenses of a specific department or program.

F. Analysis: reporting, trending, and tracking results; report analyzing.

1. Critical success factors are defined by management. They are the essential factors needed in order to continue in the business or to continue providing a service or a program.
2. Key performance indicators: balanced approach to planning and forecasting process of measuring organizational performance against plan,

ensures the ultimate financial success of the organization. Goals help to provide organization focus.

  a. In addition to profitability, areas for indicator determination may include nonfinancial measures such as growth, profitability, quality, and productivity. Examples:

    (1) Growth: 10% in new patients registered.
    (2) Profitability: achieve 3% net revenues after expenses.
    (3) Quality: decrease staff turnover to less than 15%; decrease medication errors. Increase patient satisfaction in telephone access.
    (4) Productivity: increase number of patient visits for each support staff full time equivalent employee.

  b. Variance reports: demonstrate actual results compared to the plan.

REFERENCES

American Medical Association (1999): *Physician's current procedural terminology, CPT 2000, standard edition.* Chicago, IL: Author.

Caroselli C (1996): Economic awareness of nurses: relationship to budgetary control. *Nurs Econ* 14 (5):292-298.

Cleverley W (1997): *Essentials of health care finance,* ed 4. Gaithersburg, MD: Aspen.

Goldfield N (1993): Ambulatory encounter systems: implications for payment and quality. *J Ambulatory Care Management* 16(2):33-49.

Grimaldi P (1999): Medicare increases managed care's accountability, Part 2. *Nurs Management* 30(2):10-11.

Hartley L (1998): Fiscally "fit" in a managed care system. *Nurs Econ* 29(12):23-28.

Kongstvedt P (1995): *Essentials of managed health care.* Gaithersburg, MD: Aspen.

Schmidt KM, Hart AC, Aaron WS, editors (1998): *ICD-9-CM,* vol 1,2,3. Reston, VA: St. Anthony.

West D, Hicks L, Balas A, West T (1996): Profitable capitation requires accurate costing. *Nurs Econ* 14 (3):162-170, 150.

7 Informatics

IDA ANDROWICH, PhD, RNC, FAAN
KAROLE MOUREK, PhD, RN

OBJECTIVES

Study of the information presented in this chapter will enable the learner to:

1. Define the concept of nursing informatics and list applications within ambulatory care nursing.

2. Understand the benefits and requirements for a computerized patient record (CPR).

3. Identify criteria for evaluating computer technology for use in the ambulatory setting.

4. Understand the rationale for a nursing minimum data set (NMDS) in the ambulatory setting.

5. Articulate the importance of standardized languages, particularly focusing on the NMDS nursing elements (diagnosis, intervention, outcome, and intensity).

6. Identify reasons for documentation and common documentation formats that promote nursing in ambulatory care settings.

7. Describe the potential of clinical decision support systems (CDSS) and evidence-based practice (EBP) to manage performance outcomes and enhance clinical care.

8. Identify challenges and potential benefits of telehealth, as it relates to the nurse practicing in the ambulatory care setting.

9. Understand current issues relating to privacy and confidentiality of medical record information, unique identifiers for providers and consumers, and interactive databases.

Nurses are familiar with and have always demonstrated the ability to incorporate technology into their professional practice in order to improve the quality of health care they provide. Nursing informatics is a term that came into being during the technology explosion. According to Pillar, Jacox, and Redman, technology, the practical application of science, can be classified as either information-oriented or therapeutic in use (cited in Hebda, 1998). Therapeutic technologies in the ambulatory care setting could include laser and cryosurgery, pharmacotherapeutics, and magnetic resonance imaging (MRI), as well as various electronic monitoring devices. Information technologies can be classified as either information producing or information managing.

This chapter focuses on developing a basic understanding of nursing informatics, associated information technology applications, and the issues associated with using technology to meet patient needs and to enhance health care delivery in the ambulatory care setting. Every nurse practicing today must be familiar with a range of health care information technology applications. Ambulatory care nurses will also need to understand how to best use informatics and technology to improve the quality of patient care and support professional practice, while at the same time be able to evaluate any risk to their patients or practice environment as a result of these technological applications.

DEFINITION OF NURSING INFORMATICS AND APPLICATIONS

A. Nursing informatics is defined by the American Nurses' Association as "the development and evaluation of applications, tools, processes, and structures which assist nurses with the management of data in taking care of patients or supporting the practice of nursing" (ANA, 1994, p. 3).

B. Hanna (cited in Turley, 1996) envisions a model for nursing informatics that applies theories from computer science, information science, and cognitive science and incorporates them into nursing science.

C. Conceptual basis for the understanding of information technology (Graves and Corcoran, 1989).

    1. Information is derived from data (basic facts or observations) that is organized in such a manner as to have meaning to the user.

    2. Knowledge is an evaluation or recognition of something with familiarity that is gained through experience that can put the information to use.

D. Over the past two decades professional nursing has recognized the importance of informatics in the health care arena.

    1. Automated systems in health care have existed for 30 years and were initially developed to meet the financial need for reimbursement. In the 1980s, nurses began to recognize that relevant patient information could be obtained using information technology that would support patient care delivery, nursing service administration, nursing education, and nursing research.

    2. "Information systems and health statistics deal with data which have been ordered and have a name, so that they can be counted. What has no name cannot be counted and consequently has no impact. What has an incorrect or incomplete name leads, when counted, to irrelevant data prohibiting practical use or even a sensible interpretation" (Lamberts, Wood, and Hofmans-Oakkes, 1993, p. 38).

    3. Nursing informatics is applicable in all areas of nursing: clinical practice, administration, education, and research.

        a. Nursing practice activities are supported by computers and include:

            (1) Generation of patient-focused work lists.

            (2) Computer-generated care plans.

            (3) Transmission of orders to ancillary departments.

            (4) Scheduling procedures.

            (5) Retrieving test results.

            (6) Charting medications and treatments.

            (7) Changes in the plan of care.

            (8) Documentation in discharge summaries.

            (9) Monitoring of patients through devices.

    b. A nursing administration information system has seven essential components (Saba and McCormick, 1996).

       (1) Quality management.

       (2) Personnel files.

       (3) Communication networks such as e mail.

       (4) Budgeting and payroll.

       (5) Census.

       (6) Summary reports.

       (7) Forecasting and planning.

    c. Nursing education applications include:

       (1) Computer-assisted instruction.

       (2) Computer-adaptive testing.

       (3) Distance learning.

       (4) Internet resources.

       (5) Computerized tracking of competencies.

    d. Nursing research areas supported by information technology include:

       (1) Computerized literature searches.

       (2) Complex statistical analysis of data.

       (3) Standard languages documentation strategy development.

       (4) Population-based decision support.

4. Nurses who have information science and computer science expertise combined with their health care expertise are uniquely positioned to assume roles in translating the information needs of patient caregivers to those designing the actual systems to capture patient care data.

5. All nurses need to be able to translate the data/information provided by existing systems and to evaluate it in order to promote improved patient care.

THE COMPUTERIZED PATIENT RECORD

The computerized patient record (CPR) is an "electronic patient record that resides in a system specifically designed to support users by providing accessibility to complete and accurate data, alerts, reminders, clinical decision support systems, links to medical knowledge, and other aids" (Institute of Medicine [IOM], 1991, p. 6).

    A. Uses of a CPR (adapted from IOM CPR Report).

    1. Document services provided.

    2. Foster continuity of care (serves as a communication tool).

    3. Describe diseases and causes (supports diagnostic work).

    4. Support decision-making about diagnosis and treatment of patients.

    5. Facilitate care in accordance with clinical practice guidelines.

    6. Generate reminders (e.g., preventive or health maintenance action needed).

    7. Allocate resources and assess workload.

    8. Analyze trends and develop forecasts.

B. Requirements of a CPR (adapted from IOM CPR Report).
  1. Record content.
    a. Uniform core data elements (refer to section on Nursing Minimum Data Set in Ambulatory Care on p. 101).
    b. Standardized coding systems and formats.
    c. Common data dictionary.
    d. Information on outcomes of care and functional status.
  2. Record format: integrated record with all providers, disciplines, and sites of care included.
  3. System performance standards for a computerized patient record (CPR).
    a. Rapid retrieval.
    b. 24-hour access.
    c. Easy data input.
    d. Available at convenient places.
  4. Linkages.
    a. With other information systems (e.g., laboratory, radiology, and pharmacy).
    b. With relevant literature (refer to section on Decision Support Systems on pp. 105-106 for bibliographic database and website examples).
    c. With other institutional databases and registries.
    d. Electronic transfer of billing information.
  5. Intelligence.
    a. Decision support (refer to section on Decision Support Systems on pp. 105-106).
    b. Clinician reminders.
    c. Customizable alert or alarm systems (e.g., for allergies and drug interactions).
  6. Reporting capabilities.
    a. Standard clinical reports.
    b. Customized reports.
    c. Derived documents (e.g., insurance forms and mandated reports).
    d. Trend reports and graphics.
  7. Control and access: safeguards against violations of confidentiality and unauthorized use.
  8. Training and implementation.
    a. Minimal training required for system use.
    b. Graduated implementation possible.
C. Because of the power and potential of automated, computer-based documentation, the translation of nursing documentation from the paper record to the electronic record involves more than merely translating what was done on paper to the computer.
D. Nursing Information Data System Evaluation Center (NIDSEC) (ANA, 1997) is a program established in 1995 by the American Nurses Association (ANA) Board of Directors.
  1. The mission of NIDSEC is to develop and disseminate standards pertaining to information systems that support the documentation of

nursing practice, and to evaluate voluntarily submitted information systems against these standards.
2. This mission supports the long-term goal of widespread integration of ANA-recognized languages for nursing into nursing practice, education, administration, and research.
3. NIDSEC Standards (ANA, 1997) focus on four dimensions of nursing data sets and the information systems containing them.
   a. Nomenclature (the actual terms used).
   b. Clinical content (linkages among terms).
   c. Clinical data repository (how the data are stored and made accessible for retrieval).
   d. General system characteristics (such as performance and attention to security and confidentiality).
4. These standards are published by American Nurses Publishing and entitled *NIDSEC Standards and Scoring Guidelines* (ANA, 1997) and can be obtained from the American Nurses' Association.

EVALUATION

Evaluating computer technology, particularly software, for use in ambulatory settings is an important role of the nurse manager or unit leader.
A. A major reason for dissatisfaction with software applications is unmet expectations on the part of the user. This often occurs because the ability to communicate between the domain expert in the problem domain (the nurse in the clinical area) and the domain expert in the solution domain (the programmer) is poor.
B. A number of questions that should be addressed before purchasing any software include:
   1. How much flexibility is in the software? Is it possible to customize?
   2. Can the software be modified if situations change?
   3. What type of technical support and training are available? How much will they cost?
   4. Will this software interface with other existing software? What will it take in terms of programming to build interfaces? Is the software compatible with existing hardware?
   5. What is the plan for upgrades? How much will they cost?
   6. Is the system equipped with adequate back up? Adequate security (sign-on codes or passwords)?
   7. Is the system user-friendly? This entails screen design, commands, menus, and navigation throughout the program. For example, can screens be skipped for a simple entry, or does the program require a lock-step screen-by-screen approach? Can the user go back and edit one data element without redoing the entire entry?
   8. What industry standards does the software meet? For example, Health Language 7 (HL7) is the accepted standard for messaging in health care.

NURSING MINIMUM DATA SET IN AMBULATORY CARE

A. The nursing minimum data set (NMDS) includes 16 data elements that must be collected by all nurses, for all patient encounters, across all settings (Werley and Lang, 1988).
   1. Patient elements.
      a. Age.
      b. Gender.
      c. Unique patient identifier: may be medical record number, Social Security number, or another unique means of patient identification.
      d. Payment mechanism: insurance coverage or reimbursement information.
      e. Medical diagnosis: typically coded in ICD9 coding.
      f. Disposition: refers to discharge status, not as relevant to ambulatory care setting; useful information for ambulatory care would include living arrangements (e.g., lives alone, etc.).
   2. Facility.
      a. Facility identifier: facility type or provider code.
      b. Dates of care: in ambulatory care, pertains to encounter date.
      c. Unique provider identification: this is new for nursing to have a unique provider number and with automated or computerized documentation is often the sign-on ID.
   3. Nursing care provided.
      a. Nursing diagnosis.
      b. Nursing intervention.
      c. Nursing outcome.
      d. Nursing intensity.
B. Allows for aggregation and comparison of nursing practice across settings.
C. The NMDS data elements have many elements in common with the *Uniform Hospital Discharge Data Set* (UHDDS) and the *Uniform Ambulatory Care Discharge Data Set* (UACDDS) (National Committee on Vital Health and Statistics, 1996).
D. The NMDS is designed so that a comparison of patient-centered data can be made in order to evaluate the effectiveness of nursing interventions across practice settings, across specialties, across specialty settings, and geographic boundaries.
E. The UACDDS is similar to UHDDS but is based on a patient encounter, not on an admission.
F. Other data elements are incorporated into the UACDDS (e.g., living arrangements of patient, patient's support systems, medications, and patient's ability to manage activities of daily living).

STANDARDIZED LANGUAGES

"If you cannot name it, you cannot teach it, research it, practice it, finance it, or put it into public policy."—Norma Lang, PhD, RN, FAAN (Lang, 1998)

A. Unified, not necessarily uniform, languages are necessary to document and use the nursing elements in the NMDS (diagnosis, intervention, outcomes, and intensity).

B. To support the use of multiple vocabularies and classification schemes, the American Nurses' Association (ANA) formed a committee to set criteria for an accepted nursing language and to approve languages meeting the criteria.

C. The ANA Steering Committee on Databases to Support Nursing Practice has as its goals to propose policy and program initiatives regarding nursing classification schemes, uniform nursing data sets, and the inclusion of nursing data elements in national databases.

D. The committee is now called the Committee for Nursing Practice Information and Infrastructure.

E. The Steering Committee recommended that the profession work toward the development of a unified nursing language system that would allow linking or mapping of similar terms, retaining the integrity and purpose of each specific scheme/vocabulary. This unified system would facilitate development, analysis, and use of nursing data sets.

F. The Committee also developed specific criteria for vocabularies to meet to be eligible for recognition. These criteria include:

1. Be clinically useful for making diagnostic, intervention, and/or outcome decisions.
2. Go beyond an application or synthesis/adaptation of vocabularies/classification schemes currently recognized by ANA, or present explicit rationale why it should also be recognized.
3. Be stated in clear and unambiguous terms, with terms precisely defined.
4. Have been tested for reliability of the vocabulary terms.
5. Have been validated as useful for clinical purposes.

G. As of December 1999, languages that have met these criteria and have been approved by the ANA include:

1. American College of Pathology's Systematic Nomenclature for Medicine-Reference Terminology (SNOMED-RT) (College American Pathology, 1997).
   a. A comprehensive, multiaxial nomenclature classification system.
   b. Created for the indexing of the entire medical and health care vocabulary.
2. Home Health Care Classification (HHCC) (Saba, 1997). Saba's Georgetown System for Patient Problems, Interventions, and Outcomes.
   a. Used by home care agencies in providing health care services in the home and community settings.
   b. Diagnosis and interventions vocabularies are structured identically and modifiers are used to evaluate outcomes of conditions.
   c. The diagnoses and interventions are classified according to 20 care components with 145 diagnoses and 160 interventions.
   d. The system is not copyrighted.
3. North American Nursing Diagnosis Association's (NANDA) (Jones, 1999) nomenclature for nursing diagnosis.
   a. Used by nurses to document nursing diagnoses in all settings where nursing care is delivered.

   b. Classified under 9 patterns of human response to illness and life transitions.

   c. Contains 150 nursing diagnoses with accompanying etiologies, risk factors, and defining characteristics.

   d. NANDA holds the copyright.

4. Nursing Interventions Classification (NIC) (Iowa Interventions Project, 2000), developed by a team at the University of Iowa led by McCloskey and Bulechek, is a taxonomy for classifying nursing interventions.

   a. Used by nurses in all settings where care is delivered to document nursing interventions.

   b. The third edition (2000) contains 486 interventions.

   c. The three-level taxonomy contains domains, classes, and interventions.

   d. Both direct and indirect care interventions are included.

   e. Mosby publishes and holds the copyright.

5. Nursing Management Minimum Data Set (NMMDS).

   a. Developed by Delaney and Huber (Huber, Delaney, Crossley, Memhert, and Ellerbe, 1992).

   b. For use by managers in all nursing care settings.

   c. Contains 17 defined data elements.

   d. Environment (9 elements, for example, patient population, volume, care delivery model, etc.).

   e. Nurse resources (4 elements, for example, manager demographic profile, nursing care staff demographic profile, staffing).

   f. Financial resources (4 elements, for example, payer type, budget expenses, etc.).

   g. NMMDS is copyrighted by Delaney and Huber.

6. Omaha (the Omaha VNA's system for problems, interventions, and outcomes) (Martin and Sheet, 1992; Martin, 1999).

   a. Used by nurses to describe and document care in community settings.

   b. Contains 40 nursing problems (diagnoses) and a number of associated nursing interventions and outcomes (composed of knowledge, behavior, and status subscales).

   c. The system is not copyrighted.

7. Ozbolt's Patient Care Data Set (PCDS) (Ozbolt, 1997; Ozbolt, 1999).

   a. Used by nurses to document care in all settings, but primarily developed for the acute care setting.

   b. Comprises nursing diagnoses (many are from NANDA and the HHCC), patient care actions, and nursing outcomes.

   c. Organized around the 20 care components of the HHCC with two additional components for the acute care setting.

   d. Copyright held by Ozbolt/Vanderbilt University.

8. Perioperative Nursing Data Set (PNDS) (Kleinbeck, 1996) developed by the Association of Operating Room Nurses.

   a. Used by perioperative registered nurses and surgical service managers in a variety of perioperative settings.

   b. Contains a set of specific NANDA-approved diagnoses (N=68), 127 nursing interventions, and 29 nursing outcomes, all specific to the perioperative setting.

    c. AORN holds the copyright for this data set.

  9. Nursing Outcomes Classification (NOC) (Iowa Outcomes Project, 2000), developed by a team led by Johnson and Maas at the University of Iowa.

    a. Used by nurses to document patient outcomes that are sensitive to nursing.

    b. The second edition (1999) contains outcomes for individual patients, families, and caregivers. Each outcome has a Likert–type scale to measure the degree to which the patient has attained that outcome.

    c. Mosby publishes and holds copyright for this classification.

H. Another important standardized nomenclature not yet approved by the ANA is the International Classification of Nursing (ICNP) (International Council of Nursing [ICN], 1999).

I. Standardized languages can be used for:

  1. Outcomes data collection, retrieval, analysis.

  2. Decisions about care management.

  3. Quality management and improvement.

  4. Decision support.

  5. Statistical and epidemiologic reporting (vital statistics, tumor registries).

  6. Administrative (billing, cost data).

J. In conclusion.

  1. Vocabulary is an urgent issue in nursing and nursing informatics.

  2. Vocabulary is central to the integration of patient care data and research.

DOCUMENTATION STRATEGIES

A. Health professionals document care for many reasons:

  1. To communicate care provided to all providers.

  2. To provide continuity of care; to ensure a historical, narrative record of an episode or episodes of care and the patient's responses to treatment.

  3. To document care provided or not provided for legal reasons.

  4. To facilitate reimbursement (Turley, 1996).

B. According to (Hebda, 1998) there are two approaches to automated nursing documentation—the nursing process approach and the critical pathway/ protocols approach.

  1. The nursing process approach is based on the traditional paper forms used by nurses. This format addresses multiple functions.

    a. Documents nursing admission assessment.

    b. Documents discharge instructions via menu lists.

    c. Generates nursing work list with routine scheduled activities related to care of each patient.

    d. Documents specific data such as vital signs, weights, and intake and output measurements.

    e. Provides standardized care plans for nurses to be individualized for patients.

    f. Documents nursing care in the progress note format.

    g. Documents medication administration via medication administration records (MAR).

  2. Critical pathway/protocols approach, an approach particularly popular with the rise of managed care, is an interdisciplinary approach to documentation and is based on use of critical pathways or protocols to structure documentation.

    a. Provider selects one or more critical pathways for the patient.

    b. Standard MD or other order sets are included in pathway and are automatically processed.

    c. The system is capable of tracking variances from anticipated care (critical pathway) and is able to aggregate variance information for analysis by provider.

    d. This provides feedback loop, and the information is used to improve care and client outcomes.

DECISION SUPPORT SYSTEMS (DSS)

Nurse leaders are constantly challenged to keep up with the rapidly growing and constantly changing information base relevant to their practice. Computers can assist in this process by bringing necessary information to the practicing nurse in forms that will leverage the information-seeking and decision-making processes. Nurse leaders must use all available evidence to increase the probability of "doing the right thing." In the future, institutions will be successful in the marketplace to the extent that they have comparable, reliable, relevant data for cost, utilization, and outcome studies, for guideline development, for performance management, and for identification of best practices.

  A. An automated decision support system provides an ambulatory nurse with a tool that enhances the nurse's ability to make effective and timely decisions in semistructured uncertain situations.

  B. Structure of any decision support system includes:

    1. Some type of user interface that facilitates or triggers inquiries.

    2. A knowledge base (database) containing expert information that is organized to promote decision-making.

    3. Inference engine with analytic models that can generate alternative solutions.

  C. An example of how a decision support system might operate in a clinical setting is the scheduling of immunizations.

    1. The system would ask you to input the child's age, weight, immunization history, and other pertinent facts.

    2. The database would use the information provided to compare with accepted practice standards contained in the knowledge base.

    3. Then the algorithm in the inference engine would be used to provide a recommendation for the next immunization to be scheduled.

  D. Benefits of decision support systems.

    1. Organizes and interprets a large amount of data.

    2. Standardizes decision-making criteria.

    3. Brings scarce expertise to distant sites.

    4. Provides expert level assistance to novice.

    5. Allows for capturing (extracting and documenting) knowledge of experts (Peterson and Jeselon, 1998).

E. "An intelligent health care system is a learning organization and promotes a culture of knowledge and empowerment among its members "(Tan, 1998, p. 35).

F. The computer has virtually unlimited storage and great information processing capability, whereas man has limited storage and memory, but much experience, knowledge, intuition, and judgment. We must build on both the strengths of man and the computer (Weed, 1997).

G. The trend in ambulatory patient care is to organize care around targeted patient populations (e.g., high cost or high volume). Care planning relies upon identification of best practice models from the literature that derives recommendations from large population studies.

H. Population-based decision support is one form of decision support systems. In these situations, data from a number of patients are aggregated and used to provide information to support patient care for individual patients.

I. Evidence-based nursing practice is the "conscientious, explicit, and judicious use of the current best evidence in making decisions about the care of individual patients" (Sackett, Rosenberg, Gray, Haynes, and Richardson, 1996). This same principle can be used in planning care for patient populations. Sources of evidence include:

    1. Computerized literature databases, such as the Cumulative Index of Nursing and Allied Health Literature (CINAHL) and the National Library of Medicine's (NLM) Medline.

    2. On-line, published, systematic evidence reviews such as the Cochrane Collaboration's Library of Reviews and the American College of Physicians (refer to the Bandolier site at http://www.jr2.ox.uk/bandolier/), the Agency for Health Care Policy and Research (http://www.ahcpr.gov), and CINAHL's Clinical Innovations Database (CCID) (http://www.cinahl.com).

J. The goal of evidence-based practice is (see Chapter 24):

    1. Rigorous answers for clinical questions.

    2. For patients—What is the best care option?

    3. For providers—How am I doing? How am I doing compared to others? Inside and outside the system?

    4. For the ambulatory care nursing professional—How can I improve?

TELEHEALTH ISSUES

A. Telehealth can be defined as the use of modem telecommunications and information technology to provide health care to individuals at a distance and to transmit information to provide care (Hebda, 1998).

B. Issues to be addressed in light of the increased use of distance technology for patient education, clinical diagnosis, and therapeutic interventions include:

    1. Provider credentialing—with the advent of telephone nursing practice and distance telehealth media the importance of ensuring competence and accountability, in many cases across state lines or national borders requires thoughtful consideration.

        a. The National Council of State Boards of Nursing (NCSBN) in 1997 adopted a system of mutual recognition via interstate compact (Hebda, 1998).

        b. This would allow a single licensure system for nurses practicing in more than one state (physically or electronically).

        c. The issue of multistate licensure continues to be dynamic and will need creative resolution in order to protect both the public and members of the health care professions.

    2. Information quality—few standards are available for providers and consumers to use to evaluate the quality of information that is offered on the Internet.

    3. An ambulatory care nurse can use the AAACN metric to evaluate information for use and should also teach patients to be savvy information consumers.

    4. The AAACN metric (Androwich, 1999).

        a. Accuracy—How valid and reliable does this information seem? Is it consistent with "mainstream" knowledge or is it apparent? Why not?

        b. Authorship—What is expertise and credibility of author(s)? Does the author of the information have a commercial interest in the product referenced? If so, is the commercial relationship explicit? What organization(s) is the author or site associated with? Are they credible?

        c. Attribution—Is the information referenced? Are the citations reliable and do they include experts in the area?

        d. Currency—How dated is the information? When was the information posted?

        e. Nursing Practice Relevance—Is this important to my patients? Is it a POEM? (A POEM is Patient Oriented Evidence that Matters—matters because it will require practice change.)

    5. The overall soundness of a source is evaluated based on the above criteria.

PRIVACY AND CONFIDENTIALITY/ACCREDITATION

A. The Kennedy-Kassebaum Act, *Health Insurance Privacy and Portability Act (HIPPA)*, provides safeguards for patient health care data. At minimum this means that measures are in place to protect against:

    1. Unauthorized access and harm to patient care data (system security).

    2. Accidental or intentional disclosure to unauthorized persons or unauthorized data alteration (data security).

3. Transmission of sensitive information to unauthorized recipients (data confidentiality).
4. Assurance of consistency and accuracy of data stored in data-based systems (data integrity).

B. At the Federal level the National Committee on Vital and Health Statistics (NCVHS) has been charged by congress with providing recommendations related to the degree of security needed for various types of data elements. All ANA-approved nursing vocabulary developers were invited by NCVHS to testify concerning this issue in summer 1999.

C. Joint Commission for Accreditation of Healthcare Organizations (JCAHO) (1996), Information Standards require:

1. Measures that protect information confidentiality, security, and integrity (user access, retrieval of information without compromising security or confidentiality, written policies controlling patient records, and guarding records and information).
2. Uniform definitions and methods for data capture in order to facilitate data comparison within and among health care organizations.
3. Education on principles of information management and training for system use.
4. Accurate and timely transmission of information (24-hour availability, minimal delay of order implementation, pharmacy system designed to minimize errors, and quick turnaround of test results).
5. Integration of clinical and nonclinical systems.
6. Client-specific data information: system collects and reports individual data and information that can be used to support practice, aid research, and support decision-making.
7. Aggregate data/information: system generates supports that support care, improve performance, support operations and research.
8. Knowledge-base information-literature available in print or electronic form.
9. Comparative data: system can provide information useful for comparison.

REFERENCES

American Nurses' Association (1994): *The scope of practice for nursing informatics.* Washington, DC: American Nurses Publishing.

American Nurses' Association (1997): *NIDSEC standards and scoring guidelines.* Washington, DC: American Nurses Publishing.

Androwich I (1999): Evidence-based practice: harvesting the evidence. *Chart* (March): 5.

College of American Pathology (CAP) (1997): *SNOMED International—the systematized nomenclature of medicine-reference terminology.* Northfield, IL: College of American Pathology. Available: http://www.snomed.org

Graves J, Corcoran S (1989): The study of nursing informatics. *Image,* 21(4):227-231.

HCFA Press Office (1997): *Health insurance portability and accountability act of 1996 administration simplification.* Available: http//www.ncvhs.gov

Hebda T (1998): *Handbook for nurses and health care professionals.* Menlo Park, CA: Addison Wesley Longman.

Huber D, Delaney, C, Crossley J, Memhert M, Ellerbe S (1992): A nursing management minimum data set. *J Nurs Admin* 22(7/8):35-40.

Institute of Medicine (IOM) (1991): *The computer-based patient record: an essential technology for health care.* Washington, DC: National Academy Press.

International Council of Nursing (ICN) (1999): *ICNP update—beta 1 version.* Available: http://www.icn.ch/icnpupdate.htm

Iowa Interventions Project (2000): *Nursing interventions classification (NIC),* ed 3. St. Louis: Mosby.

Iowa Outcomes Project (2000): *Nursing outcomes classification (NOC),* ed 2. St. Louis: Mosby.

Joint Commission on Accreditation of Healthcare Organizations (JCAHO) (1996): *Accreditation manual for hospitals: medical records process.* Chicago: JCAHO.

Jones D (1999): *North American Nursing Diagnosis Association (NANDA).* Philadelphia: North American Nursing Diagnosis Association (NANDA). Available: http://www.nanda.org

Kleinbeck S (1996): In search of perioperative nursing data elements. *AORN* 63(5):926-931.

Lamberts H, Wood M, Hofmans-Oakkes I (1993): *The international classification of primary care in the European community.* New York: Oxford University Press.

Lang N (1998, March 25-28): Language, Classification, and Data: *A powerbase for clinical practice: If you cannot name it. . . .* Paper presented at the AAACN 23rd Annual Conference, Atlanta, GA.

Martin K, Sheet NJ (1992): *The Omaha system: applications for community health nursing.* Philadelphia: WB Saunders.

Martin K (1999): The Omaha system: past, present, and future. On-line *J Nurs Informatics* 3(1):1-6.

Ozbolt J (1997): From minimum data to maximum impact: using clinical data to strengthen patient care. *MD Computing* 14:295-301.

Ozbolt J (1999): *The patient care data set: profile.* Nashville, TN: Vanderbilt University Medical Center.

Peterson GP, Jeselon P (1998): Health decision support systems in nursing. In Tan J, editor: *Health decision support systems.* Gaithersburg, MD: Aspen.

Saba V, McCormick K (1996): *Essentials of computers for nurses.* New York: McGraw-Hill.

Saba V (1997, May 28): *Home health care classification (HHCC) of nursing diagnoses and interventions.* Paper presented at the AMIA Spring Institute: Implementation of nursing vocabularies in computer-based systems (an invitational working conference), San Jose, CA.

Sackett D, Rosenberg WM, Gray JA, Haynes RB, Richardson WS (1996): Evidence based medicine: what it is and what it isn't. *BMJ* 312:71-72.

Tan J (1998): Health decision support systems. Gaithersberg, MD: Aspen.

Turley J (1996): Toward a model of nursing informatics. *J Nurs Scholarship* 28(1):309-313.

Weed L (1997): New connections between medical knowledge and patient care. *BMJ* 315:231-235.

Werley H, Lang N (1988): *Identification of the nursing minimum data set.* New York: Springer.

8 Legal Aspects

DEBRA ANN CLEMENTINO, JD, MS, RN

OBJECTIVES

Study of the information presented in this chapter will enable the learner to:

1. Describe the sources and types of law.

2. Discuss the legal implications of informed consent.

3. Explain patient transfer issues regulated by the Emergency Medical Treatment and Active Labor Act (EMTALA).

4. Discuss patient abandonment issues and nursing implications.

5. Describe negligence and identify reportable situations.

6. Discuss the legal aspects of documentation.

7. Explain telephone nursing practice liability issues.

8. Describe the regulation of nursing practice.

9. Explain workplace regulatory compliance issues mandated by the Equal Employment Opportunity Commission (EEOC) and the Occupational Safety and Health Administration (OSHA).

LEGAL ASPECTS OF AMBULATORY CARE NURSING

Legal issues can arise as a result of providing ambulatory nursing care to patients. It is important to understand how the law affects ambulatory nursing practice. Nurse practice acts regulate the practice of ambulatory nurses to protect the public and make ambulatory nurses accountable for their actions. This chapter is designed to provide ambulatory care nurses with basic legal knowledge and to discuss ways to perform nursing duties with an increased awareness of potentially litigious situations.

As nurse practice acts differ from state to state, it is particularly important to become familiar with the specific laws in your own state.

GENERAL OVERVIEW OF LAW

Law can be defined as standards of conduct established and enforced by the government of an organized society.

    A. Sources of law.

        1. Statutory law.

            a. Law passed by the legislature.

            b. Publications containing statutes are called codes.

            c. Federal statutory law.

            (1) Law passed by the Congress of the United States.
            (2) Federal statutes are contained in the United States Code.
        d. State statutory law.
            (1) Law enacted by the state legislature.
            (2) It is not uniform in the fifty states.
    2. Administrative law.
        a. Federal and state legislatures establish administrative agencies to make enforceable rules and regulations.
        b. Administrative agency orders.
            (1) Issued when there is a violation of an agency rule or regulation.
            (2) Have the effect of a court order.
        c. Administrative agency actions are appealable to the courts.
    3. Common law.
        a. Law derived from court decisions previously made.
        b. Usually, common law deals with issues outside the scope of statutory laws.
        c. Originally based on the unwritten laws of England and was later applied to the United States.
        d. Consists of broad principles, not rules, that adhere to fairness, reason, and common sense.
        e. Flexible principles that adapt to changes in society.
        f. States recognize common law principles today.
    4. Equity.
        a. Historically developed in England to provide an adequate remedy to an injured party when common law failed to do so.
        b. If an exception to the common law was necessary, the court of chancery developed principles based on the king's innate sense of justice and right.
        c. When common law and equity courts clashed, equity prevailed.
        d. Equity acts according to the spirit, not the letter, of the law.
        e. Equitable and common law principles are now merged in most states.
        f. Equitable principles are used in courts today.
B. Types of law.
    1. Criminal law.
        a. Criminal statutes.
            (1) Provide protection to society.
            (2) Enacted by the state and federal legislature.
            (3) Approved by the governor or the President.
        b. Two types of criminal offenses.
            (1) Misdemeanors: minor crimes.
            (2) Felonies: major crimes.
        c. Punishment imposed may range from community service work and fines to imprisonment and death.
        d. Examples of violations of criminal law by nurses.
            (1) Practicing nursing without a license.
            (2) Illegal diversion of drugs.

        (3) Intentional or unintentional patient deaths.

        (4) Assisted suicide.

  2. Civil law.

    a. Nurses more often become involved in civil rather than criminal lawsuits.

    b. Civil law deals with violations of individual rights.

    c. Disputes are resolved by a judge or a jury.

    d. Some areas of civil law include contract law, tax law, labor law, and tort law.

    e. Tort law.

        (1) A tort can be defined as a wrong or injury to an individual caused by another who had a legal duty to that individual.

        (2) A tort can be unintentional, intentional, or quasi-intentional.

        (3) Unintentional torts: negligence.

        (4) Intentional torts: assault, battery, false imprisonment, intentional infliction of emotional distress.

        (5) Quasi-intentional torts: defamation of character (slander or libel), invasion of privacy, and breach of confidentiality.

CONSENT

The consent requirement is based on the premise that every competent patient has a right to determine what will be done to his or her own body. Informed consent should be obtained prior to any medical treatment.

  A. History.

    1. Initially, the focus of consent was simply to obtain the patient's agreement prior to treatment.

    2. In the 1960s, the focus has changed to *informed* consent, obtained prior to treatment.

    3. Informed consent is required in most states.

  B. Informed consent is given if the patient receives the following information.

    1. Nature of the treatment.

    2. Benefits or outcome anticipated.

    3. Possible risks involved and the probability of each risk, if ascertainable.

    4. Alternatives to treatment.

    5. Consequences associated with refusing treatment.

  C. Exceptions to informed consent.

    1. When immediate care is required in an emergency.

    2. When disclosing the risks may result in illness, emotional distress, or failure to receive the life-saving treatment.

    3. As state law varies, the exceptions to informed consent may vary between states.

  D. Duty to obtain informed consent.

    1. The treating physician often makes the necessary disclosures and obtains the patient's informed consent.

    2. Practical considerations may necessitate the delegation of this responsibility to a nurse.

    3. The physician bears the ultimate risk of liability if informed consent is not obtained.

E. Disclosure of a health care professional's HIV status.

    1. Wide publicity followed the death of Kimberly Bergalis of Florida from AIDS, which she apparently contracted from her dentist.

    2. Some individuals question whether health care professionals must disclose their AIDS/HIV status to patients before performing invasive procedures.

    3. State courts have rather uniformly held that health care professionals must disclose their AIDS/HIV status to patients before performing any invasive treatment.

F. Legal competency to consent.

    1. Laws dealing with competency to consent, including issues such as age of majority, vary between states.

    2. The law presumes every adult is mentally competent until a court decides otherwise.

    3. Therefore, after patients have been declared mentally incompetent by a court, they are incapable of giving valid consent.

    4. Generally, a person is incompetent if they lack the ability and capacity to understand.

    5. A person may be legally incompetent for the following reasons:

       a. Unconscious or in a persistent vegetative state.

       b. Impaired brain function caused by:

          (1) Mental retardation.

          (2) Senility.

          (3) Brain damage.

          (4) Stroke.

       c. Minor who has not reached the age of majority.

          (1) Age of majority is determined by state law.

          (2) Range is between the ages of 18 and 21.

    6. Although state law varies, if the patient is legally incompetent, many state laws allow the following persons to provide consent for oneself or another person:

       a. A parent for a minor.

       b. An emancipated minor, who is a minor living independently from her/his parents and is self-supporting, may consent for herself/himself.

       c. A legal guardian of the incompetent person.

       d. A minor seeking treatment of drug abuse, sexually transmitted infection (STI), venereal disease, pregnancy and prevention of pregnancy may consent for herself.

       e. A person appointed in a living will or a durable power of attorney.

       f. Anyone standing *in loco parentis* (in the place of the parents) for a minor.

       g. Patient's next of kin.

G. Documenting consents.

    1. Both a verbal and written consent are legally effective.

2. Most states do not have a requirement that a valid consent be in writing.
3. To avoid potential liability, it is always advisable to obtain a written consent.

PATIENT TRANSFER ISSUES REGULATED BY THE EMERGENCY MEDICAL TREATMENT AND ACTIVE LABOR ACT (EMTALA)

In 1986, Congress passed the Emergency Medical Treatment and Active Labor Act (EMTALA) (see 42 U.S.C.A. sec. 1395dd) to prevent the transfer of patients from one facility to another solely based on the patient's ability to pay. This antidumping legislation prevents emergency facilities from refusing to treat and then dumping poor and uninsured patients onto the street or transferring them to another facility.

A. Protected persons: patients who come to a hospital emergency department requesting an examination or medical treatment.
B. Patients must be examined to determine if an emergency medical condition exists.
C. Emergency medical condition as defined by EMTALA: A medical condition manifesting itself by acute symptoms of sufficient severity (including severe pain) such that the absence of immediate medical treatment could reasonably be expected to result in:
  1. Placing the health of the individual (or, with respect to a pregnant woman, the health of the woman or her unborn child) in serious jeopardy, or
  2. Serious impairment to bodily functions, or
  3. Serious dysfunction of any bodily organ or part (see 42 U.S.C.A. sec. 1395dd[e][A]i-iii).
D. The definition of emergency medical condition includes women who are having labor contractions:
  1. That there is inadequate time to effect a safe transfer to another hospital for delivery, or
  2. That transfer may pose a threat to the health or safety of the woman or the unborn child (see 42 U.S.C.A. sec. 1395dd[e][B]i-ii).
E. Requirements for an appropriate transfer to another facility.
  1. The transferring hospital must have provided the necessary medical treatment within its means to minimize the risk to the health of the patient and unborn child.
  2. The receiving hospital must have the space and qualified individuals to provide the necessary care.
  3. The receiving hospital must agree to accept the transfer, provide the necessary treatment, and have an accepting physician of record.
  4. The transferring hospital must provide a copy of the patient's medical record to the receiving hospital.
  5. The transfer must be performed by competent staff and with appropriate medical supplies including life support equipment, if needed.

6. A hospital must not transfer an unstable patient unless:
   a. The patient requests a transfer in writing after he/she has been informed of the hospital's obligations and the risk of transfer, and
   b. A physician or another qualified medical personnel certifies that the benefits of care to be received at the receiving facility outweigh the increased risks to the patient if not transferred.

F. Penalties.
   1. Civil penalties may be brought against:
      a. Hospitals that violate the transfer requirements.
      b. Physicians who are responsible for the examination, treatment, and transfer of patients and violate the EMTALA requirements.
   2. A physician who repeats a gross and flagrant violation of the EMTALA requirements may be excluded from participation in the reimbursement process.
   3. EMTALA provides civil enforcement for:
      a. Any patient harmed by the hospital's violation.
      b. Any hospital that experiences a financial loss as a result of another hospital's violation.
   4. EMTALA provides protection to:
      a. Any qualified medical personnel who refuses to authorize a transfer of an unstable patient.
      b. Any hospital employee who reports a violation of an EMTALA transfer requirement.

ABANDONMENT

Abandonment is a knowing (i.e., intentional) relinquishment of the patient-provider relationship, which may be adverse to the patient.

An advanced practice nurse has a duty to provide care to patients until the relationship is legally terminated. Liability for abandonment exists when an advanced practice nurse fails to see a patient with whom a relationship exists without an acceptable reason.

A. The advanced practice nurse-patient relationship is legally terminated if:
   1. Nursing care is no longer necessary.
   2. The patient ends the relationship.
   3. The patient is transferred to another provider.
   4. The advanced practice nurse ends the relationship after adequate notice to the patient.
   5. The advanced practice nurse is incapable of providing care.

B. The patient ends the relationship.
   1. The patient should be told of the dangers of terminating care, if further treatment is needed.
      a. If requested, the patient should be referred to another provider.
      b. If requested, information necessary to ensure continuity of care should be provided to the subsequent provider.
   2. The advanced practice nurse should request that the patient provide a written verification of the termination of the relationship.

3. If the patient does not provide written verification of the withdrawal from the relationship, then the advanced practice nurse should send written verification to the patient.

C. The patient is transferred to another provider.
   1. Transfer to another provider may occur when the advanced practice nurse is unavailable due to vacation or meetings.
   2. The advanced practice nurse has a duty to identify a qualified substitute provider.

D. The advanced practice nurse ends the relationship after adequate notice to the patient.
   1. Adequate notice is given when it is in writing and allows the patient sufficient time to locate another provider.
   2. Reasons for an advanced practice nurse to end a patient-provider relationship include:
      a. Patient not complying or cooperating with treatment plans.
      b. Patient's failure to pay bills when financially able to do so.

E. If an advanced practice nurse is unable to provide care, he/she may be excused from responsibility.
   1. If ill, a replacement should be arranged, if possible.
   2. If two patients need care at the same time:
      a. Prudence must be exercised in determining priority.
      b. One patient must not be given up entirely to attend to another.
      c. Frequency of attendance of each patient is a factor that would be used to determine if one patient has been abandoned.

F. When an advanced practice nurse fails to see a patient with whom a relationship exists without an acceptable reason, liability may exist for:
   1. Breach of contract or
   2. Malpractice, if an injury occurs.

G. If a patient is instructed to call if further care is needed:
   1. The patient has the responsibility to call.
   2. Abandonment does not occur if the patient fails to call or follow instructions.
   3. However, if a patient has a known disability preventing them from being able to call, it may be necessary to follow up.
   4. If a patient is unable to provide self-care at home, an advanced practice nurse may need to consider plans for home care or placement.

H. Continuation of home health care.
   1. Ambulatory nurses may be exposed to charges of abandonment if home health services are discontinued.
   2. Home health services may be discontinued when:
      a. A source of payment no longer exists.
      b. The environment is unsafe for the ambulatory nurse.
      c. Physician orders terminate care as no longer medically necessary.
   3. If home health services are discontinued, documentation should include:
      a. Notice provided to the patient and physician.
      b. Alternative means taken to prevent endangerment to the patient,

such as identification of other available and accessible community resources.

REPORTABLE SITUATIONS

Nurses are personally liable for their own actions and have an ethical obligation to report incompetent nursing practice. During the delivery of nursing care, nurses must always seek to prevent harm to the patient and legal liability to the organization. Not all instances of incompetence require reporting, depending on state laws.

Ambulatory nurses also have an obligation to report any suspicion of neglect and abuse to the proper legal authorities, including the police. In many states, this reporting is mandatory and the reporter may remain anonymous.

- **A.** The four elements of negligence required for nursing malpractice are:
  - **1.** A duty of care is owed to the patient.
    - **a.** Duty owed is based on nursing standards of care.
    - **b.** Legal definition of scope of duty owed: what a reasonably prudent ambulatory care nurse would have done under similar or like circumstances.
  - **2.** The nurse breached that duty when nursing actions deviated from the standard of care.
    - **a.** Nursing actions were incompetent such as failure to use sterile technique during dressing changes.
    - **b.** The nurse failed to act such as failure to report an adverse reaction to the administration of a drug.
  - **3.** The patient suffered damages.
    - **a.** Physical injury.
    - **b.** Psychologic injury.
    - **c.** Financial loss.
  - **4.** The nurse's actions directly caused the patient's damages.
    - **a.** The wrongful nursing actions were the legal cause of the patient's damages.
    - **b.** The legal definition of causation: "but for" the wrongful nursing action, the patient would not have suffered damages.
- **B.** Reportable malpractice and/or quality situations may include:
  - **1.** Medication errors.
  - **2.** Patient falls.
  - **3.** Equipment injuries.
  - **4.** Failure to assess and monitor a patient's condition.
  - **5.** Failure to ensure patient safety (i.e., use of restraints).
  - **6.** Failure to confirm accuracy of physician order.
  - **7.** Failure to communicate (reporting a change in a patient's condition).
  - **8.** Improper technique or performance of treatments.
  - **9.** Failure to follow organization procedure.
  - **10.** Failure to maintain patient confidentiality.
  - **11.** Failure to complete sufficient and appropriate patient education.
- **C.** Reportable neglect and abuse situations may include:
  - **1.** Suspected child abuse.

      2. Suspected child neglect.

      3. Suspected elder abuse.

      4. Suspected elder neglect.

   D. Peer review.

      1. Reportable situations can be reviewed via an internal organizational system called peer review.

      2. Peer review in ambulatory nursing is a continuous quality improvement activity whereby nurses assess each other's care.

      3. Peer review activities are generally protected and not discoverable in a court of law.

      4. However, in some states this protection is limited to a hospital-based setting.

   E. Impaired nurses and assistance programs.

      1. Most hospitals and state licensure boards have confidential assistance programs for professionals impaired by substance abuse.

      2. These assistance programs are usually confidential and allow successful individuals to return to their professions.

THE LEGAL ASPECTS OF DOCUMENTATION

Nursing documentation has great legal significance. Often the outcome of court cases depends upon the quality of documentation. Nurses can be held liable for negligence and professional misconduct because of inadequate documentation. Failure to document has become synonymous with failure to provide nursing care.

   A. The value of adequate documentation.

      1. The medical record is legal proof of the type and quality of nursing care provided to patients.

      2. The medical record can be used as a defense against claims of negligence and failure to provide care.

      3. Adequate documentation prevents nonreimbursement by third-party payers.

   B. To be considered adequate, nursing documentation must be:

      1. Factual.

      2. Objective—never enter personal opinions.

      3. Accurate.

      4. Consistent.

      5. Timely.

      6. Complete.

   C. Legal issues on how to document.

      1. Always use ink.

      2. Never erase an entry.

      3. If an error in documentation occurs, draw a line through the error and write "error" above it with your initials.

      4. Always use the appropriate medical record or graph.

      5. Document on each line without leaving spaces between entries.

         a. Document an omission as a new entry.

         b. Avoid adding to a previously written entry.

6. Only use standard abbreviations.
7. Document legibly and clearly.

D. Legal issues on what to document.
   1. Document symptoms using the patient's own words placed in quotation marks.
   2. Document each objective observation.
   3. Document the identification and analysis of any patient problem.
   4. Document any nursing actions taken.
   5. Document the patient's response to any nursing actions.
      a. Effects of medications.
      b. Response to treatments.
   6. Document actions taken to ensure patient safety.
   7. Document only the care that you provide and never document the care provided by other nursing staff.
   8. Sign and date each and every entry.

E. Legal issues on computerized documentation.
   1. To ensure accuracy, double-check any entries (systems should include methods of providing a record of changes, additions, etc.).
   2. Do not reveal individual identification codes.
   3. Report anyone suspected of using your identification code.

TELEPHONE NURSING PRACTICE LIABILITY ISSUES

Consumers are increasingly demanding health care information and seeking advice about health care problems by telephone. Many health systems employ registered nurses to triage telephone queries and dispense health care advice. Telephone nursing practice is an area of ambulatory care nursing practice that presents an increased risk for liability. The ambulatory nurse must be aware of safeguards against legal problems resulting from telephonic health care interactions.

A. Telephone orders (see Box 8-1).
   1. Generally, telephone orders should be taken only when a physician is incapable of physically visiting the patient.
   2. Documenting the telephone order per established policies and procedures for the organization of practice.
      a. Document the order on the physician order record.
      b. Document the date, time, and write "t.o." for telephone order and record the physician's name followed by the nurse's signature.
   3. To avoid liability, determine if the physician has subsequently countersigned the telephone order within the time frame established for the organization of practice.

THE REGULATION OF NURSING PRACTICE

The nurse practice act is a statute or legislative act that regulates nursing practice in each state. Nurse practice acts may differ between states.

A. Nurse practice act.
   1. Defines nursing practice.

■ BOX 8-1

■ **SAFEGUARDS AGAINST LEGAL PROBLEMS RESULTING FROM TELEPHONE TRIAGE**

- Use medically approved protocols to establish a standard of care. Do not deviate from the protocols unless changes are in writing and approved by the appropriate medical authority.
- Document the call and advice provided. For example, if a suit is filed 3 years later claiming the nurse did not advise the mother appropriately, the nurse's position is much more defensible if the documentation shows that protocols were followed and appropriate advice was given. Documentation may include a log, a note in the patient's chart, or a recording of the call.
- Provide callers with an option to seek medical attention sooner if they do not agree with the advice or if the condition persists or worsens.
- Develop a mechanism to regularly review documentation and advice for consistency, accuracy, and quality.
- Orient and train staff in telephone triage protocols, policies and procedures, phone encounter techniques, dealing with difficult calls, and documentation.
- Measure outcomes. Conduct regular consumer satisfaction surveys. Follow up promptly on problems and quality issues.
- Establish a positive helping relationship at the outset of the call. The average call lasts approximately 6 minutes. The effectiveness of this short encounter is often dependent on skillful communication. The initial contact can often make or break the caller's confidence and satisfaction with the telephone interaction.
- Encourage the caller to briefly describe the problem and its duration, onset, and location; past medical history; medications; and allergies. Be sure to obtain the age of the person with the problem.
- Use terminology the caller can understand. Avoid medical jargon as much as possible.
- Listen carefully to the caller and avoid jumping to conclusions. Callers may mask their real concern for fear of embarrassment, particularly regarding sensitive issues such as sexually transmitted infections or mental health problems.
- Try to talk to the person with the problem, directly if possible. Direct communication is usually more reliable and inclusive than secondhand information.
- Thoroughly assess the problem before determining an action plan. The caller may underplay the symptoms and want reassurance that the problem is insignificant.
- Pay attention to the degree of anxiety and concern expressed by the caller. Remember, the telephone nurse is at a disadvantage and cannot see or touch the person. If the caller is emphatic that the person is ill even though protocols may recommend home care measures or observation while waiting for an appointment, encourage the caller to seek medical attention sooner. It is better to be overly cautious than to miss a serious condition.
- Always provide the caller with the option to call back or seek medical attention if the condition persists or worsens or new symptoms develop.
- Attend conferences, workshops, and continuing education offerings to establish competency in communication skills, assessment, and telephone triage to reduce the risk of medical-legal problems.

From Briggs JK (1997): *Telephone triage protocols for nurses.* Philadelphia: JB Lippincott, pp. 3-4.

2. Establishes nursing practice standards.
3. Defines licensure requirements.
4. Creates and empowers a board of nursing to oversee nursing practice.
5. Provides a foundation upon which to evaluate the existence of nursing malpractice.
B. The state's nursing licensing board.
   1. Receives its authority from the nurse practice act.
   2. Protects the public from uneducated, unsafe, or unethical nurses.
   3. Disciplines nurses who do not comply with standards of safe nursing practice.
   4. Collaborates with employee assistance programs for chemically or mentally impaired nurses.
C. Licensure issues across state lines.
   1. Although nursing licensure is a state function, health care is increasingly being practiced across state lines, including:
      a. Telephone triage management, in which patients are given health care advice via telephone from a person in a different state.
      b. Telemedicine, in which patients are assessed at remote locations using two-way audiovisual and computerized equipment such as stethoscopes, otoscopes, and ophthalmoscopes.
      c. Teleradiology, in which digitalized radiographic images are being sent to distant locations over telephone lines for interpretation.
   2. These technological advances present difficult licensure issues that are yet to be totally resolved. Potential answers might include:
      a. Gaining licensure in all states in which an organization does business.
      b. Development of a national licensure system.

WORKPLACE REGULATORY COMPLIANCE (EEOC AND OSHA)

Nurses and nurse managers are required to comply with regulations providing for equal opportunity and safety in the workplace. The Equal Employment Opportunity Commission (EEOC) is a federal agency that enforces regulations concerning equal opportunity. The Occupational Safety and Health Administration (OSHA) provides regulations that mandate safe working conditions.

A. The Equal Employment Opportunity Commission (EEOC).
   1. The legal regulations for providing equal opportunity are found in:
      a. Title VI and Title VII of the Civil Rights Act of 1964.
         (1) Amended by the Equal Employment Act of 1972.
         (2) Prohibits employment discrimination due to race, color, religion, sex, or national origin.
      b. Title IX of the Education Amendments of 1972.
         (1) Prohibits discrimination due to sex.
         (2) Limited to any educational program or activity receiving federal funds.
      c. Equal Pay Act of 1963.

      (1) Amended by the Education Amendments of 1972.

      (2) Requires equal pay for men and women doing substantially similar jobs.

    d. Age Discrimination in Employment Act of 1967: prohibits discrimination due to age for employees between the ages of 40 through 70.

2. An employee who has been discriminated against must:

    a. File a complaint with the EEOC within 180 days or

    b. File their complaint with a local or state agency that handles discrimination issues within 300 days.

3. After a complaint has been filed, the EEOC will:

    a. Conduct an investigation.

    b. Act as a mediator to resolve the problem, if discrimination is found.

4. If mediation is not successful, the EEOC will:

    a. File a lawsuit on behalf of the employee or

    b. Issue a "right to sue" letter that allows the employee to file a lawsuit.

5. Issuance of the "right to sue" letter:

    a. May be requested by an employee, if the EEOC has not investigated the complaint within 180 days.

    b. Does not signify that the EEOC has found discrimination.

6. If a court determines that discrimination exists, the employer may be ordered to do any of the following:

    a. Accommodate the employee, as needed.

    b. Promote the employee.

    c. Otherwise remedy whatever discrimination has occurred.

    d. Pay money damages.

    e. Pay punitive money damages, if the employer's actions were willful or reckless.

B. The Occupational Safety and Health Administration (OSHA).

  1. General information.

    a. Is a branch of the U.S. Department of Labor.

    b. Enforces the rules and regulations set forth in the Occupational Safety and Health Act of 1970.

    c. Applies to employers in all U.S. states and U.S. possessions who employ one or more persons and who engage in business affecting commerce.

    d. Exempts all local, state, and federal government employees.

    e. Uses surprise inspections and large fines to ensure compliance.

  2. Main purposes of OSHA.

    a. To ensure safe and healthy working conditions.

    b. To provide national guidelines and standards.

  3. Some examples of regulations enforced by OSHA.

    a. Standard Precautions to protect health care workers from exposure to blood and body fluid-borne pathogens.

      (1) Hepatitis B (HBV).

      (2) Virus that causes AIDS (HIV).

    b. Protective equipment requirements.

c. Inspection procedures.

d. Risk management of potentially exposed employees.

e. Lifting guidelines.

f. Respiratory guidelines.

g. Confined-space regulations.

h. Ergonomic guidelines.

i. Egress.

4. National Institute for Occupational Safety and Health (NIOSH).

a. Is a federal agency responsible for research and education.

b. Has representatives who perform inspections to ensure compliance.

5. Regulation violations.

a. Citations and penalties vary depending on the seriousness of the violation.

b. Violation citations must be posted at the worksite.

c. Employers may contest the citation.

REFERENCES

Briggs JK (1997): *Telephone triage protocols for nurses.* Philadelphia: JB Lippincott, pp. 3-4.

Emergency Medical Treatment and Active Labor Act of 42 of 1986, U.S.C.A., Title 42, sec. 1395dd.

Other Recommended Readings

American College of Emergency Physicians (1997): *Policy statement on medical direction of interfacility patient transfers.* Dallas: American College of Emergency Physicians.

Andrews M, Goldberg K, Kaplan H (1996): *Nurse's legal handbook,* ed 3. Springhouse, PA: Springhouse, pp. 238-239, 253.

Ballard DC (1999): Home health and ambulatory nursing liabilities. In Rostant DM, Cady RF, editors: *Liability issues in perinatal nursing.* Philadelphia: JB Lippincott, Williams & Wilkins, pp. 168-169.

Cady RF (1999): Telephone triage and the office nurse. In Rostant DM, Cady RF, editors: *Liability issues in perinatal nursing.* Philadelphia: JB Lippincott, Williams & Wilkins, pp. 149-155.

Catalano JT (1996): *Contemporary professional nursing.* Philadelphia: FA Davis, pp. 175, 294-300.

Creighton H (1986): *Law every nurse should know,* ed 5. Philadelphia: WB Saunders, pp. 2-4.

Huber D (1996): *Leadership and nursing care management.* Philadelphia: WB Saunders, pp. 95-97.

Marriner-Tomey A (1996): *Guide to nursing management and leadership,* ed 5. St. Louis: Mosby, pp. 211, 455-457, 473.

Rohman LW, Huber PL (1996): Health: patient rights and policing the quality of health care. In Hauser BR, editor: *Women's legal guide.* Golden, CO: Fulcrum, pp. 35-37, 41-43.

Rubert MC (1999): Patient rights. In Rostant DM, Cady RF, editors: *Liability issues in perinatal nursing.* Philadelphia: Lippincott, Williams & Wilkins, pp. 180-182.

Trandel-Korenchuk DM, Trandel-Korenchuk KM (1997): *Nursing & the law,* ed 5. Gaithersburg, MD: Aspen, pp. 110-111.

Wilkinson W, Smith L (1996): Disabilities. In Hauser BR, editor: *Women's legal guide.* Golden, CO: Fulcrum, p. 266.

9 Patient Advocacy

E. MARY JOHNSON, BSN, RN, Cm, CNA

OBJECTIVES

Study of the information presented in this chapter will enable the learner to:

1. Describe the relationship between ethical concepts and advocacy behavior.

2. Describe specific applications of advocacy behavior as it relates to ambulatory practice.

3. Discuss the importance of patient education to advocacy actions.

■■ It is the absence of health (illness) that often initiates people into using health care systems. Many, if not most, individuals have a limited view and understanding of how today's health care industry works but hold high expectations for its abilities and promise. This knowledge deficit can become apparent when illness and its unknown outcomes create individuals who feel vulnerable. The relationship between the patient and the health care team has always been described as fiduciary, meaning a relationship built on a public confidence involving trust. This trust is translated by the public (patients) to mean that the health care team will act in the best interest of the patient. It is within this trust and commitment as a profession that nursing frames decision-making and advocacy behaviors as we respond to the needs of patients and families.

Perhaps never in the history of the modern day health care system has the emphasis been greater than now for nurses to recognize and act as patient advocates in today's health care world. Identifying when and how, exploring who and what can be done as implementers of health care, may in reality, be the most critical skill nurses offer to patients.

Ethical and advocacy principles are connected through a framework of agreed concepts and actions taken on the part of an individual and/or professional organizations. The mission of the American Academy of Ambulatory Care Nursing is to advance and influence the art and science of ambulatory care nursing practice (AAACN, 1999). Within the AAACN Nursing Administration and Practice Standards (2000, p. 6), is a description of what ambulatory care nursing values. These values include a specific reference to "the opportunity to serve as patient advocate." Philosophically and organizationally, these public documents are congruent with nursing's commitment as a profession. An accepted principle of biomedical ethics includes the concept that professions must possess the knowledge, skill, and diligence to uphold the moral and legal standards of due care. Understanding how the nursing profession performs this role through ethical decision-making and advocacy behaviors is fundamental to the nursing practice in ambulatory care (Johnson, 2000).

A. **Context of Patient Advocacy.** According to Virginia Henderson, the clinical definition of nursing is: "to assist the individual, sick or well, in the performance of those activities contributing to health or its recovery (or to a peaceful death) that he would perform unaided if he had the necessary strength, will, or knowledge, and to do this in such a way as to help him gain independence as rapidly as possible" (1961, p 42).

1. Nursing profession is:
   a. Essential part of society.
   b. Dynamic and reflects the changing nature of societal need.
   c. "Owned by society" in the sense that a "profession acquires recognition, relevance and even meaning in terms of its relationship to that society, its culture and institutions, and its other members" (ANA, 1995).

2. Authority for the practice of nursing.
   a. Based on a social contract that acknowledges professional rights and responsibilities, as well as mechanisms for public accountability (ANA, 1995).
   b. Based on specific state nurse practice acts.
   c. Based on accepted standards of practice.
   d. Based on applicable state and regulatory rules.

3. People seek the services of nurses:
   a. To obtain information and treatment in matters of health and illness.
   b. To resolve problems or manage health-promoting behaviors.
   c. To identify both short and long-term health goals.
   d. To act as advocates for people dealing with barriers encountered in obtaining health care (ANA, 1995).

4. Performance of advocacy role in ambulatory setting through:
   a. Providing patient education.
   b. Providing access to care.
   c. Providing ongoing assessment of patient.
   d. Providing continuity of care.
   e. Providing informed decision making.
   f. Providing mechanisms to measure patient satisfaction.

5. AAACN values statement includes:
   a. Welcoming the opportunity to advocate appropriately for patients/families.
   b. Shared responsibility among patients, families, and other members of the health care team in all phases of health care delivery.
   c. Education to enable patients and families to understand and make informed decisions.
   d. Continuity of care.

6. Linkage of advocacy and ethics.
   a. *Advocacy*—act or process of advocating or supporting (a cause or proposal) on behalf of another (Steinmetz et al, 1997). This definition

of advocacy is similar to that found in the conceptual framework for ambulatory care nurses. The conceptual framework defines advocacy as compassion, caring, emotional support (Haas, 1998).

b. *Ethics*—a branch of philosophy dealing with the values related to human conduct, with respect to the rightness or wrongness of certain actions; and to the goodness and badness of the motives and ends of such actions; a set of moral principles or values, the principles of conduct governing an individual or a group (Steinmetz et al, 1997).

7. The linkage of ethics and advocacy principles for ambulatory nursing practice is in recognizing (understanding) that ethics provides a conceptual framework and advocacy is the appropriate actions (behaviors) in implementing decisions made on behalf of patients.

B. **Present Context of Patient Advocacy.** Today's health care system presents challenges on many fronts that require advocacy for patient/family.

1. Scientific advancement in medicine in past decade.

   a. Potential availability and application of advancements (e.g., gene therapy, transplantation, drug protocols, microscopic endoscopy applications).

   b. Allocation and rationing of medical advancements can occur as a result of:

      (1) Geographic location.

      (2) Cost to payer.

   c. Institutional decision including cost constraints/benefit analysis about specific therapies, and experimental procedures to be offered.

2. Financial issues.

   a. Governmental initiatives/decisions.

      (1) Medicare/Medicaid programs: promotion of HMO systems to elderly and poverty level populations.

      (2) Omnibus Reconciliation Bill of 1985 (COBRA): progressively decreased payments for health care delivery requiring decision making about types of services that institutions will provide to consumers.

      (3) Corporate compliance: the health care industry faces a growing challenge to conduct business, including treatment, billing, and relationships with other health care providers, in compliance with a variety of laws, regulations, and program requirements. The intention is that business practices do not cross over into intentionally designed abuse (Cantone, 1999). A recent focus of the government has been a judicial initiative to detect fraud and abuse in the Medicare/Medicaid programs. The response by institutions and individual physicians has been the development of extensive internal review and education to providers about HCFA rules and regulations. Development of systematic processes for measuring compliance with written compliance plans has also happened as a proactive response and expectation.

   b. Private sector insurers.
      (1) Shrinking fee-for-service market because of higher individual cost; this type of insurance plan allows for more choice by individual about health care options.
      (2) Proliferation of managed care insurance products has accrued throughout the country, including high-risk Medicare and Medicaid HMO plans.
         (a) Failure of these ventures has also occurred resulting in decreased access for Medicare-Medicaid populations.
         (b) HMO's decision-making approval processes can create a moral dilemma for health care providers. Decisions about what testing and consulting services are needed are currently frequently challenged/denied by HMOs.
   c. Business sector issues.
      (1) Budget constraints exist for health care dollar.
         (a) Increased co-pays, putting coverage at risk.
         (b) Decision to seek health care can be delayed putting health at risk.
         (c) Demand for quality care for insured employees requires institutional accountability for care delivery by providers.
         (d) Operational challenges, including redesign of ambulatory care operations practice patterns, primarily as a result of compressed length of stay (LOS) in hospitals.
            (i) Increased volume in ambulatory settings because of decreased LOS.
            (ii) Increased acuity in ambulatory care because of decreased LOS.
            (iii) Increased availability and incorporation of new technology.
            (iv) Increase in home care and long-term care referrals.
 3. Political response to today's health care market focused on recognizing and providing solutions involving:
   a. Securing long-term funding of Medicare/Medicaid programs.
   b. Promotion of managed care initiative including:
      (1) Defining clinical outcomes.
      (2) Application of professional practice guideline.
      (3) Ongoing quality processes and measurements in place.
   c. Increased access to health care systems.
   d. Aging U.S. population/demographics (baby boomers).
   e. Patient's Bill of Rights legislation (proposed).
   f. Rising number of uninsured Americans (approximately 44 million in 1998) (Iglehart, 1999).
   g. Prescriptive drug coverage.
 4. Quality assessment.
   a. Evaluation begins with patient rights/responsibilities (autonomy).

      b. Balance between cost and quality of care delivered.

      c. Nursing identification of and participation in evaluation of quality issues.

      d. External review agencies.

        (1) Perform reviews and monitor activities to assure consistent and reliable care.

          (a) Joint Commission on Accreditation of Healthcare Organizations (JCAHO).

          (b) American Academy Ambulatory Health Care (AAAHC).

          (c) National Commission Quality Assurance (NCQA).

          (d) American Accreditation Healthcare Commission (URAC).

          (e) Federal and state regulatory agencies.

      e. Internal review systems and improving organizational performance (IOP) begin at (JCAHO, 1999):

        (1) Clinic/unit level.

        (2) Department level.

        (3) Institutional review.

          (a) Leadership responsibility/decisions as to what areas of improvement will be reviewed and supported with resources.

          (b) Leadership has oversight responsibility to ensure that changes focus on improvement of care for patients.

C. Advocacy Opportunities. The advocacy for patients/families is best done when linked to education about both health/disease management and the health care system itself.

    1. Empowerment of the patient and family to make informed decisions.

      a. Until early 1990s, health care providers often encouraged patients to have symptoms evaluated through an office visit. This did little to affirm and reassure the decision making of the patients and families and promoted vulnerability, viewing medicine as mystifying and maybe even magical.

      b. Currently, the shift is toward a partnership between providers and educated patients (Linnell, 1998).

        (1) Shift recognizes reality of care being episodic and frequently provided by patient and/or family.

        (2) Shift requires education of patients/families to evaluate and manage illnesses through a combination of self-care, telephone management, and office visits.

        (3) Shift requires education of patient/family to support their ability to assimilate, interpret, and evaluate information for decision making.

    2. Clinical operations must be designed to safely respond to the new flow patterns and be monitored for their responsiveness.

      a. Increased outreach efforts within community. For example, Fluogen immunization at schools, churches, etc.

      b. Flexible hours for delivery of services. For example, pediatric clinics open 7 days per week.

3. Nurses' role in advocacy behaviors is based on assessment of patient needs and on organizational systems available to provide care. Skills required include:
   a. Expert clinical assessment skills.
      (1) Telephone triage.
      (2) Telephone management/case management: often proactive in focus.
      (3) Office visit: consistent assessment and reassessment.
   b. Expert intervention skills.
      (1) Understanding disease process, disease management, family dynamics, and community resources.
      (2) Understanding basic survival skills in disease management.
      (3) Lifestyle skills: current adaptation to health challenges.
      (4) Health promotion: proactive, holistic approach to lifestyle.
   c. Confident decision-making skills.
   d. Partnering skills with patients/families/health care team.
   e. Knowledge of mechanisms to coordinate care across institutions/community to provide continuity.
   f. Knowledge of the fiscal impact of care decisions.
4. Nurse plays central role in working with patients/families to assure:
   a. Right access.
   b. Right provider.
   c. Right time frame.
   d. Right level of care.
5. Patient satisfaction is a subjective data collection that responds to the perception of care delivered—understanding that perception is reality to the patient.
   a. Measurement indicators.
      (1) Patient survey feedback at provider level, unit level, institutional level.
      (2) Accreditation bodies review findings and institutional response to these findings.
      (3) Third party payers response to care provided.
      (4) Complaint resolution process in place. Units/institutions need to create atmosphere of objectivity and specific processes for this to happen. Recognizing own values and biases of health care personnel.
      (5) IOP activities at unit level measuring patient satisfaction.
   b. Customer service.
      (1) Patient perception is reality: do not underestimate this concept in terms of marketing and public relations.
      (2) Treat each patient and family with dignity and courtesy: nurse needs to recognize his or her own beliefs/values. This includes patient's family and the larger community.
   c. Techniques: promoting advocacy and customer service.
      (1) Look directly at the person.

(2) Listen quietly.

(3) Speak softly.

(4) Acknowledge issues and responsibilities.

(5) Acknowledge individuality and autonomy.

D. Future Advocacy Opportunities for Nurses in Ambulatory Care.

1. Challenge to:

   a. Advocate with current cost containment focus.

   b. Bottom line decisions.

   c. Episodic nature of patient visits.

2. Need to create opportunities for nurses to discuss and decide issues with leadership about matters such as patient complaints, IOP results, program changes.

   a. Leadership voice in operational decisions (i.e., begins at unit level and includes evaluation of current services provided and the ability to add additional new program development).

   b. Health care resources/allocation (i.e., evaluation of appropriate equipment, space, personnel, and systems to meet changing practice).

   c. Learn of opportunities from other professions.

      (1) Identify centers of excellence with quality outcomes.

      (2) Apply appropriate adaptation of results for specific environments.

      (3) Network with other professionals.

   d. Must help patients/families understand their rights and responsibilities in participating in the health care system (i.e., build trusting partnerships, choices available).

   e. Shared responsibility concept between patient/family and health care team.

      (1) Empowerment of patient/family through education.

      (2) Awareness of JCAHO intent regarding this standard.

E. Leadership Coordination. Skills necessary to organize and manage an undertaking, while moving forward on agreed goals. Ambulatory care nurses can apply these skills in their work setting and the community to benefit patients.

1. Internal operations.

   a. Consider process for integrating the Patient Self-Determination Act of 1991 (Rouse, 1991).

      (1) Requires that patients are asked about and given opportunity to decide their advance directive as relates to health care decisions.

      (2) This is mandated for acute care, skilled nursing home health care, hospice care, long-term care, and HMO settings.

      (3) This federal requirement is not required in ambulatory setting, however this discussion with primary care provider should be done as part of health care partnership/relationship, preferably over time and before a health care crisis occurs for the patient (Johnson, 2000).

      (4) Respects and values the individual patient.

    b. Participate in the design and implementation of an institutional system that provides consistent documentation of this information in patient record. Although this is extremely challenging, it is becoming more important as a result of increasing complexity of systems serving patients.

    c. For selected ambulatory patients requiring an acute care episode, begin discharge planning in ambulatory setting (i.e., crutch walking for joint replacements, introduction to specific durable medical equipment used in certain procedures).

    d. Promote increased communications between ambulatory/acute care/home care settings to improve the continuity of care for patients.

        (1) Meet periodically with most frequent providers to promote understanding of how systems work and can improve to benefit all.

        (2) Ensure flow of written communication regarding the plan of care.

2. External environment.

    a. Community education/involvement in promoting understanding of how the health care system works.

        (1) Schools: local systems and colleges (i.e., work with school board to promote preventive health curriculum).

        (2) Advocacy resources.

            (a) Internet (i.e., Advocacy in Ambulatory Care, Patient Advocate Foundation, www.patientadvocate.org).

            (b) State insurance departments.

            (c) Health Care Financing Administration (HCFA), through Peer Review Organization (PROS).

            (d) American Hospital Association—Society for Healthcare Consumer Advocacy.

            (e) Professional organizations/societies.

            (f) American Association of Retired Persons (AARP).

        (3) Church community: parish nursing programs.

    b. Professional organizations/political activism.

        (1) Professional organizations support the nurse's ability to advocate.

            (a) Create standards of care to benefit patients.

            (b) Provide ongoing education for nurses.

            (c) Publish journals and texts to support care of patients.

        (2) Professional organizations advocate directly.

            (a) Support lobbying efforts.

            (b) Propose public policy related to care.

    c. Create business opportunities.

        (1) Intermediary between patients and insurance company.

        (2) Roles within managed care organizations in quality management; specifically, evaluating indicators of quality as they relate to subscribers.

(3) Independent consultant: based on recognized expertise (i.e., redesign, accreditation process, clinical MISD systems, research, risk management/quality measurement).

(4) Independent practice as a personal, professional medical advocate to help patients determine if they are getting appropriate care (Vitanza, 2000).

REFERENCES

American Academy of Ambulatory Care Nursing (2000): *AAACN Ambulatory care nursing administration and practice standard,* ed 5. Pitman, NJ: Anthony J. Jannetti.

American Academy of Ambulatory Care Nursing (1999): AAACN fact sheet. *AAACN 1999-2000 membership directory.* Pitman, NJ: Anthony J. Jannetti.

American Nurses' Association (1995): *Nursing's social policy statement.* Washington, DC: American Nursing Press.

Cantone L (1999): Corporate compliance: critical to organizational success. *Nurs Econ* 17(1):15-19, 52.

Haas S (1998): Ambulatory care nursing conceptual framework. *AAACN Viewpoint* 20(3):16-17.

Henderson V (1961): *Basic principles of nursing care.* London: International Council of Nursing.

Iglehart J (1999): The American health care system—expenditures. *N Engl J Med* 340(1):70-71.

Johnson E (2000): Advocating for patients. *AAACN Viewpoint* 22(4):1, 6-7.

Joint Commission on Accreditation of Healthcare Organizations (1999): *1999 Hospital accreditation standards (HAS), standards, intent.* Oakbrook Terrace, IL: Author.

Linnell K (1998): Patient health education in the changing ambulatory care environment. *AAACN Viewpoint* 20(1):1-6, 8.

Rouse F (1991): Patients, providers and the PSDA. *Hastings Center Report 1991* 21(5) (Suppl. Sept/Oct):52-53.

Steinmetz S, et al, editors (1997): *Random House Webster's unabridged dictionary,* ed 2. New York: Random House.

Vitanza A (2000, March 6): Guardian angels aids those lost in medical maze. *Healthcare Monitor* pp. 1, 9.

Staffing and Workload

SHEILA A. HAAS, PhD, RN
CLARE HASTINGS, PhD, RN

OBJECTIVES
Study of the information presented in this chapter will enable the learner to:

1. Discuss methods of determining staffing requirements and skill mix in ambulatory care nursing.

2. Compare and contrast staff recruitment and retention strategies in ambulatory care settings.

3. Understand major content and methods for orientation of staff in ambulatory care nursing.

4. Discuss common methods of monitoring productivity in ambulatory care nursing.

5. Enumerate the issues and challenges with staffing and workload in ambulatory care nursing.

∎∎ The needs of ambulatory care patients are increasingly complex and the demands for care are more intense today because of both demographics and changes in length of stay for hospitalized patients. Methods of determining staffing requirements and skill mix in ambulatory care nursing have become a major concern for nurses working in ambulatory care settings. Visit volume is no longer a good predictor of the number and type of staff needed to care for ambulatory patients. Instead, numbers and types of nursing staff must be sufficient to serve both the number of patients and the complexity of their needs. Recruiting and orienting ambulatory care nurses has become a more difficult challenge as well. Ambulatory care nurses have traditionally had hospital nursing experience prior to hire into ambulatory care. As hospitals have downsized, fewer experienced hospital nurses are available to work in ambulatory care settings. Orientation and competency assessment must now include assessment of basic as well as specialty-specific competencies. Nurses practicing in ambulatory settings need to be aware of these issues as they move to new settings, or participate in the orientation of new staff.

DETERMINING STAFFING AND SKILL MIX IN AMBULATORY CARE

    A. Definitions.

        1. *Staffing* is the process of assessing patient care needs, determining and providing the appropriate number and mix of nursing personnel to meet patients' requirements for care and desired quality outcomes.

        2. *Workload* refers to the amount of patient care required in a specified period of time.

3. *Skill mix* refers to the number and types of nursing personnel assigned to care for a given patient population.
4. *Nursing personnel* typically providing that nursing care in ambulatory settings include:
   a. Registered nurses (RNs).
   b. Licensed practical nurses/licensed vocational nurses (LPNs/LVNs).
   c. Unlicensed assistive personnel (UAP).
      (1) Nurse aides/nursing assistants (NAs).
      (2) Medical technicians or medical assistants (MTs or MAs).
      (3) Receptionists.
      (4) Clerks.
   d. Advanced practice nurses (APNs).
      (1) Nurse practitioners (NPs).
      (2) Certified nurse midwives (CNMs).
      (3) Certified registered nurse anesthetists (CRNAs).
      (4) Clinical nurse specialists (CNSs).
5. *Mid-level providers* are defined in managed care organizations as APNs and physician assistants (PAs).
6. *Staffing ratio* is the ratio of nursing personnel to patients requiring care.
7. *Full-time equivalent (FTE)* refers to a full-time position or combination of positions that is equal to 40 hours of work per week.
8. *Provider* refers to a licensed independent practitioner (LIP) such as a physician or nurse practitioner.
9. *Ambulatory nursing intensity* has various definitions in the literature.
   a. Verran (1981) defined it as a combination of nursing care complexity and the time needed to do complex work.
   b. Currently to validate a definition of ambulatory nursing intensity, a Delphi study is being conducted on the dimensions of ambulatory nursing intensity (Haas, Hackbarth, Cullen, and Androwich, 2000).

B. A staffing process consists of:
   1. A precise statement of the mission of the organization and the services that patient and/or patient caregiver can expect, including the standards of care.
   2. Determination of the nursing care delivery model (i.e., primary nursing care, team, modular, case management).
   3. Determination of patient population care needs.
   4. Use of a specific method to determine the number and types of staff required to provide care.
   5. Determination of environmental factors that influence staffing (i.e., geographic layout, physician expectations).
   6. Development of assignment patterns for staff using established health care setting personnel guidelines, policy statements, procedures as well as professional standards.
   7. Determination of the scheduling process and procedures.
   8. Evaluation of quality of care provided and judgement reflecting impact of staffing via process and outcome measures.

C. Factors influencing staffing.

1. Payer mix and market factors.
   a. Level of managed care and capitation that alters incentives for various care delivery modes.
      (1) Under capitation, each patient visit adds cost.
      (2) Under capitation, cost is split among MD, RN, and overhead.
      (3) Under capitation, value of RN is in decreasing the cost per covered life including reducing the number/cost of visits.
2. The process of care delivery.
   a. Patient flow through the facility.
   b. Volume of services provided.
   c. Provider roles and practice styles.
   d. Use of midlevel providers.
   e. Availability, competency, and number of UAPs.
   f. Integration of services along the continuum of care.
   g. Availability of consult services.
3. Types of patient encounters.
   a. Scheduled vs. unscheduled.
   b. New vs. return and/or follow-up visits.
   c. Office visit vs. procedure-based.
   d. Education or counseling visit.
   e. Telecommunication contact.
   f. Referral.
4. Requirements per patient encounter.
   a. Time required for encounter.
   b. Intensity or level of skill required of provider and support staff.
   c. Both time and intensity important.
5. Interdisciplinary team function (Hastings and Haas, 1998; Hastings, 1997).
   a. Non-physician staff seen as augmenting/extending MD role.
   b. Non-physician staff seen as value-added providers of service.
6. Provider-perceived (MD, APN, PA) needs for support staff.
   a. Prior to visit.
   b. During visit.
   c. Following visit
   d. Telephone support requirements.
7. Legacy from inpatient staffing models.
   a. False assumption that each visit requires nursing care.
   b. Unnecessary application of inpatient standards for assessment and observation.
8. Use of benchmarking or comparative data to set staffing levels.
   a. Based on what exists in current practice, not necessarily what should be.
   b. Often difficult to find appropriate comparisons, because practices and settings may vary even in the same specialty.
D. Nursing intensity systems for ambulatory care.
   1. They are in developmental stages.

   2. Their purpose is to differentiate:
   a. Types of visits.
   b. Types of providers needed.
   c. Number of nursing personnel needed.
   3. Types of nursing intensity systems.
   a. *Prototype intensity systems* involve categorizing patients/patient visits into four or five categories that describe care, complexity, time required, and nursing intensity. These categories:
      (1) Are based on role dimensions and can dictate required nursing care needed (i.e., teaching, care coordination, advocacy based on role dimensions).
      (2) Can determine visit types and time.
      (3) Can predict types (RN, LPN, UAP) of personnel needed.
   b. *Factor-based intensity systems* involve use of indicators that are summed to derive the time and complexity of care required. These indicators:
      (1) Are based on activities and time needed to do each activity needed for care.
      (2) Can predict staff time required, but usually does not predict type of nursing personnel needed.
   4. In ambulatory care, nursing intensity systems cannot be used prospectively for staffing on a day-to-day basis because of visit volume, rather are used for trending retrospectively.
   5. Issues with nursing intensity systems in ambulatory care that should assist with determining staffing.
   a. *Validity:* All classification systems are dependent on instruments to measure nursing intensity. These are only valid if they truly measure or capture what they are supposed to measure: the work that nursing personnel does in ambulatory care.
      (1) No generally accepted definition or measure of nursing intensity in ambulatory care.
      (2) Role ambiguity in nursing in ambulatory care continues.
   b. *Reliability:* Any instrument designed to determine nursing intensity in ambulatory care must be used consistently by everyone; it must be user friendly and easy to use with a large visit volume.
   c. *Automation:* Given the visit volume in many ambulatory care areas, a nursing intensity system must be computerized and must have sufficient capacity to handle large volumes of data.

RECRUITMENT AND RETENTION OF NURSES IN AMBULATORY CARE

A. Definitions.
   1. *Recruitment* involves seeking, attracting ("selling the organization"), and selecting qualified candidates for positions available in a cost-effective manner.
   2. *Retention* is maintaining qualified persons in positions.

B. Requirements for recruitment and retention.
  1. Planning for numbers and types of personnel, as well as where and how to best look for new hires.
  2. Developing relationships with potential sources of new hires (i.e., schools of nursing).
  3. Attention, even during times of perceived surplus nursing personnel (shortages are cyclical).
  4. Cooperation throughout the organization to be successful; current employees "sell" the organization.
  5. In ambulatory care, recruitment entails overcoming myths and stereotypes.
    a. Ambulatory care nursing is "a piece of cake," "easy," "a vacation" compared to inpatient nursing.
    b. Ambulatory care is the place to go for straight day shifts, no evenings, nights, or weekend shifts (no longer true).
C. Recruitment planning includes:
  1. Developing a position description including responsibilities, accountabilities, and required qualifications (accurate position descriptions are more likely to result in a good match).
  2. Identifying all relevant sources of potential candidates including the use of summer internships for student nurses.
  3. Determining the optimal mode of communicating vacancies, (i.e., personnel communication, internal postings, letters, ads).
  4. Ensuring that all recruitment communication is in compliance with internal and external policies on recruitment.
  5. Validating that the compensation package is appropriate for the position and the marketplace.
  6. Coaching current employees regarding recruiting, selling, and selecting candidates.
  7. Evaluating responses to the recruiting effort and modifying it as needed.
D. Variables affecting recruitment.
  1. Competitiveness of salaries and benefits as well as perceptions of salary compression over time (perception that nurses' salaries have not consistently increased as have those of other occupational groups).
  2. Available supply of qualified nursing personnel.
    a. In a poor national economy, nurses tend to work more, as the economy improves, nurses may work fewer hours.
    b. Fewer young nurses are available, as a result of decreased enrollments related to a perceived surplus of nurses in the early 90s and attraction of other careers open to young people.
    c. The mean age of nurses is mid-40s (USDHHS, 1996).
    d. Size of the applicant pool is also influenced by specific position qualifications. Often see increased demand for specialty prepared nurses (OR, ER, critical care).
    e. Proximity to schools of nursing.
  3. Available resources for advertisements, literature, and recruiter visits to career days.

    4. Attractiveness of the work setting and perceptions about the safety of the work environment.

    5. Reputation of the organization regarding past employment practices and quality of patient care.

    6. Values related to scheduling, time available for leisure.

    7. Status of national and local economy.

    8. Reputation for work group cohesiveness.

E. Factors that attract professional nurses to ambulatory care (Hackbarth, Haas, Kavanagh, and Vlasses, 1995).

    1. Hours and schedules without rotating shifts.

    2. Challenging nature of the work (variety, rapid pace).

    3. Working with clients and families over a long period of time.

F. Factors that keep nurses working in ambulatory care (Hackbarth et al., 1995).

    1. Working with clients and families over a long period of time.

    2. Nature of the work.

    3. Seeing outcomes of care.

    4. Autonomy in practice.

    5. Coworker relationships.

    6. Teaching and health promotion.

    7. Hours (declines in importance for many nurses after working for a period of time in ambulatory care).

G. Recruitment issues for ambulatory settings.

    1. With hospital downsizing, and fewer hospital nursing positions available, fewer recruits will come to ambulatory care with inpatient experience.

    2. Ambulatory care is expanding and will require more nurses. New recruitment strategies must be considered, such as providing ambulatory settings as student clinical sites and recruiting the best and brightest.

H. Recruitment strategies for ambulatory care nursing.

    1. Enhance understanding of all nurses of the ambulatory care nurse role.

    2. Participate in venues such as certification that provide overt recognition of ambulatory care nurse expertise.

    3. Increase ambulatory care nurse participation in professional nursing organizations.

I. Retention in ambulatory care nursing positions.

    1. Requires planning.

    2. Factors that increase likelihood of retention.

        a. A planned orientation to each ambulatory care nursing role.

        b. A planned preceptor, coaching, and mentoring program for new recruits.

        c. A planned continuing development program for employees.

        d. A recognition program for individual contributions and accomplishments.

        e. Collegial working relationships.

        f. A salary and benefits that are perceived as equitable with inpatient nursing.

      g. Flexible or self-scheduling.

      h. Less role ambiguity, role stress, or role overload.

      i. Trust in the organization.

   3. Cost effective because turnover:

      a. Involves recruitment, orientation, and development costs.

      b. Affects productivity.

      c. Affects quality of care.

   4. Is often closely correlated to long-term relationships with patients and families.

ORIENTATION TO AMBULATORY CARE NURSING POSITIONS

  A. Definitions.

   1. *Orientation* is a planned process for introducing a new employee to the work setting and assessing the ability of the individual to perform basic job requirements.

   2. *Coaching* is an approach to developing individuals within an organization that falls somewhere between precepting and mentoring. It is an ongoing, face-to-face relationship whereby the coach assists the new employee to develop behaviors that will enhance success in their new role (Haas, 1992).

   3. *Competency* is the documented ability of the individual to perform job role requirements. It includes both knowledge and application of skills.

  B. Orientation programs may be brief or nonexistent in ambulatory care because of:

   1. Lack of clarity about roles.

   2. Assumption that if one has worked with the patient population in the hospital, then one has the experience necessary to work in ambulatory care.

   3. Lack of resources.

      a. Human.

      b. Texts on ambulatory care nursing.

      c. Films/computer-assisted instruction.

      d. Assessment tools for ambulatory care.

  C. Purpose of orientation program.

   1. Clarify position expectations.

   2. Provide an understanding of reporting relationships and accountabilities.

   3. Assess competence in all three ambulatory care nursing roles—clinical nursing, organizational/systems, and professional nursing.

   4. Address identified performance deficits in each of the ambulatory care nurse roles.

   5. Develop understanding of resources available in the organization and community.

   6. Socialize to the organization's culture.

7. Determine if nurse is capable of safe, independent performance.

D. Components of an orientation program.
1. History, mission, philosophy, and values of the organization.
2. Organization charts, job description for role of orientee.
3. Employee handbook or policies.
4. Completion of all personnel functions—W2 forms, life, health insurance, etc.
5. Competency assessment for nursing practice.
6. Copy of union contract, if unionized.
7. Introductions to key staff and colleagues and at least a brief discussion of their roles.

E. Competency assessment.
1. Competency assessment required of all caregivers before they can deliver care. Competency assessment is most effective when it is organized into a framework based on the role of nursing in the facility and the patient population served (Hastings, 1995).
   a. Assessment of clinical nursing role competency.
   b. Assessment of organizational/systems role competency (ability to fulfill organizational/systems role in ambulatory care, including supervision of ancillary staff).
   c. Assessment of professional nursing role competency (ability to contribute to professional advancement and ongoing improvement in the quality and delivery of care).
2. Clinical nursing role competency.
   a. The ability to apply technical skills and clinical judgement in the care of designated patient populations.
   b. Competency statements describe the knowledge and skills necessary for clinical practice within the setting.
   c. Competency requirements defined by clinical setting, role of the nurse, and patient population served.
   d. Clinical competencies include core clinical competencies (cross all sites) and specialty competencies (specifically related to patient population).
3. Organizational/systems role-based competencies.
   a. Are specific to site of employment.
   b. Include knowledge and skills needed to effectively implement roles on multidisciplinary team.
   c. Include interpersonal, collegial, and system-management competencies.
   d. Include computer applications (if appropriate).
4. Professional nursing role competencies.
   a. Include knowledge and skills necessary to advance personally and professionally within role (i.e., self-development planning).
   b. Include knowledge and skills necessary to participate and contribute to the profession (i.e., quality improvement, evaluating research findings, precepting staff).

5. The competency assessment process.
    a. Must be documented.
    b. Must be setting-specific.
    c. Must include documentation of method used to assess competencies.
        (1) Demonstrated successful completion of (i.e., CPR on manikin).
        (2) Observed in practice (i.e., successful venipuncture on a patient).
        (3) Validated via scenario/case study (i.e., nurse describes decisions and actions for a clinical emergency).
        (4) Tested (i.e., nurse passes arrhythmia recognition test).
    d. Competency assessment should be integrated into the orientation process so that the nurse has the opportunity to demonstrate new and existing skills in an orderly fashion.
    e. Figure 10-1 is a sample competency assessment form.

PRODUCTIVITY MONITORING IN AMBULATORY CARE

A. Definitions.
    1. *Productivity* is a measure of the volume of output produced related to the amount of resources consumed/used to produce the specified output.
    2. *Productivity Ratio:* Productivity = output/input (Chamberlain, 1965).
    3. *Output* is the product or service expressed in terms of dollars that are statistically adjusted to eliminate the effects of inflation.
    4. *Input* is the dollar cost of person-hours needed to produce a product or service.
    5. *Productivity in nursing* is "the relationship between the amount of acceptable output produced and the input required to achieve that output." (Jelnick and Dennis, 1976, p. 9).
    6. *Nursing outcome classification* (NOC) involves a systematic use of standards and language that identifies patient outcomes, indicators, and measurements that are responsive to nursing interventions (Johnson and Maas, 1997).
    7. *Traditional nursing productivity ratio* is hours of care required multiplied by quality and divided by hours of care expended (Dennis, Dunn, and Benson, 1980).
    8. *Efficiency* is a measure of how well work is done with respect to the use of worker time, materials, capital, or other resources (Ruh, 1982). Often, efficiency is measured by budget variances for personnel and supplies.
    9. *Effectiveness* is a measure of how well the work meets or exceeds stated goals or standards.
    10. *Outcomes* are used synonymously with results achieved from planned or unplanned interventions.
    11. *Nursing-sensitive ambulatory outcomes* are changes in the actual or potential health status, behavior, or perceptions of individuals, families, or populations that can be attributed to nursing interventions provided in an ambulatory care setting in which client-nurse contacts may be single or intermittent contacts of 23 hours or less.

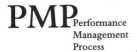 **PMP**Performance
Management
Process

 WASHINGTON
HOSPITAL
CENTER

Department/Specialty/Unit Competencies Form
Ambulatory Care

Employee name _____   Period covered _____

Employee number _____

The following values are to be used on this form:

PERFORMANCE LEVEL	METHOD OF EVALUATION

PERFORMANCE LEVEL

5 = Exceptional
4 = Exceeds standards
3 = Fully meets standards
2 = Needs improvement
1 = Unsatisfactory
NA = Not applicable

METHOD OF EVALUATION

V = Verbalizes knowledge   W = Written evaluation
D = Demonstrates skill   C = Course(s)/Class(es)
I = In-service(s)   SL = Self-learning packet
AV = Audiovisual presentation

[More than one method may be indicated]

No.	Competency to be assessed	[ ] N/A	Performance level	Method of evaluation
1.	**Assessment and triage:** Conducts a rapid, effective patient assessment to determine needs for the visit and follow-up on ongoing problems. Identifies and appropriately refers urgent/complex problems to the appropriate provider.			
2.	**IV therapy/venipuncture:** Accesses vein for the use of IV therapy or to obtain a blood sample. Maintains patency and administers IV fluid safely.			
3.	**Medication administration:** Safely administers all prescribed medications according to hospital protocol, including IV push administration.			
4.	**Nutrition:** Integrates principles of nutrition into patient assessment and the plan of care.			
5.	**Pain management:** Assesses patient's level of pain, and intervenes to reduce pain to an acceptable level of comfort.			
6.	**Wound and skin care:** Assesses current wounds and appropriately cares for wound within the clinic setting. Instructs patient of wound care and prevention at home.			
7.	**Telephone management:** Maintains skills and knowledge necessary to assess, triage, and manage patients by telephone.			
8.	**Patient education:** Incorporates principles of adult and adolescent learning into assessment of learning needs and barriers, as well as the design and delivery of patient education.			
9.	**Integrates competencies necessary to deliver optimal nursing care to patients:** • Routine prenatal care • Prenatal care with medical/obstetrical complications • Chronic disease management (diabetes, stroke, arthritis, CHF, HIV, etc.) • Outpatient surgical follow-up • ENT assessment and treatment			

_____   _____
Employee signature   Date   (Signature does not necessarily indicate agreement. An employee who wishes to do so may have written comments attached to the PMP form by submitting them in writing to the supervisor/reviewer within five (5) days of the reviewer.)

_____   _____   _____   _____
Supervisor/reviewer signature   Supervisor/reviewer name   Title   Date
                                 (Please print)

FIGURE 10-1 ■ Sample Competency Assessment Form (Copyright 1999 Washington Hospital Center, Washington, D.C.).

B. Issues with measuring productivity in nursing.
  1. Often no physical product is created in nursing. Once the service is performed, the evidence disappears (Ruh, 1982).
  2. Marked discretion in professional nursing work (planning, assessment, and evaluation) is difficult to measure.
  3. Continued difficulty with measuring quality in ambulatory care; often only measure easily quantifiable variables (i.e., immunizations).
C. Current measures of productivity in ambulatory care.
  1. Focus is on outcomes such as:
    a. Cost of care.
    b. Financial performance (cost per procedure).
    c. Satisfaction of patients and staff.
    d. Health status.
    e. Incidence of complications.
    f. Access and availability: time to next appointment.
    g. "Report card" measures: immunization rates, mammogram rates.
    h. Visit volume.
  2. Little work on measurement process productivity.
    a. Concern with increasing expectation that providers see more patients per hour is that outcomes may not be as good because the care process is shortened.
    b. Much ambiguity as to who should be involved in the care process.
D. Approaches to productivity improvement in ambulatory care.
  1. Role clarity for nursing personnel.
    a. Use personnel at levels consistent with their competence and education.
    b. Provide orientation and continuing education for staff.
    c. Involve nursing personnel in evolution of roles.
  2. Appropriate staffing ratios to achieve efficiency and effectiveness.
    a. Staffing ratios will differ related to patient population being served (i.e., oncology patients requiring high tech, teaching, and care coordination dimensions of nursing care will require more RNs and fewer UAPs in ambulatory care settings).
    b. Collaboration among nursing staff working with a given patient population.
  3. Use and evaluate effectiveness incentives to enhance productivity such as gain sharing, which is a program where employees receive a portion of revenues gained as monies saved through specified efforts of employees.
  4. Use automation to enhance effectiveness: the computerized patient record, databases.
  5. Use of standardized nursing languages: North America Nursing Diagnosis Association (NANDA), Nursing Intervention Classification (NIC), Nursing Outcome Classification (NOC), Omaha System, and Saba Home Healthcare Classification B (see Chapter 7) to capture data on nursing process and outcomes.
  6. Use performance appraisal and coaching to enhance effectiveness.

ISSUES AND CHALLENGES WITH STAFFING AND WORKLOAD

A. Assumption that methods used in inpatient settings will work as well in ambulatory care mandates that we:
1. Develop, implement, and evaluate a simple yet valued and reliable nursing intensity system for ambulatory care to track and trend the demand for numbers and types of ambulatory care nursing personnel.
2. Develop, implement, and evaluate process and outcome measures that demonstrate the impact of different nursing staff mixes.
3. Develop, implement, and evaluate ambulatory care productivity measures.
   a. Measures need to capture the unique contribution of nurses and other providers on the interdisciplinary team.
   b. Data should be easily entered, preferably as a part of routine documentation.
      (1) Embed the nursing minimum data set elements in encounter form data.
      (2) Embed NIC and NOC coding in nursing documentation (Johnson and Maas, 1997).
   c. Select measures of processes and outcomes over which providers (nurses) have control.
   d. Select measures that are easily understood by those being evaluated.
   e. Select measures that are compatible with corporate mission and measures.
B. The characteristics of ambulatory care nursing have changed as patients coming to ambulatory settings are sicker and there has been an increase in capitation that alters the incentives for providers and requires that we:
1. Develop, implement, and evaluate strategies to enhance work group effectiveness.
2. Develop, implement, and evaluate staffing ratios for specific patient populations.
3. Develop, implement, and evaluate orientation programs and competency assessment for ambulatory care nursing personnel.
4. Develop retention strategies that assist with retention of competent nursing personnel.

REFERENCES

Chamberlain N (1965): *The labor sector.* New York: McGraw-Hill.

Dennis L, Dunn M, Benson G (1980). *An empirical model for measuring nursing in acute care hospitals.* Chicago: Medicus Systems.

Haas S, Hackbarth D, Cullen P, Androwich I (2000): *Defining nursing intensity in ambulatory care.* Research at analysis phase.

Haas S (1992). Coaching: developing key players. *J Nurs Administration* 22(6):54-58.

Hackbarth D, Haas S, Kavanagh J, Vlasses F (1995): Dimensions of the staff nurse role in ambulatory care: Part I—Methodology and analysis of data on current staff nurse practice. *Nurs Econ* 13(2):89-98.

Hastings C (1997): The changing multidisciplinary team. *Nurs Econ* 15(2):106-108, 105.

Hastings C (1995): Orientation and competency assessment in ambulatory care, AAACN Workshop: Role transitions into ambulatory care nursing. Orange, CA, and Oakland, CA, November.

Hastings C, Haas S (1998): Update on the AAACN/MGMA staffing study, and Strategies for managing patient satisfaction, concurrent session. American Academy of Ambulatory Care Nursing Annual Conference, Atlanta, March.

Jelnick R, Dennis L (1976): *A review and evaluation of nursing productivity.* DHEW Publication No. (HRA). Bethesda, MD: U.S. Department of Health, Education, and Welfare.

Johnson M, Maas M (1997): *Nursing outcomes classification (NOC): Iowa outcomes project.* St. Louis: Mosby.

Ruh W (1982): The measurement of white collar productivity. *National Productivity Review.* Autumn, 16-26.

U.S. Department of Health and Human Services (1996): *The registered nurse population.* Rockville, MD: Health Services and Resource Administration, Bureau of Health Professionals, Division of Nursing.

Verran J (1981): Delineation of ambulatory care nursing practice. *J Ambulatory Care Management* 4(2):1-13.

THE CLINICAL NURSING ROLE IN AMBULATORY CARE

11

Primary Care/Family Health Care Nursing

CAROL JO WILSON, PhD, RN, CS, FNP
GAIL DELUCA, MS, RN, CS, FNP

PATIENT PROTOTYPES

Family Health Promotion and Disease Prevention ▪ Domestic Violence ▪ Substance Abuse ▪ Nutrition and Eating Disorders ▪ Teen Issues

OBJECTIVES

Study of the information presented in this chapter will enable the learner to:

1. Know the clinical guidelines for regular health screening.

2. Describe assessment techniques for domestic violence.

3. Identify resources for substance abuse.

4. Utilize nutritional status assessment tools to assess and provide resource referral for common nutritional disorders.

5. Appraise the most common teen issues, identifying screening methods and resource referrals.

▪▪ Health care in America is undergoing revolutionary changes at an increasingly accelerated pace. In the 19th century, health focused on illnesses caused by unsanitary conditions and epidemics. As our agrarian culture became industrialized, the populace looked to employers and then to the government to provide basic necessities such as health care. Following World War II, acute illness care moved from the home into the hospital. The 1960s saw the federal government addressing inequities in health care with the implementation of Medicare and Medicaid. Today we are still struggling with many of the same societal ills such as poverty, lack of education, and class differences that have historically plagued the world.

Health care in the 21st century will be focused on prevention and health promotion within communities and home care. Indeed, the comprehensive plan for U.S. health care, *Healthy People 2010,* is aimed at increasing life span and access to preventive services while decreasing disparities in health (USDHHS, 2000). This chapter will present family health promotion and address current issues facing families today including domestic violence, sexual abuse, eating disorders, substance abuse, and various teen issues.

Central to any health promotion is the client's internalization, recognition, and willingness to make the changes that will positively affect overall health. Prochaska and Velicer (1997) have proposed six stages of change through which a client progresses when faced with altering most lifestyle patterns. Assessing the stage of change in the client can assist the ambulatory care nurse in creating specific interventions focused to move the client further along the health continuum.

The stages of change include precontemplation, contemplation, preparation, action, maintenance, and termination. In the precontemplation stage, the client does not possess or express the desire to change. Targeted actions by the ambulatory care nurse for this stage could include education about the benefits that change will bring. In the next stage, contemplation, the client is weighing the benefits of change and intends to initiate the change within the upcoming 6 months. For continued progression, actual or perceived pain or loss associated with the change must be reduced. Toward the end of the contemplation stage, benefits must exceed the loss associated with the targeted change. Once the client makes the change, he is in the action stage. Here, assistive strategies include reduction in cues associated with the problematic behavior, reinforcement of the negatives associated with the old behavior, and review of successful tactics associated with the positive change. In the maintenance stage, the client has incorporated the change into his lifestyle but continues to apply all processes leading to his successful change, thus preventing relapse. Finally, in the termination stage the client experiences no temptation from the previous behavior and has fully incorporated the new behavior into his lifestyle. Few people achieve this stage; consequently it is realistic for clients to have a lifetime goal of maintenance (Prochaska and Velicer, 1997).

Lifestyle changes can have an enormous impact on disease prevention. When contemplating the numbers of health problems responsive to lifestyle modification, understanding the stages of change is crucial to health promotion and goal attainment described in *Healthy People 2010.*

FAMILY HEALTH PROMOTION AND DISEASE PREVENTION

Family health is "a dynamic changing relative state of well-being, which includes the biological, psychological, spiritual, sociological, and cultural factors of the family system" (Hanson and Boyd, 1996, p. 177). Development of family nursing as an entity has progressed over the centuries as a result of a variety of societal changes. The family has become the focus of theory development, research, and policy-making (ANA, 1991; DHHS, 1991). Many professional organizations have been developed to support and educate the family. Consumers are increasingly knowledgeable and interested in health promotion. The relationship between stress and illness, the importance of wellness care (rather than disease-focused care), and the need to treat the whole person are increasingly recognized as essential elements in society today.

The family may be viewed as context for the individual, client, system, or component of society. The family unit teaches health/illness beliefs, values, and behaviors. It is known that family functioning affects an individual's health, and an individual's lifestyle, practices, and health affect the family. Promotion of family health is important to society. Nurses in ambulatory settings can influence the family's quality of life with health promotion.

A. Assess/screen/triage. Of the dozens of family assessment tools, several focus on health and health promotion:

1. Family APGAR (Smilkstein, 1978).
2. Family assessment tool: Family health care plan (Stanhope and Lancaster, 1992).
3. Family genogram and eco-map (Hartman, 1978).
4. Family hardiness index (McCubbin and Thompson, 1987).
5. Family health promotion-protection plan (Pender, 1987).
6. Friedman family assessment model (Friedman, 1992).

B. Primary, secondary, tertiary prevention.

1. Primary prevention includes health promotion and specific measures to keep people free from disease and injury (see Care Management and Patient Education sections below).
2. Secondary prevention consists of early detection, diagnosis, and treatment.
3. Tertiary prevention includes recovery and rehabilitation and specific measures to minimize disability and increase functioning.

C. Referral to social services, community resources, support groups, churches, legal aid, and shelters.

D. Care management.

1. Conduct regular health screening.
   a. Screen blood pressure, height, weight, and tobacco and/or substance use at every visit.
   b. Clinical breast examination (yearly) and breast self-examination (monthly).
   c. Mammogram (yearly after age 50).
   d. Pap smear.
   e. Clinical testicular examination (yearly) and testicular self-examination (monthly).
   f. Immunizations
   g. Fecal occult blood test.
   h. Lipid panel.
   i. Physical examination (every 5 years).
2. Support pro-family legislation.
3. Provide continuity of care over time for families.

E. Patient education.

1. Life-lengthening habits.
   a. No tobacco use.
   b. No alcohol or only in moderation.
   c. 7 to 8 hours of sleep nightly.
   d. Regular, frequent, nutritionally dense small meals.
   e. Daily breakfast.

      f. Normal weight.

      g. Moderate, regular exercise.

   2. Self-responsibility and care.

   3. Awareness of effects of stress.

   4. Environmental awareness.

      a. Sanitation/personal cleanliness.

      b. Hazards in home/work.

F. Advocacy: Many organizations can help educate and support family health.

   1. American Alliance for Health, Physical Education, Recreation, and Dance, (703) 476-3400, *www.AAHPERD.org*

   2. National Council on Family Relations, (612) 781-9331, *www.NCFR.org*

   3. National Health Information Clearinghouse, (800) 336-4797, *www.NHIC-NT.HEALTH.org*

G. Telephone practice.

   1. Provide information on how to contact provider.

   2. Be available by phone, beeper, and/or e-mail.

   3. Guided self-care/nurse telephone triage and consultation.

H. Documentation.

   1. Include subjective and objective data as well as interventions and outcomes in documentation of care.

   2. Include prevention in SOAPP notes (extra P for prevention).

I. Outcome management.

   1. Reduction of preventable diseases.

   2. Improved quality of life.

   3. Increased communication and functioning within the family.

   4. Absence of dysfunctional coping behaviors.

J. Protocol: See *Clinician's Handbook of Preventive Services* (USPHS, 1998) for each professional organization's recommended schedule for health screening.

DOMESTIC VIOLENCE

Domestic violence is an issue of power and control involving physical, emotional, sexual, and/or economic abuse in an adult intimate relationship, perpetuated primarily by men (95%) against women. Components of domestic violence may involve physical battering, sexual assault or coercion, psychological intimidation, isolation, physical restraint, and financial exploitation. In the United States, approximately 25% of women have been abused by current or former partners and 50% of women who are killed are killed by partners (Dunphy, 1999). Domestic violence is the single major cause of injury to women; most seek health care for stress-related conditions rather than trauma in the primary care setting.

    There is no common factor such as age, socioeconomic status, ethnic or racial group, or religious affiliation that is associated with domestic violence. Certain contributing factors include past history of abuse, poor self-image and communication skills, need for power/control over another, jealousy, alcohol and/or drug abuse. Many relationships are characterized by a cycle of tension-building, abusive event, and honeymoon phase. Child abuse and neglect is any physical or mental nonaccidental injury to a child or any failure to provide a child with adequate food, clothing, shelter, supervision, and care (Uphold and Graham, 1998). Approximately 600,000 cases of physical abuse and 1.4 million cases of child neglect are reported each year (Uphold and Graham). Certain contributing factors include past history of abuse, low income, increased stress, and alcohol and drug abuse. In addition, the child being male, handicapped, fussy as an infant, or slow to develop increases the likelihood of abuse or neglect.

A. Assess/screen/triage.

1. Screen for abuse at every health visit. Explain that you ask all patients these questions because so many are abused and you need to know to offer assistance.

2. Ask the patient directly about abuse without the partner or parents present.

3. Ask the SAFE questions.

   a. Stress/safety: What stresses are in the relationship? Do you feel safe?

   b. Afraid: Do you feel afraid at times? Have you ever been threatened, abused, or forced into sexual intercourse?

   c. Friends/family: Are they aware of your situation? Can they help?

   d. Emergency plan: Do you have a safe place to go? Do you need help?

B. Primary, secondary, tertiary prevention.

1. Primary prevention: Educate about domestic violence and child abuse.

2. Secondary prevention.

   a. Screen for domestic violence.

   b. Screen for common accompanying psychological problems such as depression, anxiety, suicidal ideation, and drug abuse.

   c. Screen for withdrawal, role reversal, habit disorders, inappropriate dress, peer problems, poor hygiene, failure to thrive, sexual acting out (children), and financial and marital difficulties.

   d. Recognize the most common physical injuries of abuse are contusions, fractures, lacerations, abrasions, burns, and sprains and involve the head, eyes, neck, and torso (bathing suit pattern).

   e. Recognize that patients with chronic pain and/or headaches, sleep and appetite disturbances, fatigue, palpitations, dizziness, sexual problems, and frequent STIs/UTIs may have a root cause of abuse.

   f. Be alert to an inconsistent, inadequate, vague, or contradictory explanation of the injury.

   g. Suspect abuse if a long interval has occurred between the time of the injury and the victim seeking help.

   h. Look for the presence of injuries in various stages of healing.

3. Tertiary prevention.

   a. Follow up to build a trusting relationship.

   b. Educate as to the chronicity and repetitive nature of the cycle of abuse.

   c. Employ a multidisciplinary approach with a domestic violence counselor, psychologist, or social worker.

C. Clinical procedures.
   1. Assess for immediate danger.
   2. Assess for life-threatening injuries.
   3. Assess and treat injuries and current wounds.
   4. Measure height, weight, vital signs.
   5. Assess skin, eyes, head, neck, torso.
   6. Assess genitalia. (The majority of children who have been abused have no detectable genital injury).
D. Referral.
   1. Reporting is mandatory if abuse involves children (less than 18 years of age), the elderly, or disabled adults.
   2. Reporting is mandatory if the injuries are from a dangerous weapon, if there is high risk for serious injury, or if the adult victim's mental capacity is questionable.
   3. Referral to community resources such as local shelters, hotline numbers, legal and financial services, child protection services is essential.
E. Care management.
   1. Validate the woman's or child's experiences.
   2. Explore options.
   3. Advocate a safety plan.
      a. Detailed escape plan.
      b. Savings.
      c. Preparations to leave.
   4. Build on patient's strengths and avoid victim-blaming.
   5. Respect adult patient's right to self-determination.
   6. Provide support, reassurance, and confidentiality.
   7. Provide information about community resources.
F. Patient education.
   1. Educate about disease process, signs and symptoms, treatment, and prevention strategies.
   2. Reinforce that domestic violence/child abuse is a crime and the victim is not at fault.
G. Advocacy.
   1. National Domestic Violence Hotline, (800) 799-7233, (800) 333-SAFE, *www.NDVH.org*
   2. Pennsylvania Coalition Against Domestic Violence (National Resource Center on Domestic Violence), (800) 537-2238, *www.PCAVD.org*
   3. National Coalition Against Domestic Violence, (202) 745-1211, *www.NCADV.org*
   4. National Child Abuse Hotline, (800) 422-4453.
   5. Center for the Prevention of Sexual and Domestic Violence, (206) 634-1903, *www.CPSDV.org*
   6. National Center on Elder Abuse, (202) 898-2586.
H. Telephone practice.
   1. Arrange for follow-up by phone either directly or through a friend or relative.

2. If caller is being victimized, assess the danger and call 911.

I. Documentation.

   1. Record patient's description of how the injury occurred (stories that change over time suggest abuse).

   2. Record all findings in nonjudgmental, factual language, understanding the chart is a legal document.

J. Outcomes.

   1. Improved quality of life.

   2. Elimination of the attacks.

   3. Able to reach safe environment.

   4. Children are not perpetuating the cycle.

SUBSTANCE ABUSE

Substance abuse is a maladaptive pattern of substance use leading to clinically significant impairment or distress as manifested by one or more of the following occurring within a 12-month period: recurrent substance use resulting in a failure to fulfill major role obligations at work, school, or home; recurrent substance use in situations in which it is physically hazardous; recurrent substance-related legal problems; and/or continued substance use despite having persistent or recurrent social or interpersonal problems caused by or exacerbated by the effects of the substance (DSM-IV, 1994). The cause may be genetic, psychological, sociocultural, or learned behavior. About 10% to 16% of primary care patients have substance abuse problems (Dunphy, 1999).

A. Assess/screen/triage.

   1. CAGE questionnaire.

   a. Have you felt a need to Cut down on drinking or taking a substance?

   b. Have you felt Annoyed by yourself or others about drinking or taking substances?

   c. Have you felt Guilty about drinking or taking substances?

   d. Have you had to drink or take substances first thing in the morning (Eye opener)?

   2. MAST: Michigan Alcoholism Screening Test.

   3. AUDIT: Alcohol Use Disorders Identification Test.

   4. Ask about frequency, quantity, maximum used in one day, and last time the substance was used.

   5. Be alert to early signs of substance abuse.

   a. Gradual and unexplained deterioration in scholastics or unexplained school absences.

   b. Increased difficulties with parents or peers.

   c. Increased frequency of accidents.

   d. Personality changes such as irritability and depression.

   e. Weight loss or gain.

   f. Difficulty concentrating.

B. Primary, secondary, tertiary prevention.

   1. Primary prevention.

      a. Ask about alcohol, tobacco, and recreational drug use at every visit.

      b. Educate about drugs, alcohol, and tobacco in schools, clinics, and mass media.

  2. Secondary prevention.

      a. Contract with patient for timeline to quit. Utilize stages of change for best results.

      b. Teach about techniques and medications to stop abuse.

      c. Reinforce changing behavior.

  3. Tertiary prevention.

      a. Attend support groups.

      b. Participate in individual and/or family counseling with a psychiatrist or addiction specialist.

      c. Participate in in-house drug treatment program.

C. Clinical procedures.

  1. Alcohol.

      a. Laboratory values.

         (1) High macrocytic anemia (MCV).

         (2) High gamma glutamyl transferase.

         (3) High serum amylase.

      b. Pharmaceutical treatment.

         (1) Naltrexone (Revia) diminishes craving for alcohol.

         (2) Disulfiram (Antabuse) yields severe adverse effects when combined with alcohol.

  2. Tobacco.

      a. Cessation techniques.

         (1) Set a date to quit.

         (2) Inform family and friends.

         (3) Set goals.

         (4) Have a support person available.

      b. Pharmaceutical treatment.

         (1) Nicotine patch.

         (2) Nicorette gum.

         (3) Bupropion (i.e., Wellbutrin, Zyban, or Wellbutrin SR).

         (4) Nicotrol NS (nasal spray).

         (5) Nicotrol inhaler.

  3. Illicit substances: Dependent on type of substance abused.

D. Referral.

  1. Alcoholics Anonymous, (212) 870-3400, *www.alcoholicsanonymous.org*

  2. Al-Anon World Service Office, (800) 356-9996, *www.alanon.alateen.org*

  3. Rational Recovery, (530) 621-2667, *www.rational.org/recovery*

  4. Narcotics Anonymous, (818) 773-9999, *www.na.org*

  5. National Cancer Institute, Cancer Information Service, (800) 4-CANCER

  6. American Academy of Family Physicians, AAFP Stop Smoking Kit, (800) 274-2237, *www.AAFP.org*

  7. American Cancer Society, (800) 227-2345, (800) ACS-2345, *www.cancer.org*

  8. American Lung Association, (800) 586-4872, *www.lungusa.org*

E. Care management.
   1. Maintain acceptance of the patient.
   2. Provide ongoing support.
F. Patient education.
   1. Inform that change may take several attempts.
   2. Teach about negative consequences of continuing addictive behavior.
   3. Stress positive results associated with quitting addictive behavior.
G. Advocacy.
   1. National Clearinghouse for Alcohol and Drug Information, (800) 729-6686.
   2. Support clean air legislation.
   3. Decrease accessibility of addictive substances to children and teens.
   4. Lobby for less media visibility for tobacco and alcohol in billboards, magazines, and sporting events.
H. Telephone practice. Have a support person or group available by beeper for support.
I. Documentation. Record subjective and objective information along with the nursing assessment and treatment plan.
J. Outcome.
   1. Substance-free or reduced substance lifestyle.
   2. Increased quality of life and relationships.
   3. Positive relationships with others.
   4. Personal satisfaction with choices.

NUTRITION AND EATING DISORDERS

Of the ten leading causes of death, five are related to poor diet. Adequate nutrition is crucial to the maintenance of health and prevention of major chronic diseases. This is achieved by intake of the five basic food groups as well as regular exercise.

Optimal health benefits occur from regular exercise completed in either 30 minutes of continuous activity or an accumulation of 30 minutes daily in divided activity at least four days per week. Both aerobic weight bearing exercises as well as strengthening resistance exercises contribute to cardiovascular health, maintenance of ideal body weight, and prevention of bone demineralization with resultant osteoporosis. Endurance for aerobic types of activities can be increased gradually over time and provide excellent benefit (Uphold and Graham, 1998).

The food guide pyramid (Figure 11-1) provides a visual key to the proper dietary balance of the five food groups. Key to good nutrition is balance of a variety of dietary intake with caloric expenditure to maintain a healthy body weight. Good nutrition is achieved by consuming at least the minimum number of recommended servings from each food group each day. The base of the pyramid contains foods with the greatest number of servings per day while the tiny tip of the pyramid depicts the small portions reserved for fats and sweets.

Proper adaptation of the pyramid into eating habits necessitates understanding of portion or serving size. In order for patients to familiarize themselves with proper portion size, food measurement may be utilized until visual inspection of portion

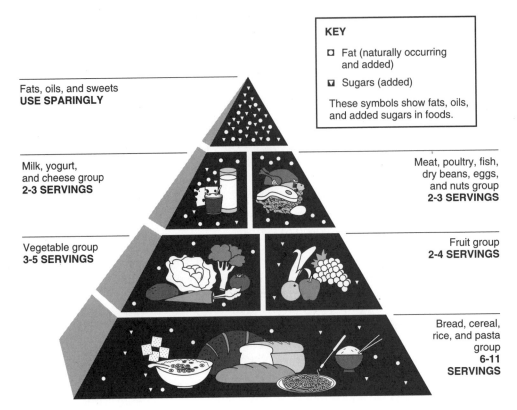

FIGURE 11-1 ■ Food Guide Pyramid (Source: U.S. Department of Agriculture.)

size can be estimated. The bread and pasta group is the largest group and requires 6 to 11 servings per day. One serving from this group includes one slice of bread, one ounce of cereal, or one half cup of rice, pasta, or cooked cereal. Thus a dinner serving of pasta may account for three or four servings. A serving of fruit (recommended two to four servings per day) is equivalent to one medium piece of whole fruit, one half cup of chopped, cooked, or canned fruit, or 3/4 cup of fruit juice. The deep colored vegetables are nutrient-dense and contain fiber and micronutrients essential to health, therefore, vegetable consumption should be highly encouraged (Cummings, 2000). One cup of raw, 1/2 cup of cooked, or 3/4 cup of vegetable juice corresponds to one serving (recommended three to five servings per day). The meat and poultry group (recommended two to three servings per day) provides protein and amino acids necessary for muscle growth. Two or three ounces of meat, chicken, or fish constitute one serving. Also included in this food group are beans, eggs, and nuts. One egg, 1/2 cup of cooked beans or two tablespoons of peanut butter constitute one serving. The dairy group provides the greatest source of calcium essential to skeletal integrity and has major significance in adolescents, pregnant, and postmenopausal women (Cummings, 2000). One cup of milk or yogurt or 1 1/2 ounces of cheese establish one serving (recommended two to three servings per day). The caloric and fat content can be reduced by low fat dairy choices. The tip of the pyramid is reserved for fats, oils, and sweets. No serving size is supplied for this group but caution is recommended to use this group sparingly.

Although proper diet and exercise is well accepted as methods to achieve health and diminish risk for certain diseases, disturbances in eating patterns exist. The following section will address common eating disorders and obesity.

Anorexia Nervosa and Bulimia Nervosa

Anorexia nervosa (AN) and bulimia nervosa (BN) are two common types of eating disorders predominantly found among middle and upper class adolescent young women in developed countries. Prevalence in this population is about 1% for AN and 3% for BN (Uphold and Graham, 1998). Both disturbances are characterized by an exaggerated, intense fear of becoming obese. AN is identified by self-induced food restriction, stemming from an extreme fear of weight gain resulting in a body weight of less than 85% of the minimal normal weight for age and height (American Psychiatric Association, 1994). Half of bulimics are of normal weight (Bomar, 1996), and thus may be more difficult to identify. In BN, a faulty compensatory action is used to prevent weight gain resulting in binge/purge cycling occurring at least twice weekly for 3 months (Dunphy, 1999; Uphold and Graham). Although not completely understood, these eating disorders are thought to be multifactorial and may include physiologic components, depression, family dynamics, and/or sociocultural pressures including unrealistic concepts of beauty and body size.

    A. Assess/screen/triage.
        1. Demographic/psychological profile.
            a. Adolescent or young adult female.
            b. Upper or middle socioeconomic class.
            c. Exaggerated fear of becoming fat.
            d. Perfectionistic, intelligent, overachieving, self-critical (AN).
            e. Competitive, emotionally reactive, coexisting mood disorders, impulsivity (BN).
        2. Symptom assessment.
            a. Preoccupation with weight loss/excessive exercise habits.
            b. Underweight (AN) or normal to slightly overweight (BN) for height.
            c. Denial of the seriousness of current body weight (AN).
            d. Self-evaluation based on body size/shape.
            e. Secondary amenorrhea (at least 3 missed cycles) (AN).
        3. Risk factor assessment.
            a. Obtain history.
                (1) Weight gain/loss or weight cycling.
                (2) Perception of body size.
                (3) Eating patterns (unusual patterns, food choices, eating in isolation).
                (4) Self-destructive behaviors.
                (5) Exercise patterns.
                (6) Past or current psychiatric history.
            b. Evaluate for suicidal intent.

B. Primary, secondary, tertiary prevention.
   1. Primary prevention.
      a. Communication skills and demonstrated caring within the family.
      b. Emphasis on psychosocial development rather than appearance (Dunphy, 1999).
   2. Secondary prevention.
      a. Restoration or maintenance of ideal body weight.
      b. Balanced diet with adequate caloric consumption.
      c. Symptom recognition.
      d. Involvement of a multidisciplinary team approach.
   3. Tertiary prevention.
      a. Multidisciplinary team management including the primary health provider, mental health professional, and other religious or community resources as necessary.
      b. Outpatient or inpatient management depending on the severity of the disorder.
      c. Resource referral.
C. Collaboration/resource identification and referral.
   1. Anorexia Nervosa and Related Eating Disorders Association, PO Box 5102, Eugene, OR 97405, (541) 344-1144, *www.anred.com*
   2. National Association of Anorexia Nervosa and Associated Disorders, PO Box 7, Highland Park, IL 60035, (847) 831-3438, *www.anad.org*
   3. The National Eating Disorders Organization, 6655 South Yale Avenue, Tulsa, OK 74136; (918) 481-4044; *http://www.laureate.com*
   4. The American Anorexia/Bulimia Association, 293 Central Park West, Suite 1R, New York, NY 10024; (212) 501-8351; *http://members.aol.com/amanbu*
D. Care management.
   1. Coordination of the multidisciplinary team.
   2. Reinforcement of the multidisciplinary team's recommendations.
   3. Goal attainment of normalized weight and/or body image.
   4. Demonstration of calm, supportive, caring attitude.
E. Patient education.
   1. Communication skills and demonstrated caring within the family (Dunphy, 1999).
   2. Emphasis on psychosocial development rather than appearance (Dunphy).
   3. Maintain regular meal plans.
   4. Ideal body weight.
   5. Chronicity of the disorder.
F. Telephone practice.
   1. Evaluate exacerbation or resolution of behaviors.
   2. Assess deviation or compliance with the therapeutic plan.
   3. Evaluate suicidal intent.
   4. Provide emotional support, educational assistance as needed.
G. Communication/documentation: Document subjective and objective data along with the nursing assessment and treatment plan.

H. Outcome management.
    1. Adequate caloric consumption resulting in achievement of ideal body weight.
    2. Realistic body image.

Obesity

Obesity affects approximately one third of the American population and is a growing epidemic. Simply, obesity is body fat in excess of that needed for metabolic function. Although it affects both genders, all age groups (though incidence increases with age), and every socioeconomic status, it has a disproportionate prevalence among certain ethnic groups. Obesity is a chronic disorder with multifactorial etiologies and is a risk factor for other disorders including degenerative joint disease, hypercholesterolemia, type 2 diabetes, hypertension, and heart disease. Although obesity can certainly be related to medications and/or endocrine disturbances, in most instances risk factors for the development of obesity include genetic predisposition, sedentary lifestyle, and diets high in calories and fats. Cyclical weight gain and weight loss (yo-yo syndrome) may be seen in obesity.

Measurements defining obesity include a body weight 120% of ideal (Dunphy, 1999), or a body mass index (BMI) equal to or greater than 27 (Uphold and Graham, 1998). Persons with greater than 100% excess body weight are considered morbidly obese. It should be noted that weight should be measured on a balance or electrical scale with minimal clothing. Other measurements estimate adipose deposition patterns. Most commonly used for this purpose is the waist–hip ratio (WHR). The importance of increased WHR values (greater than 1.0 for men or 0.8 for women) is to predict future risk of diabetes, hypertension, heart disease, and stroke.

  A. Assess/screen/triage.
    1. Height, weight. Review the record for weight history over the past 6 months and past year, noting any patterns or trends.
    2. BMI:

$$\frac{\text{weight (kilograms)}}{\text{height (meters)}^2}$$

    3. WHR:

$$\frac{\text{abdominal girth (centimeters)}}{\text{hip circumference (centimeters)}}$$

    4. Pinch test (Dunphy, 1999).
      a. Measured midtriceps, subscapular, buttocks, thigh, lower chest wall.
      b. Excessive fat accumulation is a pinch volume greater than 1 inch.
    5. Relative weights (Dunphy, 1999).
      a. Men: 106 pounds plus 6 pounds for each inch of height over 5 feet.
      b. Women: 100 pounds plus 5 pounds for each inch of height over 5 feet.
    6. Bioelectric impedance analysis.
      a. Estimates percent of body fat.
      b. May have up to 10% error.
  B. Primary, secondary, tertiary prevention.

1. Primary prevention.
   a. Identification of at-risk individuals.
   b. Benefits and obesity prevention for nonobese family members and children.
   c. Patient education.
      (1) Maintenance of ideal body weight (IBW).
      (2) Accurate interpretation of food label content.
      (3) Balanced dietary intake following the food guide pyramid (see Figure 11-1).
      (4) Avoidance of obesity-related disease.
      (5) Lifelong chronicity of the disease.
      (6) Regular exercise to increase caloric demand, lessen bone demineralization, and prevent lean tissue loss.
2. Secondary prevention.
   a. Early detection and diagnosis.
      (1) Height and weight trends.
      (2) WHR.
      (3) BMI.
      (4) Electrical impedance.
   b. Identification of maladaptive behaviors contributing to obesity.
      (1) Food as a coping mechanism.
      (2) Food as a reward.
   c. Identification of environmental cues to eat.
   d. Encouragement of lifestyle changes (see Nutrition and Eating Disorders).
   e. Follow general dietary guidelines.
      (1) Increase nutrient-dense, low calorie, high fiber foods.
      (2) Increase water consumption to eight glasses per day.
      (3) Increase sources of complex carbohydrates (without added sugar or fat).
      (4) Slowly increase fiber between 25 to 40 grams per day.
      (5) Limit sources of concentrated sugars.
      (6) Limit fat intake to less than 30% of the total calories.
      (7) Limit after-dinner snacking.
      (8) Limit alcohol intake.
3. Tertiary prevention.
   a. Balanced diet incorporating the recommended daily dietary allowances.
   b. Daily caloric deficit achieving a one- to two-pound weight loss per week.
      (1) Caloric deficit calculation: (IBW in kilograms × 30) − (500 to 1000 calories)
      (2) Initial exercise goal of 20 minutes four times weekly.
      (3) Maintenance exercise goal of 30 minutes, four times per week.
   c. Behavior modification techniques.
      (1) Goal setting and goal visualization.

(2) Food journal identifying foods eaten and emotions associated with each meal or snack.
  d. Support groups.
   (1) Weight Watchers.
   (2) Take Off Pounds Sensibly (TOPS).
   (3) Overeaters Anonymous.
  e. Pharmacologic interventions. These interventions may augment weight loss, but behavioral change is paramount for permanent results.
   (1) Antidepressants.
   (2) Appetite suppressants.
   (3) Antiobesity drugs.
  f. Surgical interventions.
C. Clinical procedures.
 1. Pharmacologic therapies.
 2. Surgical interventions such as gastric bypass, partial gastrectomy, or gastroplasty (Dunphy, 1999).
 3. Psychotherapeutic interventions.
D. Resource identification and referral (Uphold and Graham, 1998).
 1. TOPS, (800) 932-8677, *tops.org*
 2. Overeaters Anonymous, (708) 346-0000, *www.region5oa.org/chicago*
 3. Weight Watchers, (800) 651-6000, *www.weightwatchers.com*
 4. University of Alabama at Birmingham Eat Right Nutrition Information Service Hotline, (800) 231-DIET.
 5. Weight Control: Losing Weight and Keeping it Off, American Academy of Family Physicians, 8880 Ward Parkway, Kansas City, MO 64114-2797; (800) 944-0000; *http://www.aafp.org*
 6. National Organization of Mall Walkers, PO Box 191, Hermann, MO 65041, (573) 486-3945.
 7. Walking Test, The Rockport Walking Institute, 220 Donald Lynch Boulevard, PO Box 480, Marlboro, MA 01752, (508) 485-2090, *www.rockport.com*
E. Care management.
 1. Calm, supportive milieu of acceptance.
 2. Coordination of the professional team.
 3. Reinforcement that multiple failures precede success.
F. Patient education. See section B.1.c on page 162.
G. Communication/documentation: Document subjective and objective data along with the nursing assessment and treatment plan.
H. Outcome management.
 1. Achievement of IBW.
 2. BMI between 18.5 and 24.9.
 3. Enhanced sense of well-being.
 4. Improved quality of life through incorporation of permanent behavioral changes into lifestyle.
 5. Improvement in obesity-related disorders.

TEEN ISSUES

Teenage years, ages 13 through 21, a transitional stage of development between childhood and adult, conjures up an array of emotions, ideas, and new insights as the adolescent transcends a new area of growth. Profound changes occur in physiologic as well as psychologic development. The primary task of adolescent development is to evolve personal identity through integration of childhood experiences as well as new task mastery. These tasks include development of a personal identity with development of analytical thinking skills, a sexual identity, personal values, and greater independence, with intensified peer relationships (Jarvis, 2000).

In the United States, a cultural norm exists valuing both the family and protection of the adolescent from premature acquisition of adult responsibilities; however, this norm does not exist across cultures, especially those that are non-European (Kotch, 1997). Variances in cultural expectations of teen development are noted by different theorists. Hall, one theorist describing the second decade, identifies turbulence and conflict associated with teenage years, whereas other theorists such as Benedict and Mead view these years as potentially serene if teens were acculturated into the adult role by society (Jarvis, 2000). Thus, ambivalence felt by society toward this age group may create a tendency toward trivialization of the developmental and health issues specific to teens (Kotch). Wide disparities in economic status and family composition (single or two parent homes), among adolescents exist in differing ethnic groups within the United States itself, posing special needs. Poverty increases the risk of poor adolescent transitions, school problems, incarceration, unwanted pregnancies, and difficulty gaining employment (Kotch).

In addition to the declining influence of the family and increasing sovereignty of the peer group, the media, especially music and television, has major negative influences in adolescent development. Prolonged television viewing has been associated with poor academic performance, increased obesity, aggressive behavior, and socialization of the teen into the market economy (Kotch, 1997). Involvement with television encourages social isolation in teens with resultant poorer socialization and coping skills and places them at risk for depression.

Physically, female development may begin as early as 8 years old, with menarche occurring on an average at 12.5 years. In males, testicular enlargement occurs between 10.5 and 13.5 years. The wide continuum of development affects the adolescent's self-concept as there is keen awareness of secondary sex characteristic emergence among peers. Although the physical health of adolescents is generally excellent, health risks are prevalent and mainly result from judgment errors. Immature judgment and impulsivity places the teen at increased risk for accidents, substance abuse (drugs, alcohol, and tobacco), unplanned pregnancies, or sexually transmitted infections (Jarvis, 2000). The leading causes of death in this age group are injuries from motor vehicle accidents or unintentional injuries, homicide, and suicide (Jarvis).

Understanding the physical and psychological changes occurring throughout the second decade in life creates an ideal situation for the ambulatory care nurse to provide guidance to adolescents, potentially influencing future health outcomes. By understanding their need for availability, flexibility, confidentiality, and honesty, the ambulatory care nurse through his/her sensitivity to the specific needs of this age group can engage the adolescent in health promoting behaviors.

A. Assess/screen/triage.
   1. Assess risks associated with socioeconomic position.
   2. Assess the integrity and influence of the family structure.
   3. Assess the number and relationships of friends and peer group.
   4. Integrate parent or teacher reports to create a global view of the teen.
   5. Screen for abuse and/or neglect.
   6. Observe for changes in behavior or dress.
   7. Utilize the acronym: HEADSS to establish a baseline assessment.
      a. Home.
         (1) Family constellation.
         (2) Position among siblings.
         (3) Relationship with and among family members.
      b. Education.
         (1) Grade level.
         (2) Respect for rules.
         (3) Grades or academic achievement.
         (4) Problems associated with the school.
      c. Activities.
         (1) Fun and leisure.
         (2) Friends, best friend.
         (3) Organized sports or activities.
         (4) Weekend activities.
         (5) Amount of television/Internet use.
      d. Drugs.
         (1) Ask with the caregiver absent.
         (2) Use direct, open-ended questions.
      e. Sex: Same method as for drugs.
      f. Suicide.
         (1) Assess by directly asking if the teen has ever had thoughts of killing him/herself.
         (2) Assess feelings of hopelessness and "nobody understanding" (Fenstermacher and Hudson, 1997).
         (3) Assess for anxiety, learning disorders, and low self-esteem (Fenstermacher and Hudson).

B. Primary, secondary, tertiary prevention.
   1. Primary prevention (Jarvis, 2000).
      a. Education.
         (1) Sexual behavior: safe sex, condom usage, abstinence, high-risk behaviors, contraception.
         (2) Substance abuse: tobacco use, underage drinking, illicit drug use.
         (3) Safety: seatbelts, safety sporting gear, bicycle/motorcycle helmets, storage/removal of firearms, reduction of impulsivity.

   (4) Informed choice on health care decisions.

   (5) Parent skills training.

  b. Health screening.

   (1) Height, weight, blood pressure.

   (2) Papanicolaou, chlamydia, gonorrhea if sexually active.

   (3) HIV if high-risk sexual behavior or history of street drug use.

   (4) Diet intake: decrease fast and fatty foods, increase calcium intake.

  c. Immunizations: Tetanus-diptheria booster, hepatitis B, MMR, varicella, rubella.

  d. Depression/suicide screen.

  e. Access to confidential contraception.

  f. After-school care or activities.

 2. Secondary prevention.

  a. Early detection and treatment.

  b. Referral for medical, educational, and social services for teen mothers.

  c. Counseling intervention.

  d. Provision of crisis center or hotline information.

  e. Community resources.

 3. Tertiary prevention.

  a. Multidisciplinary team intervention.

  b. Medical treatment and follow-up as indicated.

   (1) Possible hospitalization (Fenstermacher and Hudson, 1997).

   (2) Antidepressant medication.

C. Collaboration/resource identification and referral.

 1. Utilization of school nurse, school counselors.

 2. Identification of positive significant adult relationship (other than parent).

 3. Identification of religious support through teen's local church or minister.

 4. Youth programs: Big Brother/Big Sister programs, YMCA/YWCA programs, church sponsored programs.

D. Care management.

 1. Interview the adolescent without the parent present.

 2. Foster development of the nurse-patient relationship through honesty, consistency, trust, confidentiality, and enhancement of self-esteem.

E. Patient education: Refer to section B. 1. a on page 165.

F. Advocacy.

 1. Include the adolescent in all aspects of decision-making.

 2. Support legislation to establish curfew laws.

 3. Support the establishment of after-school activity programs.

 4. Support neighborhood watch programs.

 5. Support efforts to reduce television violence.

 6. Become involved in adolescent's life and surrounding community.

G. Telephone practice.

 1. Assurance of confidentiality.

    2. Provision of schedule of availability.

    3. Respectful demeanor.

H. Communication/documentation: Document subjective and objective data along with the nursing assessment and treatment plan.

I. Outcome management.

    1. Comfort with self-identity.

    2. Attain desired level of education.

    3. Reduction in teen suicide, pregnancy, injury, and sexually transmitted infection.

    4. Creation and maintenance of positive interpersonal relationships.

    5. Realistic self-view, including strengths and weaknesses.

REFERENCES

American Nurses' Association (ANA) (1991): *Nursing's agenda for health care reform.* Washington, DC: Author.

American Psychiatric Association (APA) (1994): *Diagnostic criteria from DSM-IV.* Washington, DC: Author.

Bomar PJ (1996): *Nurses and family health promotion: concepts, assessment and interventions,* ed 2. Philadelphia: WB Saunders.

Cummings S (January 31, 2000): *Taking charge of your own health: a nutrition perspective.* Website: *http://www.mgh.harvard.edu/depts/DIETETIC/article.htm*

Department of Health and Human Services (DHHS) (1991): *Healthy people 2000.* Washington, DC: Author.

Dunphy LMH (1999): *Management guidelines for adult nurse practitioners.* Philadelphia: FA Davis.

Fenstermacher K, Hudson BT (1997): *Practice guidelines for family nurse practitioners.* Philadelphia: WB Saunders.

Friedman MM (1992): *Family nursing: theory and practice,* ed 3. Norwalk, CT: Appleton & Lange.

Hanson SMH, Boyd ST (1996): *Family health care nursing: theory, practice & research.* Philadelphia: FA Davis.

Hartman A (1978): Diagrammatic assessment of family relationships. *Social Casework* 59:456-476.

Jarvis C (2000): *Physical examination and health assessment,* ed 3. Philadelphia: WB Saunders.

Kotch JB (1997): *Maternal and child health: programs, problems and policy in public health.* Gaithersburg, MD: Aspen.

McCubbin HI, Thompson AI (1987): *Family assessment inventories for research and practice.* Madison, WI: University of Wisconsin.

Pender NJ (1987): *Health promotion in nursing practice,* ed 2. Norwalk, CT: Appleton & Lange.

Prochaska JO, Velicer WF (1997): The transtheoretical model of health behavior change. *Am J Health Promotion* 12(1):38-48.

Smilkstein G (1978): The family APGAR: A proposal for a family function test and its use by physicians. *J Family Practice* 6:1231-1239.

Stanhope M, Lancaster J (1992): *Community health nursing: process and practice for promoting health.* St Louis: Mosby.

Uphold CR, Graham MV (1998): *Clinical guidelines in family practice,* ed 3. Gainesville, FL: Barmarrae Books.

U.S. Department of Agriculture (USDA) (January 31, 2000): *The food guide pyramid: a guide to daily food choices.* Available: *http://www.nal.usda.gov:8001/py/pmap.htm*

U.S. Department of Health and Human Services (USDHHS), United States Public Health Service (2000). *Healthy People 2010: National health promotion and disease prevention objectives* (conference edition, in two volumes). Washington, DC: U.S. Government Printing Office. Available: *www.health.gov/healthypeople*

U.S. Public Health Services (USPHS) (1998): *Clinician's handbook of preventive services,* ed 2. McLean, VA: International Medical Publishers.

12 Pediatrics

Compiled by LINDA SCHNEIDER, BSN, RN

PATIENT PROTOTYPES

Well Child ■ Child with Asthma ■ Child with Sickle Cell Disease ■ Child with Attention Deficit Hyperactivity Disorder

OBJECTIVES

Study of the information presented in this chapter will enable the learner to:

1. Discuss health promotion strategies, anticipatory guidance, and screening procedures associated with promoting wellness and enhancing developmental growth throughout childhood.

2. Describe the role of the nurse in the primary, secondary, and tertiary prevention of asthma in children.

3. Discuss the use of long-term control and quick relief therapy in the treatment of asthma.

4. Discuss the nurse's role in assessing, intervening, and evaluating nursing care for the many complications associated with sickle cell disease in children.

5. Discuss the nurse's role in the diagnosis and treatment of children with attention deficit hyperactivity disorder.

■■ The trend in pediatric medicine is to move children out of the hospital and into outpatient settings. We are therefore seeing an enormous growth in child health care outside the hospital. The medical community is continuously exploring avenues to treat a myriad of diagnoses in a variety of outpatient settings. These settings include private offices, satellite clinics, clinics attached to hospitals, and outpatient treatment areas within the hospital.

Although the acutely ill child is still seen in the hospital, a wide range of diagnoses is treated in the outpatient setting. However, no matter what the diagnosis, the common thread is providing developmentally appropriate care in a family-centered environment.

Four areas have been chosen that span a broad range of issues. Experts in the respective fields have explored each area.

WELL CHILD

Marianne Buzby, MSN, RN, CRNP

The majority of children are born healthy. Routine health maintenance visits promote wellness and enhance developmental growth throughout childhood. These visits incorporate health promotion strategies, anticipatory guidance, and screening procedures.

A. Assess/screen/triage.
   1. Parent interaction with infant.
   2. History.
     a. Parental concerns.
     b. Health status since last visit.
     c. Nutrition, elimination, and sleep patterns.
     d. Behavioral characteristics.
     e. Allergies.
     f. Medical history including prenatal history.
     g. Family history.
   3. Growth parameters: measure and plot on age and gender appropriate growth curve; document percentile. Growth is a key indicator of overall nutritional status and some hormone function. Over time, children grow at a velocity that follows a curve like those on established growth curves. Special growth curves are available for premature infants and infants with specific genetic disorders (Barness, 1993).
     a. Length.
       (1) Newborn-infant: recumbent position on flat surface. Increases 50% by 1 year old (Johnson and Blasco, 1997).
       (2) Toddler: transition to standing height after second birthday and plot on 2 to 18-year-old growth curve. Length doubles by 4 years old (Johnson and Blasco, 1997). Average linear growth 2.5 inches per year (Colson and Dworkin, 1997).
     b. Weight.
       (1) Newborns lose up to 10% of birth weight initially, but should regain that weight within first 2 weeks of life. Average weight gain is 20 to 30 grams/day in the first 6 weeks of life. Weight doubles by 5 months, triples by 12 months, quadruples by 2 years old (Johnson and Blasco, 1997).
       (2) Toddlers gain about 5 pounds per year (Colson and Dworkin, 1997).
     c. Head circumference.
       (1) Newborn-infant: measure broadest part of the head, across forehead, and occipital protuberance. Average growth is 1 cm/month for first year (Johnson and Blasco, 1997).
       (2) Toddler: last measurement is at 2-year-old visit, unless an abnormality has been identified. Average growth is 2 cm during second year of life (Johnson and Blasco, 1997). Between 2 and 12 years of age increase is about 2.5 cm (Colson and Dworkin, 1997).

■ TABLE 12-1
■ ■ **Average Heart Rate and Respiratory Rate of Infants and Children**

	Heart Rate/Min. (Average)	Respiratory Rate/Min. (Average)
Newborn	90-190 (140)	30-60 (35)
Infant (1 month to 1 year old)	80-160 (160)	20-40 (30)
Toddler (1 to 3 years old)	70-150 (110)	20-40 (25)
Preschooler (4 to 5 years old)	80-120 (100)	20-40 (22)
Early school-age (6 years old)	65-125 (98)	20-25 (20)
Middle school-age (10 years old)	65-110 (90)	15-25 (18)

Adapted from Bickley LS, Hoekelman RA (1999): *Bate's guide to physical examination and history taking*, ed 7. Philadelphia: Lippincott Williams & Wilkins; Fox JA, editor (1997): *Primary health care of children.* St. Louis: Mosby.

    d. Vital signs: heart rate, respiratory rate, blood pressure vary with age. Influenced by temperature, anxiety, pain, illness.
      (1) See Table 12-1 for average heart rates and respiratory rates.
      (2) Temperature of 38° C (100.4° F) or higher in an infant 0 to 36 months old is considered a fever (Burns, Barber, Brady, and Dunn, 1996). Rectal thermometer is most accurate method; tympanic membrane thermometers have variable reliability.
      (3) Blood pressure varies with age and sex of the child.
        (a) Four extremity blood pressures should be obtained at least once during infancy.
        (b) Begin to routinely measure blood pressures at age 3 years.
        (c) Plot results on standard pressure curve for boys and girls.
        (d) Select appropriate cuff size; if cuff is too small blood pressure readings are falsely elevated and too large a cuff results in falsely low blood pressure readings (National High Blood Pressure Education Working Group, 1996).
  4. Developmental assessment: Areas of development include physical, psychosocial, cognitive, language, fine motor, and gross motor development. Using an approach to children and their parents that is grounded in the developmental level of the child allows the nurse to maximize the anticipatory guidance opportunities with parents and minimize the child's anxiety during the visit.
    a. Newborn-infant (Burns, et al., 1996; Johnson and Blasco, 1997).
      (1) Psychosocial stage of trust vs. mistrust.
      (2) Sensorimotor stage of cognitive development: progresses from innate infant reflexes to object permanence and goal-directed behaviors.
      (3) Language: understands simple commands, responds with gestures to "bye-bye," babbles, has one word with meaning, imitates animal sounds.
      (4) Primitive reflexes disappear and actions become more purposeful. Motor development is cephalocaudal. Fine motor

development focuses on feeding self finger foods, using cup and spoon.

    (5) Gross motor development: rolls, sits, crawls.

  b. Toddler (1 to 3 years old) (Burns, et al., 1996; Colson and Dworkin, 1997).

    (1) Psychosocial stage of autonomy vs. shame/doubt.

    (2) Sensorimotor stage of cognitive development: begins to understand causality and uses memory for problem solving.

    (3) Language: follows commands, understands more reasoning, names pictures, names body parts, asks simple questions.

    (4) Fine motor development: scribbles, removes clothes, begins to use fork, builds with blocks.

    (5) Gross motor development: walks well, climbs, throws ball, jumps.

  c. Preschooler (4 to 5 years old) (Burns, et al., 1996; Sturner and Howard, 1997 a & b).

    (1) Psychosocial stage of initiative vs. guilt.

    (2) Preoperational stage of cognitive development: magical thinking, egocentrism, symbolic play.

    (3) Language: recognizes coins, responds to 3 action commands, tells stories, asks "how" questions.

    (4) Fine motor development: copies, cuts with scissors, dresses self, pours from a small pitcher.

    (5) Gross motor development: pedals tricycle, balance on one foot improves, able to catch a large ball.

  d. School-age (6 to 11 years old) (Burns, et al., 1996).

    (1) Psychosocial stage of industry vs. inferiority.

    (2) Concrete operational stage of cognitive development: concrete thinking, understands concepts of relation and ordering.

    (3) Language: learns how to ask for help; learns simple concepts of health maintenance (diet, hygiene, rest), and begins to take responsibility for health.

    (4) Motor development: daily exercise, participation in sports and hobbies.

B. Primary, secondary, tertiary prevention.

  1. Newborn screening.

    a. Screening tests included vary according to state law.

    b. All states offer blood test screening for phenylketonuria (PKU) and congenital hypothyroidism.

    c. Screening for tryosinemia, cystic fibrosis, toxoplasmosis, maple syrup urine disease (MSUD), and hemoglobinopathies are available.

    d. Newborn should be receiving protein feedings for at least 24 hours prior to blood tests.

  2. Vision screening: Vision screening is incorporated into the physical examination for the newborn-infant and toddler age groups; tracking an object, coordinated eye movements, and red light reflex.

    a. Screening for strabismus at any age includes corneal light reflex, cover/uncover test.

    b. Standard testing for visual acuity begins at 3-year-old visit, repeat at every well-child visit to follow.

    c. By age 3 years, vision is 20/40; by age 5-years vision is 20/30; by age 7 vision is 20/20.

    d. Screening results that are below average or demonstrate a line discrepancy between eyes should be referred (Bickley and Hoekelman, 1999).

  3. Auditory screening: Response to sound and language development are baseline; hearing screening for healthy newborn-infants.

    a. The AAP and Joint Committee on Infant Hearing recommended universal newborn hearing screening programs to detect hearing loss in infants before 3 months of age and intervene before 6 months of age (Task Force on Newborn and Infant Hearing, 1999).

      (1) Observation of behavioral response to sound is unreliable.

      (2) Screening should be done before discharge, while the infant is sleeping.

      (3) Formal newborn hearing screening has been legislated in more than 20 states (Garganta and Seashore, 2000).

    b. Begin pure tone audiometry at 3 years of age.

    c. Repeat at every well-child visit.

  4. Tuberculin screening: based on degree of risk.

    a. Children who live in high prevalence areas or have uncertain histories of exposure should have periodic screening between 4 to 6 years and 11 to 16 years of age.

    b. Annual screening is recommended for children at high risk including those exposed to confirmed or suspected TB, recent immigrants from/or travel to endemic countries, children with HIV, children who are incarcerated.

    c. Mantoux test containing 5 tuberculin units of purified protein derivative (PPD) placed intradermally is preferred (Peter, 1997).

  5. Lead toxicity screening: based on degree of risk.

    a. Assess risk for lead poisoning beginning at 6 to 9 months of age through 6 years of age.

    b. Structured questionnaires are available (American Academy of Pediatrics, 1997).

  6. Cholesterol screening: Selective screening is recommended.

    a. Children whose parent has hypercholesterolemia (>240 mg/dl) should have a baseline total cholesterol level.

    b. Children whose grandparent or parent has a history of cardiovascular disease before the age of 55 should have a baseline serum lipid profile; should be drawn after a 12-hour fast (Barness, 1993; Burns, et al., 1996).

    c. Age at initial screening is controversial; as young as 2 years old has been recommended (American Academy of Pediatrics, 1997).

7. Urine screening: Frequency of testing varies among the preventive health care guidelines.
   a. At a minimum, urine screening is recommended at 5 years of age and once during adolescence (American Academy of Pediatrics, 1997).
   b. Screening includes glucose, protein, red and white blood cells, bacteria, and bacterial breakdown products.

8. Anemia screening: Frequency of testing varies among the preventive health care guidelines.
   a. At a minimum, anemia screening is recommended once by 9 months of age *and*
   b. During adolescence (American Academy of Pediatrics, 1997).

9. Routine dental care.
   a. As soon as primary teeth erupt, regular brushing with a child-size soft-bristle brush should begin.
   b. The first dental visit is recommended as early as 1 year of age and continues at 6 month follow-up intervals (American Academy of Pediatrics, 1997).

10. Immunizations.
    a. Refer to Centers for Disease Control and Prevention (CDC) website (www.cdc.gov) or the American Academy of Pediatrics Committee on Infectious Diseases for the most current recommendations (2000).
    b. Modifications in the schedule are made often, especially related to minimal dosing intervals and immunizations in special situations.

C. Clinical procedures.
   1. Blood pressure.
      a. Select appropriate cuff size (National High Blood Pressure Education Program Working Group, 1996; Bickley and Hoekelman, 1999).
         (1) Bladder width should cover approximately 75% of the length of upper arm or thigh.
         (2) Bladder length should cover 80% to 100% of the upper arm or thigh circumference. Bladder ends should not overlap.
      b. One elevated blood pressure reading does not necessarily indicate hypertension. A series of blood pressure readings should be obtained over a period of weeks when evaluating hypertension.
      c. Dinemapp readings tend to be slightly higher than manual blood pressure readings.
   2. Vision screening tests (Fox, 1997).
      a. Preschooler.
         (1) Visual acuity tests: Allen figures, Sjogren hand, tumbling E, HOTV.
         (2) Ishihara or Hardy-Rand-Rittler for color perception.
      b. School-age child.
         (1) Visual acuity tests: Allen figures, HOTV chart, tumbling E, Snellen.
         (2) Ishihara for color perception.
   3. Auditory screening tests (Fox, 1997).

     a. Newborns (Garganta and Seashore, 2000).

        (1) Auditory Brainstem Response (ABR): assesses cochlea and auditory nerve function, and brainstem auditory pathways. Detects sensorineural and central hearing loss.

        (2) Transient Otoacoustic Emissions (TOAE): assess middle ear and cochlea function. Detects conductive and sensorineural hearing loss.

        (3) ABR and TOAE may be done individually or in combination.

     b. Preschooler.

        (1) Play audiometry.

        (2) Pneumatic otoscopy: assess mobility of tympanic membrane, allowing for more accurate diagnosis of otitis media.

        (3) Tympanometry: assess middle ear pressure and TM compliance.

     c. School-age.

        (1) Pure tone audiometry: each ear should be tested at 500, 1000, 2000, and 4000 Hz. Air conduction hearing threshold levels of greater than 20 dB at any frequency requires additional evaluation.

        (2) Pneumatic otoscopy: assess mobility of tympanic membrane, allowing for more accurate diagnosis of otitis media.

        (3) Tympanometry: assess middle ear pressure and TM compliance.

4. Developmental screening: Determines which children require a more in-depth assessment.

     a. Ongoing assessment with screening at all well-child visits is essential.

     b. Denver-II Developmental Screening Test is the most widely used (Needlman, 2000).

     c. Early Screening Inventory and Ages and Stages Questionnaires (ASQ) are brief developmental assessment tools covering multiple domains.

     d. Early Language Milestone Scale (ELM) and the Clinical Linguistic and Auditory Milestone Scale (CLAMS) assess language milestones.

5. Tuberculosis screening (Peter, 1997).

     a. Mantoux test is recommended for screening because of its specificity and sensitivity. 0.1 ml of purified protein derivative (PPD) is administered intradermally to produce a wheal. The area is assessed for induration 48 to 72 hours following the injection.

     b. Reactive results.

        (1) Children at least 4 years old with no risk factors and induration of at least 15 mm.

        (2) Children less than 4 years old or children with a positive history for risk factors and induration of at least 10 mm.

        (3) Children with close contact exposure to TB, HIV, or evidence of TB disease and induration of at least 5 mm.

6. Lead toxicity screening.

     a. Venous samples are more reliable than capillary samples. Blood lead levels are more sensitive and specific than erythrocyte protoporphyrin levels.

7. Urine screening.
   a. First void of the day is most concentrated and contains the most bacteria and bacterial breakdown material.
   b. Bagged urine specimens: if results suggest bacteriuria, a repeat specimen should be obtained via catheterization or suprapubic tap.
   c. Midstream urine specimens most desirable. Clean with a mild soap prior to void.
8. Anemia screening.
   a. Finger stick: first drop of blood should be wiped off and discarded. Allow the area to dry and do not "milk" the next drop of blood as this may alter the sample.
   b. Venous sampling.
9. Immunizations.
   a. Appropriate storage.
   b. Mixing and administering immunization.
   c. Techniques: IM injections in children < 2 years should be given in anterolateral aspect of thigh; deltoid is acceptable in school-age children.

D. Care management.
   1. Visit schedule (American Academy of Pediatrics, 1997).
      a. Newborn-infant: newborn, 2 to 4 days, 2 to 4 weeks, 2 months, 4 months, 6 months, 9 months, 12 months.
      b. Toddler: 15 months, 18 months, 24 months.
      c. Preschooler: 3, 4, 5 years of age.
      d. School-age: 6, 8, 10, 11 years of age.
   2. Immunizations.
      a. Maintain appropriate immunization schedule with attention to minimum intervals between doses and between giving different vaccines.
      b. Knowledge of which preparations/combinations of vaccines are available.
      c. Benefit/risk of each immunization; informed consent.
      d. Side effects of each immunization.
   3. Anticipatory guidance as described in patient education.

E. Patient education.
   1. Nutrition.
      a. Newborn/infant.
         (1) Breastfeeding or standard infant formula alone is adequate until 4 to 6 months old.
            (a) Solely breast-fed infants who are dark skinned or have little access to sunlight may require vitamin D supplements.
            (b) Supplemental formula feedings are not necessary and may interfere with breast milk supply.
            (c) Encourage mothers to express breast milk before or after feedings, and while at work, and freeze for supplemental feedings (Boynton, Dunn, and Stephens, 1998).

(2) Bottle feeding.
    (a) Clarify proper formula preparations; available in 3 different forms—ready to feed, liquid concentrate, powder.
    (b) Review feeding technique: never prop bottle; hold baby in upright position; burp frequently; do not use microwave to warm formula.
    (c) Average formula intake is 24 to 32 ounces per day. (Fox, 1997).
(3) Infants are developmentally ready to start solids (baby food) on a spoon between 5 and 6 months old.
    (a) Assess readiness: fairly steady head control, beginning to sit, open mouth when spoon touches lip, minimal tongue protrusion when food enters mouth, majority of food stays in mouth and is swallowed (Morris, 1992).
    (b) Purpose of baby foods is to introduce new oral textures and promote oral motor development.
    (c) Introduce one food every 3 to 4 days, starting with 1 tsp of iron fortified rice cereal. Advance to between 1/3 cup and 1/2 cup total, divided into 2 feedings. Advance to 3 to 4 tbsp of fruits and vegetables per day by one year of life (Boynton, et al., 1997).
    (d) Fruit juice should be limited to 4 ounces per day.
    (e) Early introduction of solid foods may increase risk of allergies.
(4) Introduce cup at 6 to 9 months; wean from bottle by 12 to 15 months.
(5) Introduce whole cow's milk at 1 year old. Dietary fat is required for neurologic development until 2 years old when low fat milk can be introduced.
(6) No honey until 12 months old because of risk of botulism Peter, 1997).
(7) Avoid foods such as nuts, popcorn, hot-dogs, grapes, raw vegetables that pose a risk for choking in this age group.
(8) Fluoride, iron, and multiple vitamin supplements vary depending on dietary intake.

b. Toddler.
(1) Include foods from 5 major food groups.
    (a) Adjust serving size for age; one tbsp of each food per year of life. (Figure 12-1, USDA, 1999.)
    (b) Offer 3 meals and 3 snacks per day.
(2) Decreased appetite associated with growth deceleration is common between 15 to 18 months old.

c. Preschooler.
(1) Physical growth rate decreases and child becomes more interested in feeding self, but overall less interested in eating as a result of decreased appetite.

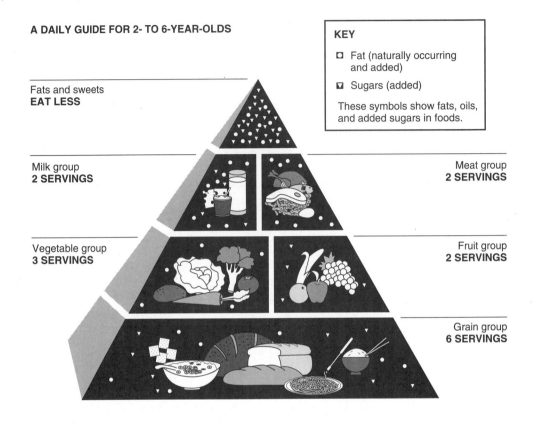

A DAILY GUIDE FOR 2- TO 6-YEAR-OLDS

KEY

▢ Fat (naturally occurring and added)

◪ Sugars (added)

These symbols show fats, oils, and added sugars in foods.

Fats and sweets
EAT LESS

Milk group
2 SERVINGS

Meat group
2 SERVINGS

Vegetable group
3 SERVINGS

Fruit group
2 SERVINGS

Grain group
6 SERVINGS

WHAT COUNTS AS ONE SERVING?

Grain group
1 slice of bread
½ cup of cooked rice or pasta
½ cup of cooked cereal
1 ounce of ready-to-eat cereal

Vegetable group
½ cup of chopped raw
or cooked vegetables
1 cup of raw leafy vegetables

Fruit group
1 piece of fruit or melon wedge
¾ cup of juice
½ cup of canned fruit
¼ cup of dried fruit

Milk group
1 cup of milk or yogurt
2 ounces of cheese

Meat group
2 to 3 ounces of cooked lean
meat, poultry, or fish.

½ cup of cooked dry beans, or
1 egg counts as 1 ounce of lean
meat. 2 tablespoons of peanut
butter count as 1 ounce of
meat.

Fats and sweets
Limit calories from these.

Four- to 6-year-olds can eat these serving sizes. Offer 2- to 3-year-olds less, except for milk.
Two- to 6-year-old children need a total of 2 servings from the milk group each day.

FIGURE 12-1 ■ Food Guide Pyramid for Young Children. (Source: U.S. Department of Agriculture.)

(2) Milk intake decreases to 16 to 24 ounces/day.

(3) Offer small, frequent meals; 3 meals and 2 snacks.

   d. School-age.

(1) Reinforce healthy food choices; balanced meals, healthy snacks.

2. Elimination (Burns, Barber, Brady, and Dunn, 1996).

   a. Newborns and infants usually stool after feedings.

(1) Normal variation: 1 stool per week to 7 stools/day; especially if breast-fed.

(2) Typically, breast-fed babies' stools are soft, seedy, and mustard in color.

(3) Formula-fed infants have more pasty stools.

(4) Should urinate a minimum of 6 times in 24 hours.

   b. Toddlers: become psychologically and physiologically ready to toilet train between 18 to 30 months.

(1) Daytime control is usually accomplished before nighttime control.

(2) Urinate 8 to 14 times a day.

   c. Preschooler: occasional accidents occur.

   d. School-age.

(1) Stooling patterns range from 3 times a day to once every 2 to 3 days.

(2) Bladder capacity is similar to an adult's; voiding 6 to 8 times a day.

3. Sleep (Ferber, 1985).

   a. Newborn-infant (AAP Task Force on Infant Sleep Position and SIDS, 2000).

(1) Up to 6 months of age, infant has one long sleep period, 6 to 8 hours; total sleep time 14 to 16 hours/day. Side lying or supine position.

(2) 6 to 12 months: long sleep period approximately 8 hours; total sleep time 10 to 15 hours/day.

(3) Supine, lowest risk position for SIDS, is preferred.

(4) Place infant in crib meeting the CPSC standards with a firm mattress and tight fitting sheets to avoid entrapment.

(5) Avoid soft bedding, pillows, and toys in the crib; and waterbeds, sofas, and soft mattresses that may create a risk of suffocation.

(6) Avoid overheating of the infant.

(7) Cosleeping is not recommended, especially when mother smokes or uses other mood altering substances, because of increased risk of entrapment, overlying, and suffocation resulting from entanglement and gas trapping beneath bedding.

   b. Toddler.

(1) Total sleep time 10 to 12 hours/day; including one nap.

(2) Bedtime rituals aid child to settle down to sleep.

(3) Nightmares and night terrors common problem.

    c. Preschooler.
      (1) Total sleep time 8 to 12 hours/day; naps gradually diminish.
      (2) Nightmares more predominant than night terrors.
    d. School-age.
      (1) Total sleep time 8 to 10 hours/day.
  4. Developmental issues.
    a. Newborn-infant: parent-infant attachment; stranger anxiety; separation anxiety.
    b. Toddler: discipline; temper tantrums; sibling rivalry; thumb-sucking.
    c. Preschooler: increasing need for peer play; interest in gender differences.
    d. School-age: development of friendships; increased self-awareness and body image issues; prepubertal issues. Academic achievements in school.
  5. Dental (Fox, 1997).
    a. Newborn-infant: primary incisors erupt between 6 to 9 months.
    b. Toddler: first molars erupt between 12 to 14 months, cuspids between 16 to 18 months, second molars between 20 to 24 months.
    c. School-age: begin to lose primary teeth and permanent teeth erupt.
  6. Injury prevention is a function of understanding normal child development and anticipating the risks that these new skills create.
    a. Falls.
    b. Burns.
    c. Suffocation.
    d. Drowning.
    e. Aspiration.
    f. Car safety.
  7. Vaccine information sheet.
  8. Alternate childcare options: in-home child care, family daycare, formal daycare, preschool, after-school programs.
F. Advocacy.
  1. Remove barriers to preventive health care services: high cost of services, transportation to services, child care needs for siblings.
  2. Increase limited primary care resources: mental health care, car seat safety programs.
  3. Increase awareness of free and low-cost health insurance available for children, such as Child Health Intervention Program (CHIPS), and early intervention services.
  4. Refer to Women Infant Children (WIC): supplemental nutrition for children birth through 5 years of age, pregnant women, and nursing mothers who meet eligibility guidelines, and for children with special nutritional needs.
  5. Increase awareness of community resources that parents can access themselves: church, school, public utility companies.
G. Telephone practice (Schmitt, 1999).
  1. Purpose: to provide high quality, safe care; triage calls to determine if the

child needs to be seen, and if so how urgently; and to support appropriate care of children in the home.

2. Components of the telephone encounter.

   a. Greeting; identification of person on the phone as well as the service they represent.

   b. History taking.

   c. Decision making/triage.

   d. Implementing the triage decision.

      (1) Recommendation: activate Emergency Medical Services (EMS) immediately, see immediately (ED or office), see within 24 hours, see within 2 weeks (chronic, recurrent symptoms), home care.

      (2) Negotiation: parent understands and is able and willing to carry out recommendation.

      (3) Follow-up.

3. Resources: computer-based protocols driven by questions, textbooks, parent information sheets. Availability of multilingual personnel.

H. Communication/documentation.

   1. Growth data must be properly documented on age- and sex-appropriate growth charts as well as in the visit record.

   2. Immunization documentation includes date of vaccination, manufacturer and lot number of vaccine, name and title of person administering the vaccine. Access to Immunization Registry to promote vaccination at every opportunity.

   3. Allergies to medications, food products, and environmental factors with a description of the reaction.

   4. All phone contacts with families should be clearly documented in the patient's record.

   5. "No Show" documented in patient record and method for communicating with family (written or via phone) to reschedule.

   6. Awareness of cultural issues.

   7. Awareness of language and reading skills of population.

I. Outcome management.

   1. Follow up on issues discussed at previous visit.

   2. Build on child's current developmental level to assess effectiveness of previous interventions and anticipate future needs.

J. Protocol development/usage.

   1. American Academy of Pediatrics (AAP), *Guidelines for Health and Supervision III*, (1997).

   2. Office of Disease Prevention and Health Promotion, *Clinician's Handbook of Preventive Services: Put Prevention into Practice*, (1998).

   3. National Center for Education and Child Health, *Bright Futures: Guidelines for Health Supervision of Infants, Children, and Adolescents*, editors M Green and JS Palfrey, (2000).

   4. Early and periodic screening, diagnosis, and treatment program.

   5. Telephone triage management.

CHILD WITH ASTHMA

Marcia Winston, MSN, RN, CRNP

Asthma is the most common chronic disease of childhood. It is found in all age groups. The basic precepts of asthma are the same, but consideration of a child's developmental level is a key part of the assessment in order to assure optimal care. The diagnosis of asthma is being made with increasing frequency in children although at the same time it is often overlooked. Asthma on both a chronic and acute basis is primarily managed in the outpatient/ambulatory setting. It is repeatedly misunderstood, often misdiagnosed and undertreated. According to Wong (1999), "The overall goal of asthma management is to prevent disability, to minimize physical and psychologic morbidity, and to assist the child in living as normal and happy a life as possible" (p. 1504).

Primarily, it is important to understand exactly what asthma is. Asthma is frequently confused with allergies, upper respiratory tract infections, bronchitis, and pneumonia. Asthma consists of chronic airway inflammation. Chronically inflamed airways are both hypersensitive and hyperreactive to triggers. Triggers include viral infections such as upper respiratory tract infections, animals, dust, mold, cockroaches, smoke, pollution, exercise, cold air, and other conditions like gastroesophageal reflux, sinus disease, and postnasal drip. Exposure to triggers leads to airway smooth muscle contraction, bronchoconstriction, and symptoms. Secondly, it is necessary to be cognizant of the various ways in which asthma can present in addition to understanding the pathophysiology of asthma and etiology of the symptoms. The most common symptoms are coughing, wheezing, shortness of breath, and a feeling of chest tightness or chest pain. It is important to understand that some children may only have occasional coughing while others have daily coughing (which may occur in spasms), wheezing, shortness of breath, and chest discomfort.

Thirdly, knowledge of asthma treatment is essential. Asthma treatment is divided into two classifications. The long-term-control or preventive maintenance medications consist of the antiinflammatory agents. In order for these medications to work optimally, they must be administered daily whether or not symptoms are present. Quick-relief therapy is used to provide symptom relief and treat acute exacerbations. Quick-relief medications are usually administered on an as-needed basis. It is crucial that the nurse understand these concepts for control of inflammation (long-term control therapy) and bronchospasm (quick-relief therapy).

A. Assess/screen/triage.
   1. Respiratory assessment: perform at each visit for acute or chronic management.
      a. Observe symptoms.
      b. Check vital signs and respiratory rate.
      c. Observe child's behavior and activity level. Child may be restless, apprehensive, or sit upright in three point/orthopneic position.
      d. Assess level of work of breathing for accessory muscle use, retractions, and nasal flaring.
      e. Auscultate the lungs for adventitious breath sounds and air move-

ment. Expiratory phase may be prolonged. Wheezing may or may not be heard depending on the intensity of bronchospasm and obstruction of air movement as a result of increased airway inflammation.

   f. Check oxygen saturation by pulse oximetry.

   g. Obtain patient symptom history.

   h. Inquire when the symptoms started, whether they are worse night or day, what possibly triggered the symptoms, whether the child is ill otherwise (fever, vomiting, diarrhea, etc.), what action the parent/caretaker has taken to relieve the symptoms, and whether it helped.

   i. Assess parent/caretakers' ability to recognize their child's signs and symptoms of an impending exacerbation.

   j. Children who experience repeated exacerbations and/or have poorly controlled asthma may develop a barrel chest because of air trapping, elevated shoulders, and increased accessory muscle use (Wong, 1999).

   k. Review peak flow diary.

2. Assess impact of asthma on quality of life.

   a. Is the child's activity level/tolerance or endurance for activities of daily living, play, or exercise/sports affected?

   b. Does play/activity/excitement trigger symptoms: coughing, wheezing, shortness of breath, chest discomfort, fatigue to any degree that the child is unable to keep up with peers or has to stop to rest?

   c. Does the parent/caretaker restrict the child's participation in gym or sports?

   d. Is the child's or the parent/caretaker's sleep interrupted by symptoms or the need for extra treatments during the night?

   e. Is the child absent from school excessively or is school performance affected?

   f. Is the parent/caretaker missing a lot of work in order to care for the child and take him/her to appointments?

   g. Is the child growing and developing appropriately? Any problems with growth and development, such as obesity can complicate asthma.

   h. Is the child tolerating his/her medications or treatments?

   i. Does the parent have a prescription plan to cover the cost of medications and insurance coverage for equipment?

   j. Have the parents/caretakers identified the child's triggers and what measures have been taken to avoid or control them?

3. Determine level of asthma severity (Table 12-2) as per National Asthma Education and Prevention Program Expert Panel Report 2 (EPR-2), 1997, in order to prioritize educational goals, define individualized asthma management plan, and determine appropriate level of nursing intervention.

B. Primary, secondary, tertiary prevention.

1. Primary prevention for asthma.

   a. Inquire about the presence of cigarette smokers in the home. Environmental cigarette smoke is a known trigger of asthma, but it also possibly precipitates asthma in those predisposed to developing it.

■ TABLE 12-2
■ ■ **Classification of Severity of Asthma**

	Clinical Features Before Treatment*		
	Symptoms†	**Nighttime Symptoms**	**Lung Function**
STEP 4 Severe Persistent	■ Continual symptoms ■ Limited physical activity ■ Frequent exacerbations	Frequent	■ FEV_1 or PEF ≤60% predicted ■ PEF variability >30%
STEP 3 Moderate Persistent	■ Daily symptoms ■ Daily use of inhaled short-acting beta$_2$-agonist ■ Exacerbations affect activity ■ Exacerbations ≥2 times a week; may last days	>1 time a week	■ FEV_1 or PEF >60% <80% predicted ■ PEF variability >30%
STEP 2 Mild Persistent	■ Symptoms >2 times a week but <1 time a day ■ Exacerbations may affect activity	>2 times a month	■ FEV_1 or PEF ≥80% predicted ■ PEF variability 20-30%
STEP 1 Mild Intermittent	■ Symptoms ≤2 times a week ■ Asymptomatic and normal ■ PEF between exacerbations ■ Exacerbations brief (from a few hours to a few days); intensity may vary	≤2 times a month	■ FEV_1 or PEF >80% predicted ■ PEF variability <20%

Source: National Heart, Lung and Blood Institute (1997): National Institutes of Health Publication No.: 97-4051.
*The presence of one of the features of severity is sufficient to place a patient in that category. An individual should be assigned to the most severe grade in which any feature occurs. The characteristics noted in this figure are general and may overlap because asthma is highly variable. Furthermore, an individual's classification may change over time.
†Patients at any level of severity can have mild, moderate, or severe exacerbations. Some patients with intermittent asthma experience severe and life-threatening exacerbations separated by long periods of normal lung function and no symptoms.

    b. Refer parents/caretakers or patients who smoke to smoking cessation programs.
  2. Secondary prevention for asthma.
    a. Ask about the presence of triggers in the home.
    b. Teach trigger control measures (Table 12-3).
    c. Encourage sound health practices.
    d. Instruct parents/caretakers and children about the importance of proper hand washing to prevent the spread of infections.
    e. Monitor each child's height and weight.

■ TABLE 12-3
■ ■ **Common Asthma Triggers and Avoidance Strategies**

Trigger	To Avoid
Domestic dust mite allergens (so small they are not visible to the naked eye)	Wash bed linens and blankets once a week in hot water and dry in a hot dryer or the sun. Encase pillows and mattresses in airtight covers. Remove carpets, especially in sleeping rooms. Use vinyl, leather, or plain wooden furniture instead of fabric-upholstered furniture.
Tobacco smoke (whether the patient smokes or breathes in the smoke from others)	Stay away from tobacco smoke. Patients and parents should not smoke.
Allergens from animals with fur	Remove animals from the home, or at least from the sleeping area.
Cockroach allergen	Clean the home thoroughly and often. Use pesticide spray, but make sure the patient is not at home when spraying occurs.
Outdoor pollens and mold	Close windows and doors and remain indoors when pollen and mold counts are highest.
Indoor mold	Reduce dampness in the home; clean any damp areas frequently.
Physical activity	***Do not avoid*** physical activity. Symptoms can be prevented by taking a short- or long-acting inhaled beta$_2$-agonist or sodium cromoglycate before strenuous exercise.

Source: National Heart, Lung and Blood Institute (1997): National Institutes of Health Publication No.: 97-4051.

(1) Use growth charts to assess development.
(2) Inform families about the complications of obesity and teach proper/age appropriate nutrition.
   f. Children need regular exercise.
     (1) For patients with exercise-induced bronchospasm,* review the importance of administering medications as prescribed before exercise and then warming up for about 15 minutes.
     (2) Patients at any level of severity may have symptoms triggered by exercise.
     (3) As per the EPR-2 (1997), exercise-induced bronchospasm may be a signal of inadequate treatment. A step up in treatment and certainly further evaluation are warranted.
     (4) Recommendations for preexercise treatment should be part of every patient's asthma management plan.
   g. Review all patients' immunization status and recommend yearly flu vaccination for patients with asthma.
  3. Tertiary prevention for asthma.
   a. Emphasize the importance of long-term control therapy.
   b. Teach symptom monitoring.

---

*Note the term exercise-induced asthma is sometimes used to imply a condition separate from asthma.

    c. Teach peak flow monitoring as appropriate.
       (1) It can be a reliable tool for children 5 years of age or older.
       (2) Establish each child's personal best expiratory flow rate; it is the highest number (or maximum rate of exhalation expressed as liters per minute) that the patient can achieve when they are well.
       (3) Define the patient's green, yellow, and red zones.
         (a) The green zone is 80% to 100% of the personal best.
         (b) The yellow zone is 50% to 80% of the personal best.
         (c) The red zone is 50% or below of the personal best.
       (4) The rationale for peak flow monitoring is that the peak flow rate can drop into the yellow zone indicating an impending exacerbation before the onset of signs or symptoms so that the action plan can be initiated.
    d. Establish that parents/caretakers know how and when to implement their child's action plan.
       (1) Knowing how to recognize the signs and symptoms of worsening asthma.
       (2) How to treat worsening asthma as well as how and when to seek medical attention or take rescue action.
       (3) These instructions should be given to the family in writing as part of the child's asthma management plan.
       (4) The plan should include routine treatment, preexercise treatment and an action plan for exacerbations.

C. Clinical procedures.
   1. Medication administration for acute asthma exacerbation.
    a. Give bronchodilators, usually albuterol diluted in normal saline, via nebulizer or metered dose inhaler (MDI) via spacer as prescribed.
    b. Administer oral corticosteroids as prescribed (1 to 2 mg/kg/day in two divided doses for 3 to 10 days, with maximum dose 60 mg/day).
    c. Perform and document respiratory assessment and peak flow rate (children ≥5 years of age) before and after administering treatments.
    d. Prepare to send child home if improved.
    e. Specify a plan for follow-up.
    f. Give specific instructions outlining steps the parent/caretaker is to do if child worsens.
    g. If the child worsens or does not respond to treatment (no improvement in breath sounds or symptoms, hypoxia/oxygen requirement, or other complicating condition) send the child to the emergency room.

D. Care management.
   1. Coordination of care: work with the parent/caretaker to meet the goals of treatment within the context of the child's development, environment, home routine, school/daycare, activities, and insurance coverage.
    a. As per the EPR-2, 1997, the goals of treatment are:
       (1) Prevent chronic and bothersome symptoms (such as nocturnal cough).

(2) Maintain normal pulmonary function (≥80% of predicted peak flow rate).

(3) Maintain normal participation in activities/exercise/sports.

(4) Prevent breakthrough symptoms, exacerbations, emergency room visits, and hospitalizations.

(5) Provide optimal pharmacotherapy with the least amount of side effects and expense.

(6) Ask about the patient/family's priorities and organize/plan care to meet their needs and expectations with asthma management.

  b. In order to meet these goals at each visit reassess:

(1) For the signs and symptoms of asthma (quantify and qualify).

(2) Review peak flow record.

(3) Quality of life/functional status (number of days of school missed, sleep disruption or decreased activity level as a result of symptoms).

(4) Acute exacerbations (requiring intervention with action plan and use of quick-relief medication or prednisone).

(5) Adherence to the management plan and whether the parent/caretaker was able to obtain all medication and equipment as prescribed (occasionally pharmacies and payers make inappropriate substitutions).

(6) Level of communication between nurse, parent/caretaker, and patient and the family's level of satisfaction with care.

2. Provide every child with a written individualized asthma management/action plan.

  a. The written asthma management plan includes name, dose, how and when to administer each medication, peak flow monitoring instructions/parameters (if appropriate).

  b. How/when to take rescue action and call the doctor or go to the emergency room.

  c. Clarify that the parent/caretaker makes a plan to educate others involved in the child's care such as school nurse, teacher, coach, babysitter, daycare personnel, and other backup family members.

3. Supply the parent/caretaker with resource materials. Section J, 1 on page 196.

E. Patient education: as per the EPR-2, 1997, five key messages are to be included in patient education.

  1. Basic facts about asthma.

  2. Roles of medications.

  3. Skills: inhaler/spacer use, self-monitoring (symptom or peak flow monitoring).

  4. Environmental (trigger) control measures.

  5. When and how to take rescue actions (including written individualized asthma management/action plan).

    a. Include the following interventions in order to meet the goals of education and promote optimal self-parent/caretaker management.

(1) Explain the concept of chronic airway inflammation and bronchospasm.

(2) Define the roles of medication: long-term control agents (antiinflammatory agents) and quick relief agents (bronchodilators) (Tables 12-4 and 12-5 outline the stepwise approach to therapy and treatment recommendations for each level of severity).

(3) Identify the patient's long-term control medication(s) by name (brand and generic) and emphasize that they must be taken whether or not symptoms are present (Table 12-6).

(4) Identify the patient's quick-relief medication (brand name and generic) and that the goal is to use it only on an as-needed basis to relieve breakthrough symptoms (see Table 12-6). Caution parents/caretakers not to give over-the-counter cough (especially cough suppressants) or cold medications.

(5) Determine the best way to administer medications to each individual patient: oral, inhaler via spacer, dry powder device, or nebulizer according to patient's developmental level, level of asthma severity, medication formulation, availability, cost, and convenience.

(6) Demonstrate proper medication administration techniques. Have the patient, parent/caretaker return the demonstration. Regularly reevaluate the child's and parent/caretaker's medication administration technique.

(7) Teach symptom monitoring and peak flow monitoring (if applicable).

(8) Teach environmental/trigger control measures. Help the parent/caretaker prioritize control measures.

(9) Agree upon a daily management plan and action plan for exacerbations.

  (a) Identify when to use the action plan including when to call the office or go to the emergency room.

  (b) Give instructions in writing.

F. Advocacy actions/implications for nurses as per the National Asthma Education and Prevention Program (NAEPP), (1997).

  1. Be familiar with the real costs (both financial and psychosocial) of asthma care to patients in your community.

  2. Identify available community resources (social services, government-sponsored programs, and voluntary organizations) to help meet the financial needs of patients. Some communities have summer camps for children with asthma, where they receive education and medical supervision.

  3. Assess whether prescribed medications, treatments, equipment, diagnostic procedures are covered by the patient's insurance.

  4. If necessary contact the payer and be prepared to provide documentation explaining why the medication, treatment, equipment, or diagnostic procedure is medically necessary.

Text continued on p. 194

■ TABLE 12-4
■ **Stepwise Approach for Managing Infants and Young Children (5 Years of Age and Younger) With Acute or Chronic Asthma Symptoms***

	Long-Term Control	Quick Relief
STEP 4 Severe Persistent	Daily anti-inflammatory medicine. ■ High-dose inhaled corticosteroid with spacer/holding chamber and face mask. ■ If needed, add systemic corticosteroids 2 mg/kg/day and reduce to lowest daily or alternate-day dose that stabilizes symptoms.	Bronchodilator as needed for symptoms (see Step 1) up to 3 times a day.
STEP 3 Moderate Persistent	Daily anti-inflammatory medication. *Either:* ■ Medium-dose inhaled corticosteroid with spacer/holding chamber and face mask *Or, once control is established:* ■ Medium-dose inhaled corticosteroid and nedocromil *Or:* ■ Medium-dose inhaled corticosteroid and long-acting bronchodilator (theophylline).	Bronchodilator as needed for symptoms (see Step 1) up to 3 times a day.
STEP 2 Mild Persistent	Daily anti-inflammatory medication. *Either:* ■ Cromolyn (nebulizer is preferred; or MDI) or nedocromil (MDI only) ■ Infants and young children usually begin with a trial of cromolyn or nedocromil *Or:* ■ Low-dose inhaled corticosteroid with spacer/holding chamber and face mask.	Bronchodilator as needed for symptoms (see Step 1).

Continued

■ TABLE 12-4
■ ■ **Stepwise Approach for Managing Infants and Young Children (5 Years of Age and Younger) With Acute or Chronic Asthma Symptoms*—cont'd**

	Long-Term Control	Quick Relief
STEP 1 Mild Intermittent	No daily medications needed	Bronchodilator as needed for symptoms ≤2 times a week. Intensity of treatment will depend upon severity of exacerbation (see component 3-Managing Exacerbations). *Either:* ■ Inhaled short-acting beta₂-agonist by nebulizer or face mask and spacer/holding chamber. *Or:* ■ Oral beta₂-agonist for symptoms. With viral respiratory infection ■ Bronchodilator q 4-6 hours up to 24 hours (longer with physician consult) but, in general, repeat no more than once every 6 weeks. ■ Consider systemic corticosteroid if 　■ Current exacerbation is severe. 　*Or:* 　■ Patient has history of previous severe exacerbations.

Step down
Review treatment every 1 to 6 months. If control is sustained for at least 3 months, a gradual stepwise reduction in treatment may be possible.

Step up
If control is not achieved, consider step up. But first: review patient medication technique, adherence, and environmental control (avoidance of allergens or other precipitant factors).

Source: National Heart, Lung and Blood Institute (1997): National Institutes of Health Publication No.: 97-4051.
NOTE:
■ The stepwise approach presents guidelines to assist clinical decision making. Asthma is highly variable; clinicians should tailor specific medication plans to the needs and circumstances of individual patients.
■ Gain control as quickly as possible; then decrease treatment to the least medication necessary to maintain control. Gaining control may be accomplished by either starting treatment at the step most appropriate to the initial severity of their condition or by starting at a higher level of therapy (e.g., a course of systemic corticosteroids or higher dose of inhaled corticosteroids).
■ A rescue course of systemic corticosteroid (prednisolone) may be needed at any time and step.
■ In general, use of short-acting beta₂-agonist on a daily basis indicates the need for additional long-term-control therapy.
■ It is important to remember that there are very few studies on asthma therapy for infants.
■ Consultation with an asthma specialist is *recommended* for patients with moderate or severe persistent asthma in this age group. Consultation should be *considered* for all patients with mild persistent asthma.

■ TABLE 12-5

■ ■ **Stepwise Approach for Managing Asthma in Adults and Children Older Than 5 Years of Age: Treatment**

	Long-Term Control	Quick Relief	Education

STEP 4
Severe Persistent
	Daily medications:
	Anti-inflammatory: inhaled corticosteroid (high dose)†
	
	And:
	    Long-acting bronchodilator: either **long-acting inhaled beta$_2$-agonist,** sustained-release theophylline, or long-acting beta$_2$-agonist tablets
	
	And:
	    Corticosteroid tablets or syrup long term (make repeat attempts to reduce systemic steroids and maintain control with high-dose inhaled steroids)
		Short-acting bronchodilator: **inhaled beta$_2$-agonists** as needed for symptoms.
		Intensity of treatment will depend on severity of exacerbation; see component 3–Managing Exacerbations.
		Use of short-acting inhaled beta$_2$-agonists on a daily basis, or increasing use, indicates the need for additional long-term control therapy.
			Steps 2 and 3 actions plus:
			Refer to individual education/counseling.

STEP 3
Moderate Persistent
	Daily medication:
	Either:
	    Anti-inflammatory: inhaled corticosteroid (medium dose)
	Or
	    Inhaled corticosteroid (low-medium dose) and add a long-acting bronchodilator, especially for nighttime symptoms; either **long-acting inhaled beta$_2$-agonist,** sustained-release theophylline, or long-acting beta$_2$-agonist tablets.
		Short-acting bronchodilator: inhaled **beta$_2$-agonists** as needed for symptoms.
		Intensity of treatment will depend on severity of exacerbation; see component 3–Managing Exacerbations.
		Use of short-acting inhaled beta$_2$-agonists on a daily basis, or increasing use, indicates the need for additional long-term-control therapy.
			Step 1 actions plus:
			Teach self-monitoring.
			Refer to group education if available.
			Review and update self-management plan.

Continued

■ TABLE 12-5
■ ■ **Stepwise Approach for Managing Asthma in Adults and Children Older Than 5 Years of Age: Treatment—cont'd**

	Long-Term Control	Quick Relief	Education
STEP 3—cont'd Moderate Persistent	If needed: Anti-inflammatory: **inhaled corticosteroids (medium-high dose)** *And* **Long-acting bronchodilator,** especially for nighttime symptoms; either *long-acting* inhaled **beta₂-agonist,** sustained-release theophylline, or long-acting beta₂-agonist tablets.		
STEP 2 Mild Persistent	One daily medication: **Anti-inflammatory:** either **inhaled corticosteroid** (low doses) or **cromolyn or nedocromil** (children usually begin with a trial of cromolyn or nedocromil). Sustained-release theophylline to serum concentration of 5-15 µg/mL is an alternative, but not preferred, therapy. Zafirlukast or zileuton may also be considered for patients ≥12 years of age, although their position in therapy is not fully established.	Short-acting bronchodilator: inhaled **beta₂-agonists** as needed for symptoms. Intensity of treatment will depend on severity of exacerbation; see component 3-Managing Exacerbations. Use of short-acting inhaled beta₂-agonists on a daily basis, or increasing use, indicates the need for additional long-term- control therapy.	Step 1 actions plus: Teach self-monitoring. Refer to group education if available. Review and update self-management plan.
STEP 1 Mild Intermittent	No daily medication needed.	Short-acting bronchodilator: inhaled **beta₂-agonists** as needed for symptoms. Intensity of treatment will depend on severity of exacerbation; see component 3-Managing Exacerbations. Use of short-acting inhaled beta₂-agonists more than 2 times a week may indicate the need to initiate long-term-control therapy.	Teach basic facts about asthma. Teach inhaler/spacer/ holding chamber technique. Discuss roles of medications. Develop self-management plan. Develop action plan for when and how

to take rescue actions, especially for patients with a history of severe exacerbations.
Discuss appropriate environmental control measures to avoid exposure to known allergens and irritants. (See Component 4).

Step up
If control is not maintained, consider step up. First, review patient medication technique, adherence, and environmental control (avoidance of allergens or other factors that contribute to asthma severity).

Step down
Review treatment every 1 to 6 months; a gradual stepwise reduction in treatment may be possible.

Source: National Heart, Lung and Blood Institute (1997):* National Institutes of Health Publication No.: 97-4051.

*NOTE:

■ The stepwise approach presents general guidelines to assist clinical decision making; it is not intended to be a specific prescription. Asthma is highly variable; clinicians should tailor specific medication plans to the needs and circumstances of individual patients.

■ Gain control as quickly as possible; then decrease treatment to the least medication necessary to maintain control. Gaining control may be accomplished by either starting treatment at the step most appropriate to the initial severity of the condition or by starting at a higher level of therapy (e.g., a course of systemic corticosteroids or higher dose of inhaled corticosteroids).

■ A rescue course of systemic corticosteroids may be needed at any time and at any step.

■ Some patients with intermittent asthma experience severe and life-threatening exacerbations separated by long periods of normal lung function and no symptoms. This may be especially common with exacerbations provoked by respiratory infections. A short course of systemic corticosteroids is recommended.

■ At each step, patients should control their environment to avoid or control factors that make their asthma worse (e.g., allergens, irritants); this requires specific diagnosis and education.

■ Referral to an asthma specialist for consultation or comanagement is *recommended* if there are difficulties achieving or maintaining control of asthma or if the patient requires Step 4 care. Referral may be *considered* if the patient requires Step 3 care (see also component I-Initial Assessment and Diagnosis).

†Preferred treatments are in **bold** print.

■ TABLE 12-6
■ ■ **Asthma Medications***

Long-Term Control Medications	Quick-Relief Medications
Mast cell stabilizer/antiinflammatories: cromolyn sodium (Intal) and nedocromil (Tilade) both available as metered dose inhalers (MDIs) and nebulizer solution[†]	*Short-acting beta₂-agonists:* albuterol (Proventil, Ventolin, Xopenex)[†] available as oral syrup and tablets, MDIs, nebulizer solution; others include bitolterol (Tornalate), metaproterenol (Alupent), pirbuterol (Maxair), terbutaline (Brethaire, Brethine)
Inhaled corticosteroids all available as MDIs except as noted: beclomethasone (Beclovent, Vanceril, Vanceril DS), budesonide (Pulmicort Turbuhaler), Rotadisk 50 µg, 100 µg, 250 µg, triamcinolone (Azmacort)	*Anticholinergics:* ipratropium bromide (Atrovent) MDI and nebulizer solution
Leukotriene modifiers available in tablets: montelukast (Singulair)[†], zafirlukast (Accolate), zileuton (Zyflo)	*Systemic corticosteroids[†]:* prednisolone (Pediapred and Prelone syrups) and prednisone tablets
Long-acting beta₂-agonists: salmeterol (Serevent MDI and Diskus)	
Methylxanthines: theophylline	
Systemic corticosteroids: prednisolone (Pediapred and Prelone syrups) and predinisone tablets	

*Generic name followed by brand name in parentheses
[†]Indicates medications commonly used in children.
Note: Review product information for more details about dosing, age specifications, precautions, contraindications, interactions, and side effects.

    G. Telephone practice.
       1. For asthma sick calls.
         a. Identify the main symptom(s).
         b. Ask about the onset and duration of the symptom(s).
         c. Assess level of respiratory distress: ask about respiratory rate, retractions, accessory muscle use, work of breathing, activity level/tolerance, any change in level of alertness or ability to talk and carry on a conversation. If possible talk to the child or have the child sing a song to determine presence of dyspnea or increased work of breathing.
         d. Ask the caller what action has been taken to treat the symptom(s) and be specific.
           (1) For example, if the parent reports that they are giving nebulizer treatments, then ask questions and document precisely: child given albuterol 0.25 ml in NaCl via nebulizer every 6 hours for the last 48 hours.
           (2) Assess whether treatments have been helpful.

(3) Also ask if the child is taking any other medications or if over-the-counter medications have been tried.

(4) If the patient monitors peak flow, inquire about peak flow rate before and after treatment.

(5) Compare to baseline and determine zone: green, yellow, or red.

    (a) Assess for symptom(s) indicating other conditions that also need evaluation: fever, vomiting, diarrhea, rash, pain, change in mental status or injury.

    (b) Collaborate with physician to plan treatment and determine level of care: increase treatments, keep child inside in air conditioning during hot weather, change medication/prescribe medication (burst of oral prednisone), arrange to see the patient in the office, or instruct the parent/caretaker to take the child to the emergency room.

    (c) Advise the parent/caretaker to call back as needed with any questions or concerns, if the child doesn't improve or if condition worsens.

H. Communication.

    1. Assess for common fears and misconceptions that can lead to poor adherence and increased symptoms.

      a. The misunderstanding that asthma is caused by an emotional problem.

      b. The lack of understanding of chronic inflammation and the need for ongoing treatment even when there are no symptoms.

      c. Asthma medications are addictive or can lose their effectiveness over time. One of the most common mistakes made in asthma management is delaying the start of treatment, to wait to see if it will get better or go away on its own. Another common problem is not replacing MDIs frequently enough and using an empty inhaler. If the medication is taken daily at recommended doses, then most MDIs last a month.

      d. Activities/exercise should be restricted.

      e. Inhaled or oral corticosteroids are the same as anabolic steroids and even if they are different, all steroids are dangerous.

      f. Asthma exacerbations occur suddenly without warning.

      g. Medication administration via nebulizer is superior to MDI/spacer.

I. Outcome management.

    1. Document specify/quantify breakthrough symptoms.

    2. Document number of courses of oral corticosteroids.

    3. Record number of emergency room visits and hospitalizations.

    4. Document number of school days missed by the patient and workdays lost by the parent/caretaker because of asthma.

    5. Consider referral to an asthma specialist (pediatric pulmonologist or pediatric allergist) as per EPR-2 for patients with a history of:

      a. A life-threatening exacerbation.

      b. Child not meeting the goals of asthma therapy after 3-6 months of treatment.

        c. Signs, symptoms, or response to treatment are atypical.

        d. Presence of other complicating conditions. Other/additional diagnostic testing is indicated.

        e. Adherence problems.

        f. Child has severe persistent asthma or has been treated with two or more bursts of oral corticosteroids in 1 year or requires daily oral corticosteroids.

J. Protocol development/usage.

    1. Resources for protocol development.

        a. National Heart, Lung and Blood Institute (301)-251-1222
National Institutes of Health
P. O. Box 30105
Bethesda, MD 20824-0105
http://www.nhlbi.nih.gov/nhlbi/nhlbi.htm

        b. The American Lung Association 1-800-LUNG USA
1740 Broadway
New York, NY 10010
http://www.lungusa.org

        c. Allergy and Asthma Network/Mothers of Asthmatics 1-800-878-4403
3554 Chain Bridge Road, Suite 200
Fairfax, VA 22030-2709
http://www.podi.com/health/aanma

        d. Asthma and Allergy Foundation of America 800-7 ASTHMA
1125 15th Street NW, Suite 502
Washington, DC 20005
http://www.aafa.org

CHILD WITH SICKLE CELL DISEASE

Ellen Butensky, MSN, RN, C-PNP

Sickle cell disease is an inherited hemoglobinopathy in which an amino acid substitution results in the production of abnormal hemoglobin. This results in shortened red blood cell survival (hemolysis) and, in times of stress, polymerization of red blood cells (sickling) which in turn leads to vasoocclusion, tissue infarction, necrosis, and pain. Patients experience crises or acute episodes of varying frequency and severity and often spend much time in the hospital. They are at risk for many long-term complications and death. Transmission is autosomal dominant. Sickle cell trait occurs when the individual inherits one sickle cell beta globin gene and one normal beta globin gene. These individuals generally have normal hemoglobin concentrations and their red blood cells do not sickle except under extreme circumstances The prevalence of sickle cell disease per 100,000 individuals is 289 African Americans, 5.3 Hispanics, 7.6 Asians, 36.2 Native Americans, and 1.7 Caucasians (U.S. Department of Health and Human Services, 1993c).

Child with Sickle Cell Disease: Acute

A. Assess/screen/triage.
  1. Fever.
    a. Infection.
      (1) High risk of infection, particularly with encapsulated organisms as a result of functional asplenia.
      (2) Leading cause of death in infants and young children (Buchanan, 1994).
      (3) Most common pathogens: *Streptococcus pneumoniae, Haemophilus. influenzae, Salmonella* (Gribbons, Zahr, and Opas, 1995).
      (4) Salmonella most common cause of osteomyelitis (Buchanan, 1994).
      (5) Assess for signs of URI, UTI, pain, otitis media (OM), sinusitis, pneumonia, pharyngitis, osteomyelitis, meningitis, gastroenteritis. Often there is no detectable focus (Buchanan, 1994).
      (6) Prompt medical attention for all episodes of fever regardless of clinical picture. Without therapy, illness progresses rapidly to cardiovascular collapse and, often, disseminated intravascular coagulation (Buchanan, 1994).
    b. Aplastic crisis.
      (1) Viral suppression of red blood cell production which, in combination with the already shortened life span of red blood cells leads to profound anemia (Gribbons, et al., 1995); temporary bone marrow aplasia.
      (2) Most often caused by parvovirus B19 (McVie, 1998).
      (3) Assess for exposure to others with viral illness, heart rate, gallop, color, dyspnea, splenic sequestration.
    c. Acute chest syndrome (ACS).
      (1) Any acute illness with a new pulmonary infiltrate on chest x-ray (Lane, 1996).
      (2) Second most common cause of hospitalization; responsible for up to 25% of deaths (Vichinsky, et al., 1997).
      (3) Occurs in 15% to 34% of patients (Gribbons, et al., 1995).
      (4) If infectious, may be caused by *S. pneumoniae, H. influenzae, Staphylococcus aureus, Klebsiella, Mycoplasma, Chlamydia* (Lane, 1996).
      (5) In one study, 3.5% of cases associated with bacteremia, most often in children under 2 years of age (Vichinsky, et al., 1997).
      (6) Noninfectious precipitating factors include poor ventilation (as a result of narcotics or anesthesia), overhydration resulting in pulmonary edema, or fat emboli from extended bed rest (Lane, 1996).
      (7) Assess for fever, rhinorrhea, dyspnea, cough, chest pain (point tenderness suggestive of vasoocclusive crisis [VOC]), breath sounds, pulse oximetry (compare to baseline), sinus tenderness, cardiac exam.

2. Pain
   a. Vasoocclusive crisis (VOC)/painful episode.
      (1) Most frequent acute episode.
      (2) Obstructed blood flow leads to decreased perfusion and oxygen delivery, resulting in pain, distal ischemia, and infarction (Gribbons, et al., 1995).
      (3) The most common cause of hospitalization (Gribbons, et al., 1995)
      (4) Young children tend to have dactylitis (hand-foot syndrome); older children tend to have more abdominal/back pain; pain can be anywhere (Gribbons, et al., 1995).
      (5) May be precipitated by infection, acidosis, hypoxia, dehydration, exposure to extreme cold, psychologic factors; often no precipitating factor can be identified (Gribbons, et al., 1995).
      (6) Assess for history of trauma, duration and quality of pain (does it feel like typical crisis pain?), fever, alleviating and aggravating factors, any medications taken, and response.
      (7) Consider work-up for infection, particularly if antipyretics have been given for pain (Ander and Vallee, 1997).
   b. Acute chest syndrome (ACS).
   c. Splenic sequestration (SS) (see section 4 below).
   d. Gallstones (see section 3 below).
   e. Avascular necrosis (AVN).
      (1) Changes in the bone, most often the femoral head or humerus, as a result of repeated infarction (Gribbons, et al., 1995).
      (2) Assess for pain, decreased range of motion, refusing to bear weight.
   f. Stroke (CVA) (see section 6 on the next page).
   g. Chronic leg ulcers.
      (1) Multifactorial etiology; thought to be the result of marginal blood supply to the skin, localized edema, and minor trauma.
      (2) Most commonly found in the ankle area.
      (3) Secondary infection common.
      (4) Leads to significant pain and immobility (Eckman, 1996).
3. Jaundice: gallstones.
   a. Bile stones from increased bilirubin as a result of chronic hemolysis; may lead to acute cholecystitis, pancreatitis, obstructive jaundice with ascending cholangitis (Al-Salem and Qaissruddin, 1998).
   b. Found in approximately 17% to 55% of patients; incidence increases with age (Al-Salem and Nourallah, 1997).
   c. Assess for RUQ pain, fever, jaundice.
4. Enlarged spleen: splenic sequestration.
   a. "Sludging" of red blood cells in microcirculation leads to rapid enlargement of the spleen, large volumes of blood are pooled causing hemoglobin to drop rapidly; platelets may be sequestered as well, leading to thrombocytopenia (Lane, 1996).

      b. Occurs in up to 30% of patients (Embury, Hebbel, Mohandas, and Steinberg, 1994).

      c. Almost all cases occur before age 6, with majority occurring before age 2, but cases have been reported in infants and older children and adults (Embury, et al., 1994).

      d. Approximately 50% will have recurrent episodes (Embury, et al., 1994).

      e. Assess spleen size and compare to baseline; assess color, activity level, heart rate, gallop, blood pressure.

   5. Priapism.

      a. Prolonged, painful erection caused by congested blood between the corpora spongiosum and cavernosum (drainage obstruction leads to engorgement, edema, and inflammation) (Gribbons, et al., 1995).

      b. May be stuttering, minor, or major (Hakim, Hashmat, and Macchia, 1994).

         (1) Stuttering: multiple episodes lasting less than 3 hours, several times a week for more than 4 weeks; usually self-limiting.

         (2) Minor: isolated or infrequent episodes lasting less than 3 hours; usually self-limiting.

         (3) Major: prolonged (usually lasting more than 12 hours), often preceded by stuttering or minor episode, often requires hospitalization.

      c. Assess stuttering versus sustained; length of time; therapies that have worked in the past; time of last void; dysuria; engorgement; presence of penile pain; rule out testicular torsion.

   6. Neurologic symptoms: cerebrovascular accident (CVA).

      a. An acute, clinically evident neurologic event: hemorrhagic (more common in older patients) or thrombotic (Lane, 1996).

      b. Thrombotic more common and occurs most often in the internal carotid, middle cerebral, or anterior cerebral arteries (Lane, 1996).

      c. Occlusion of blood vessels may cause transient symptoms or permanent neurologic dysfunction (Adams, 1994).

      d. Occurs in 6% to 15% of children with sickle cell disease, most often in those under the age of 10 years (Gribbons, et al., 1995).

      e. Complete neurologic exam; rule out VOC (point tenderness), sinusitis, otitis media, migraine.

      f. Most common presenting symptom is hemiparesis; others include seizures, dysphagia, ataxia. Coma suggests hemorrhage. Headache often precedes stroke but is only a reliable predictor if accompanied by vomiting or change in level of consciousness (Adams, 1994).

B. Primary, secondary, tertiary prevention.

   1. Primary.

      a. Penicillin prophylaxis (Pen VK 125 mg po bid 3 months to 5 years; 250 mg po bid over 5 years).

      b. Encourage fluids.

      c. Prevent exposure to cold, dehydration, and high altitudes.

      d. Routine immunizations including pneumococcal, influenza vaccines.

  2. Secondary.

      a. Rapid treatment.

      b. Consult with hematology team.

      c. Parent education.

  3. Tertiary.

      a. Coordinated care with multidisciplinary team.

      b. Rehabilitation, physical therapy, occupational therapy as needed.

C. Clinical procedures.

  1. Fever/infection: altered in thermodynamics; risk for infection.

      a. Complete blood count, reticulocyte count, blood culture; urinalysis/urine culture, chest x-ray, throat culture, lumbar puncture, stool culture, nasopharyngeal aspirate, as indicated by symptoms.

      b. Antibiotics as indicated by findings; minimum of good strep coverage: ceftriaxone or ampicillin, macrolides (erythromycin, clarithromycin, azithromycin), erythromycin if penicillin allergy; treat for bacteremia even if focus is found.

      c. Consult with hematology team regarding need for inpatient management versus outpatient management (must meet low-risk criteria; requires adequate follow-up, patient/family compliance, ability to contact family, availability of transportation for patient to return to the ED if necessary) (Platt, 1997).

  2. Vasoocclussive crisis (VOC): altered comfort: pain.

      a. Complete blood count, reticulocyte count, blood/urine/stool/throat culture, x-ray of chest/extremity/hips, amylase/lipase, abdominal ultrasound, refer for surgical consult based on symptoms.

      b. If all other causes ruled out, treat pain; prompt analgesic therapy, liberal fluid replacement (intravenously if necessary); use combination of oral opioid and nonsteroidal antiinflammatory; for severe pain, administer opioid at fixed intervals for steady state relief rather than as needed (Steinberg, 1999).

      c. Frequent assessments with developmentally appropriate pain scales.

      d. If pain is severe and not responding to oral analgesics, refer to acute care setting for intravenous opioids.

      e. Refer to pain management team if chronic/constant pain.

  3. Splenic sequestration: risk for fluid volume deficit.

      a. Complete blood count, reticulocyte count, fluid bolus 10 ml/kg; measure spleen size every hour.

      b. Refer for inpatient management for possible blood transfusion if spleen size increases or cardiovascular compromise (Embury, et al., 1994).

      c. If recurrent episodes, may need splenectomy.

  4. Acute chest syndrome (ACS): risk for altered gas exchange.

      a. Complete blood count, reticulocyte count, chest x-ray, nasopharyngeal aspirate based on symptoms; monitor oxygen saturation and compare to baseline; arterial blood gas if indicated.

      b. Avoid overhydration.

      c. Refer for inpatient management.

  5. Cerebrovascular accident (CVA): risk for injury related to tissue damage. Immediate referral for imaging and inpatient management.

  6. Aplastic crisis: risk for impaired gas exchange; risk for altered tissue perfusion.

      a. Complete blood count, reticulocyte count, blood culture, type and cross, isolate.

      b. Refer for inpatient management if anemia is severe, child is acutely ill, or cardiovascular compromise.

  7. Priapism: altered comfort.

      a. Complete blood count, reticulocyte count, fluid bolus 10 ml/kg, analgesic therapy.

      b. If no response, refer to acute care setting for possible blood transfusion and further management (Hakim, et al., 1994).

  8. Gallstones: altered comfort.

      a. Liver function tests/bilirubin profile, abdominal ultrasound to rule out cholecystitis.

      b. Pain management.

      c. Refer for inpatient management if febrile.

      d. If recurrent, may need cholecystectomy.

  9. Avascular necrosis (AVN): altered mobility.

      a. X-rays, pain management.

      b. Refer for inpatient management if pain is severe; if outpatient management is indicated, refer for follow-up treatment including bracing or, if unsuccessful, surgery (Gribbons, et al., 1995).

  10. Chronic leg ulcers: altered skin integrity.

      a. Zinc sulfate 55-110 mg po tid (children) or 220 mg po tid (adults) to promote wound healing.

      b. Refer for inpatient management if signs of cellulitis.

      c. May require skin grafts if resistant to therapy.

D. Collaboration/resource identification and referral.

  1. Local comprehensive sickle cell disease center for family support group.

  2. Sickle Cell Disease Association of America, 200 Corporate Point, Suite 495, Culver, CA, 90230, 1-800-421-8453, www.sicklecelldisease.org

  3. Social workers.

  4. Internet support groups/resources.

      a. Queenslibrary.org: links to national associations and general information.

      b. Defiers.com: patient-run site and chat room.

      c. Sickle.FHCRC.org: information regarding transplantation.

      d. Rarediseases.info.nih.gov: information regarding clinical trials.

      e. AHCPR: www.ahcpr.gov

  5. U.S. Department of Health and Human Services Public Health Services publications (U.S. Department of Health and Human Services Public Health Services, 1993a).

    E. Care management.
        1. Coordinate care with hematology, pain management team, surgery, neurology, urology, orthopedics, transfusion/pheresis team, social work, nutrition, ED, ophthalmology.
        2. During hospitalization, maintain contact with inpatient staff and provide baseline information and keep home care services up to date on status.
        3. Multidisciplinary team meetings as needed; implement mechanism for feedback from consults such as standard, carbon-copied consult forms, patient notebook.

    F. Patient education.
        1. Fever/infection.
            a. Temperature taking.
            b. Prompt attention if symptoms worsen.
        2. Vasoocclusive crisis (VOC).
            a. Medication regimen.
            b. Side effects.
            c. Myths surrounding addiction: low risk, not an indication not to treat.
            d. Adjunct methods of pain management (distraction, massage, imagery).
            e. Behavior issues.
            f. Pain may last up to a few weeks.
            g. Incentive spirometry to prevent ACS if decreased mobility.
        3. Splenic sequestration.
            a. Measuring spleen: tongue depressor placed at left costal margin and marked at spleen edge.
            b. Symptoms of worsening anemia.
            c. Encourage fluids.
        4. Acute chest syndrome (ACS).
            a. Medication regimen: complete course of antibiotic.
            b. Encourage fluids.
            c. Incentive spirometry, mobilization.
            d. Pain management.
        5. Cerebrovascular accident (CVA).
            a. Rehabilitation needs.
            b. Transfusion therapy: goal to keep hemoglobin S level below 30% (Adams, et al., 1998).
            c. Chelation therapy: subcutaneous infusion of deferoxamine over 8-10 hrs per day.
        6. Aplastic crisis.
            a. Symptoms of worsening anemia.
            b. Isolate from pregnant women because of small risk of stillbirth.
        7. Priapism.
            a. Dispelling myths: not caused by sexual arousal.
            b. May lead to sterility.
            c. Surgical intervention (shunt or prosthesis) may be indicated.
        8. Gallstones.

        a. Pain management.

        b. Signs of increasing bilirubin.

        c. Cholecystectomy may be indicated.

   9. Avascular necrosis (AVN).

        a. Pain management.

        b. Rest.

        c. Bracing or surgery may be indicated.

  10. Chronic skin ulcers.

        a. Pain management.

        b. Importance of bed rest and elevation.

        c. May take 6 weeks to 6 months to heal; recurrence common.

  11. Retinal changes.

        a. Vasoocclusion within the eye may cause retinopathy.

        b. Routine screening for the first year of life; annual eye exams thereafter.

  12. Psychosocial.

        a. Appropriate, accurate information to decrease the potential for unrealistic expectations for treatment and cure as well as feelings of guilt and anger surrounding the diagnosis.

        b. Need for adequate genetic counseling for the parents and the patient when age appropriate.

G. Advocacy.

   1. Research.

   2. Blood donation.

   3. Policy regarding parents' work absence, child's absence from school, and need for home tutoring.

   4. Early use of pain relief measures during frequent blood draws (i.e., local anesthetic, distraction, imagery, relaxation).

H. Telephone practice.

   1. Triage: Algorithms that can provide guidance can be found in the U.S. Department of Health and Human Services clinical practice guidelines, *Sickle cell disease: Screening, diagnosis, management and counseling in newborns and infants.* Publication 93-0562 (U.S. Department of Health and Human Services Public Health Services, 1993c) and *The pediatric acute care handbook* (Lieh-Lai, Asi-Bautista, and Ling-McGeorge, 1995).

        a. Fever/infection: if fever greater than 101° F (38.5° C), schedule for urgent visit; if severely ill, refer to acute care setting (U.S. Department of Health and Human Services Public Health Services, 1993c).

        b. VOC: instruct to take medication usually taken for pain; if no relief, schedule for urgent visit; if patient is in severe pain, consider referral to acute care setting for continuous narcotic infusion (U.S. Department of Health and Human Services Public Health Services, 1993c).

        c. Splenic sequestration: schedule urgent visit; if severe lethargy, decreased level of consciousness, severe pallor, refer to acute care setting for possible blood transfusion (U.S. Department of Health and Human Services Public Health Services, 1993c).

    d. ACS: if mild respiratory symptoms only and no fever, instruct to encourage fluids, rest, use vaporizer, bulb syringe in infants/toddlers; if fever and/or moderate symptoms, schedule urgent visit; if difficulty breathing, refer to acute care setting (U.S. Department of Health and Human Services Public Health Services, 1993c).

    e. CVA: for headache only, schedule urgent visit; for severe headache, other neurologic symptoms, refer to acute care setting (U.S. Department of Health and Human Services Public Health Services, 1993c).

    f. Aplastic crisis: if mild cold symptoms and no fever, encourage fluids, rest; if febrile and mild symptoms, schedule urgent visit; if severe pallor, lethargy, decreased level of consciousness, refer to acute care setting (U.S. Department of Health and Human Services Public Health Services, 1993c).

    g. Priapism: if associated with no other symptoms or mild symptoms, schedule urgent visit; if associated with fever, severe pallor, refer to acute care setting (National Institutes of Health; National Heart, Lung and Blood Institute, 1995).

    h. Gallstones: if jaundice noted, schedule urgent visit; if jaundice associated with fever or pain, triage as any patient with fever or VOC (National Institutes of Health; National Heart, Lung and Blood Institute, 1995).

    i. AVN: if nonambulatory, pain or limited range of motion of a joint, schedule urgent visit; otherwise triage as any patient with VOC (National Institutes of Health, National Heart, Lung and Blood Institute, 1995).

2. For patients managed in ambulatory setting and sent home.

    a. Follow-up status and retriage if no improvement/symptoms worsen.

    b. Inform patient/family of any lab or diagnostic test results.

    c. Maintain contact with home care nurse if applicable.

    d. Refer to acute care setting if indicated (i.e., abnormally low hemoglobin, positive culture).

I. Communication/documentation.

  1. Complete history including length of symptoms, measures taken prior to seeking medical attention, assessment/lab results, baseline assessment and lab values.

J. Outcome management.

  1. Fever/infection: response to antibiotics without allergy.

  2. VOC: good pain control with minimal use of pain medications; no development of ACS.

  3. Splenic sequestration: response of spleen size to interventions versus need for splenectomy.

  4. ACS: response to treatment without need for supplemental oxygen.

  5. CVA: response to rehabilitation; compliance with transfusion and chelation therapy.

  6. Aplastic crisis: avoid need for transfusion or good response to transfusion; prevention of repeated cases.

7. Priapism: response to treatment versus need for surgical intervention.
8. Gallstones: adequate pain control; response to treatment versus need for cholecystectomy.
9. AVN: adequate pain control; response to treatment versus need for surgery.

K. Protocol development/usage.
   1. Develop protocols for each complication based on practice of local multidisciplinary team.
   2. Refer to U.S. Department of Health and Human Services Public Health Services reference guide: *Sickle cell disease: Screening, diagnosis, management and counseling in newborns and infants,* Publication 93-0563 (U.S. Department of Health and Human Services Public Health Services, 1993b).

Child with Sickle Cell Disease: Chronic

Recent advances in care, education, and overall understanding of the disease have improved outcomes with recent data indicating that 85% to 90% of patients survive to age 20 and the median age at death is 42 for males and 48 for females (Platt, et al., 1994).

A. Assess/screen/triage.
   1. Evaluate frequency of acute episodes managed at home, pain medications taken, school attendance, activity level.
   2. Assess medication compliance.

B. Primary, secondary, tertiary prevention.
   1. Primary.
      a. Genetic counseling.
      b. Prenatal screening.
   2. Secondary.
      a. Immunizations.
      b. Encourage fluids.
      c. Prevent infection.
      d. Avoid exposure to cold, high altitudes (flying in unpressurized airplanes); avoid contact sports if enlarged spleen.
      e. Medic Alert bracelet.
   3. Tertiary.
      a. Routine medical care.
      b. Patient and family education.
      c. Strategies to foster adherence to treatment.

C. Clinical procedures (Jackson and Vessey, 1996).
   1. Complete blood count, reticulocyte count, blood pressure monitoring every 6 months.
   2. Liver function tests, urinalysis, BUN, creatinine, oxygen saturation annually.
   3. Vision/hearing screening, nutrition evaluation annually after age 10.
   4. EKG/ECHO every 1 to 2 years.

     5. Chest x-ray biannually after age 5.

D. Collaboration/resource identification and referral—refer to Acute section starting on page 201.

E. Care management.

     1. Coordination of care with multidisciplinary team.

     2. Collaborate with school/daycare (teachers and nurses).

F. Patient education (Jackson and Vessey, 1996).

     1. Routine medications (penicillin, folate, hydroxyurea, if indicated).

     2. Toilet training may be more difficult because of inability to concentrate urine and increased volume; allow for increased access to bathrooms.

     3. Issues around missing school; need for home tutoring.

     4. Adolescents: puberty is delayed but normal; impotence in males.

     5. Family planning/pregnancy: genetic counseling; need to refer for high risk monitoring.

     6. Psychosocial: parents missing work days, living with a chronic illness and adjusting to its effects, guilt due to genetic nature of disease.

G. Advocacy.

     1. Newborn screening: currently in 43 states (Day, Brunson, and Wang, 1997).

     2. Policy: regarding parents missing work; home tutoring for children.

     3. Research: gene therapy; bone marrow transplant.

     4. Blood donation.

     5. Supporting child if seeking care outside of primary clinic.

H. Telephone practice.

     1. Keep patient/family informed of laboratory/diagnostic test results.

     2. Schedule follow-up laboratory tests if abnormal values.

     3. Refer for rehabilitation services if tests indicate need (i.e., abnormal x-rays in AVN).

     4. Arrange and coordinate routine transfusion therapy if indicated (i.e., after discharge with CVA; multiple episodes of any complication).

     5. Maintain contact with visiting nurse, school nurse, daycare provider as indicated.

I. Communication/documentation.

     1. Close contact with specialists to coordinate care and keep accurate track of the frequency and number of episodes of complications.

     2. Accurate transfusion record and any antibodies that have developed.

     3. Trend of laboratory/diagnostic tests to maintain updated baseline hemoglobin, reticulocyte count, liver function tests, positive blood culture pathogen genotypes, pulse oximetry, Doppler results, x-ray findings.

J. Outcome management.

     1. Overall health and frequency of crises—evaluate need for transfusion therapy, hydroxyurea, bone marrow transplant.

K. Protocol development/usage.

     1. Develop protocol for primary care of children with sickle cell disease.

2. Refer to U.S. Department of Health and Human Services clinical practice guideline (U.S. Department of Health and Human Services Public Health Services, 1993c).

CHILD WITH ATTENTION DEFICIT HYPERACTIVITY DISORDER

Lisa Harvatine Ingalls, MSN, RN, CRNP

Inattention, hyperactivity, and impulsivity are behavioral characteristics found in varying degrees in all children. Attention deficit hyperactivity disorder (ADHD) is diagnosed when these characteristics occur to a degree that interferes with the child's academic and interpersonal development, and are not caused by another medical, neurologic, psychiatric, or educational factors. The degree of severity is highly variable. It affects 3% to 5% of school-age children—boys four times more often then girls. It is estimated that 50% to 70% of children with ADHD will still meet criteria as adolescents, and 8% to 33% will still meet criteria as adults (Mercugliano, Power, and Blum, 1999). The typical presentation varies with the age of the child. A preschooler may present with hyperactivity, being "difficult," needing constant supervision, tantrums, and aggression. The early school-age child often presents as inattentive, hyperactive, and not learning the school routines or basic academic skills. A school-age child often appears inattentive, overactive, underachieving, has messy work, and peer problems. In the adolescent, the presenting problems are often work avoidance; underachievement; inattentiveness; and problems with authority, parents, and peers (Mercugliano, et, al., 1999). The etiology of ADHD is unclear. It is suspected to be a combination of both neurobiologic and genetic factors. Studies of twins, siblings, and families have provided evidence of a genetic component (Biederman, et al., 1992).

ADHD is a behavioral diagnosis. No medical test is available to either confirm or exclude the diagnosis of ADHD. Information is gathered in the form of interviews and rating scales from several different sources. Gathering information from several sources is important to avoid bias from a setting that has inappropriate demands. Several different types of rating scales are used to gather information. Wide-range rating scales provide an assessment of many areas of functioning including ADHD symptoms, externalizing behaviors, internalizing behaviors, and peer functioning. Narrow-range rating scales assess attention, hyperactivity, impulsivity, and behavioral problems that coexist with ADHD. The rating scales have been standardized and can be scored based on age group and sex. The diagnosis of ADHD is based on meeting criteria outlined in the *Diagnostic and Statistical Manual of Mental Disorders* (4th edition, 1994).

   A. ADHD consists of either 1 or 2.

   1. Six (or more) of the following symptoms of inattention have persisted for at least 6 months to a degree that is maladaptive and inconsistent with developmental level.

    a. Inattention.
      (1) Often fails to give close attention to details or makes careless mistakes in schoolwork, work, or other activities.
      (2) Often has difficulty sustaining attention in tasks or play activities.
      (3) Often does not seem to listen when spoken to directly.
      (4) Often does not follow through on instructions and fails to finish schoolwork, chores, or duties in the workplace (not because of oppositional behavior or failure to understand instructions).
      (5) Often has difficulty organizing tasks and activities.
      (6) Often avoids, dislikes, or is reluctant to engage in tasks that require sustained mental effort (such as schoolwork or homework).
      (7) Often loses things necessary for tasks or activities (e.g., toys, school assignments, pencils, books, or tools).
      (8) Is often easily distracted by extraneous stimuli.
      (9) Is often forgetful in daily activities.
  2. Six (or more) of the following symptoms of hyperactivity-impulsivity have persisted for at least 6 months to a degree that is maladaptive and inconsistent with developmental level.
    a. Hyperactivity.
      (1) Often fidgets with hands or feet or squirms in seat.
      (2) Often leaves seat in classroom or in other situations in which remaining seated is expected.
      (3) Often runs about or climbs excessively in situations in which it is inappropriate (in adolescents or adults, may be limited to subjective feelings of restlessness).
      (4) Often has difficulty playing or engaging in leisure activities quietly.
      (5) Is often "on the go" or often acts as if "driven by a motor."
      (6) Often talks excessively.
    b. Impulsivity.
      (1) Often blurts out answers before questions have been completed.
      (2) Often has difficulty awaiting turn.
      (3) Often interrupts or intrudes (e.g., butts into conversations or games).
B. Some hyperactive-impulsive or inattentive symptoms that caused impairment were present before age 7 years.
C. Some impairment from the symptoms is present in two or more settings (e.g., at school or work and at home).
D. Clear evidence of clinically significant impairment in social, academic, or occupational functioning must be present.
E. The symptoms do not occur exclusively during the course of a pervasive developmental disorder, schizophrenia, or other psychotic disorder and are not better accounted for by another mental disorder (e.g., mood disorder, anxiety disorder, dissociative disorder, or a personality disorder).

Medication is one of the most used and effective treatments for ADHD. Long-term studies show that a combination of medication and psychosocial interventions is most beneficial (Brown, Vought, and Elksnin, 1996). The most common classes of medications used are stimulants such as methylphenidate (Ritalin), dextroamphetamine (Dexedrine), mixed amphetamine salts (Adderall), and pemoline (Cylert). Other medications used to treat ADHD instead of or in combination with stimulants include certain antihypertensives (clonidine, guanfacine), and antidepressants (tricyclics, selective serotonin reuptake inhibitors, bupropion).

A. Assess/screen/triage.

    1. Parent interview.

        a. History of presenting concern.

        b. Medical and developmental history.

        c. School history including academic skills, need for remediation, and classroom functioning.

        d. Social and family history including behavior towards parents and siblings, compliance with household chores, and completion of self-care activities.

    2. Child interview.

        a. Physical examination.

        b. Observation of motor coordination, language skills, and social style.

        c. Assessment of emotional and behavioral characteristics.

    3. School data.

        a. Rating scale completion by classroom teacher.

        b. Accuracy of seatwork and classroom behavior.

        c. Review of report cards and results of academic testing.

    4. Previous treatments and their effectiveness.

        a. Counseling and behavior management training.

        b. Current medication and dosing schedule.

B. Primary, secondary, tertiary prevention.

    1. Primary prevention.

        a. Recognize children who need a less stimulating environment.

        b. Provide clear guidelines of expectations at home and school.

        c. Provide consistent rewards/consequences for actions.

        d. Give one instruction at a time and make eye contact while giving the instruction.

    2. Secondary prevention.

        a. Medications.

        b. Nonpharmacologic interventions.

            (1) Parent training.

                (a) Preferential seating.

                (b) Homework book.

                (c) Home/school communication.

                (d) Organizational skills.

                (e) Concrete reinforcement.

                (f) Tutoring.

    3. Tertiary prevention.
        a. Educational consultant.
        b. Individualized education program.
C. Clinical procedures.
    1. Assessment of current concerns including home and school issues.
    2. Review of current treatment and effectiveness.
    3. Physical examination.
        a. Vital signs.
        b. Growth parameters.
        c. Vision and hearing screening.
        d. Respiratory, cardiac, and neurologic systems.
    4. Medication trial.
        a. Trial over several weeks.
        b. Obtain written feedback from classroom teacher each week of the trial.
        c. Obtain parent and patient verbal feedback.
        d. Review of side effects.
        e. Schedule follow-up appointment after completion of the trial.
    5. Stimulants: Ritalin, Dexedrine, Adderall, and Cylert.
        a. Titration of medication is needed to determine the optimal dose.
        b. Effective for up to 90% of children with ADHD; improves symptoms of inattention, hyperactivity, and impulsivity.
        c. Side effects.
            (1) Stomachache, decreased appetite, rebound headache, increased heart rate and blood pressure, tics, irritability, exacerbation of moodiness, sleep difficulties, and slowing of growth.
            (2) Ritalin has rare side effects of neutropenia, thrombocytopenia, and eosinophilia.
            (3) Cylert has a risk of chemical hepatitis and rare fulminant liver failure. Monitoring of liver function is recommended, but does not predict the onset of hepatitis or liver failure.
        d. Ritalin, Dexedrine, and Adderall are Schedule II controlled substances and must be prescribed according to state law.
    6. Nonstimulant medication if contraindicated, poor responder, or serious side effects from stimulants.
    7. Antihypertensive agents: clonidine (Catapres), and guanfacine (Tenex).
        a. Treats symptoms of overactivity, overreactivity, and impulsivity.
        b. Used in combination with stimulants to limit rebound and insomnia.
        c. Side effects.
            (1) Sedation, lethargy, hypotension, orthostatic signs, headache, constipation, EKG changes, and arrhythmias.
            (2) Monitoring includes regular labs, CBC with differential and chemistry panel, and EKG.
    8. Tricyclic antidepressants: desipramine (Norpramine), imipramine (Tofranil), amitriptyline (Elavil), clomipramine (Anafranil), and nortriptyline (Pamelor).

        a. Improve mood and decrease hyperactivity.

        b. Improve attention, but less effective than stimulants.

        c. Side effects.

           (1) Cardiotoxicity requiring regular EKG monitoring.

           (2) Anticholinergic effects, blood dyscrasias, drowsiness, sleep changes, headache, stomachache, anxiety, dizziness, and orthostatic hypotension.

    9. Bupropion (Wellbutrin).

        a. Improves ADHD symptoms and conduct problems.

        b. Side effects.

           (1) Agitation, dry mouth, insomnia, headache, weight loss, nausea, vomiting, constipation, tremor, and rash.

D. Collaboration/resource identification and referral.

    1. Psychologic interventions.

        a. Identify providers with expertise working with children and families with ADHD.

        b. Implementation of therapy must be behavioral approach; cognitive therapy is not effective for children with ADHD.

        c. Goals of therapy.

           (1) Provide emotional support.

           (2) Improve the parent-child relationship.

           (3) Behavior management strategies to increase appropriate behavior.

           (4) Provision of successful environmental manipulation, decreasing external stimuli, reducing alternatives, encouraging desired patterns of behaviors, and controlling diet (Whaley and Wong, 1997).

E. Care management.

    1. Management over the long term has the greatest impact on outcome.

    2. Monitoring performance of the child's functioning in the family, the community, in school, and with peers.

    3. Goals of treatment.

        a. Educate the child, family, and classroom teacher about the child's ADHD and related problems.

        b. Set achievable goals and reasonable expectations.

        c. Increase structure and positive feedback.

        d. Improve academic achievement.

        e. Improve home behavior and family relations.

F. Patient education.

    1. Basic information about ADHD.

        a. No medical test available to confirm diagnosis.

        b. ADHD does not result from poor parenting.

        c. ADHD symptoms are beyond the control of the child.

    2. Treatment involving counseling and medications can be effective.

    3. Medication effects and side effects.

        a. Periodic trial off medications to assess current effect.

    4. Frequency of follow-up visits.

    5. Keep all medications in a secure location to decrease the risk of abuse or overdose.

G. Advocacy.

  1. Support parent as ultimate child advocate.

  2. Children with ADHD may receive special services at schools that are protected by federal laws.

    a. Individuals with Disabilities Education Act of 1990 (IDEA) (PL 101-476).

      (1) Established the principle of free, appropriate education in the least restrictive environment for all children with disabilities, the right to due process, appropriate assessment, and that each child with a disability have an Individualized Education Plan.

      (2) Children with ADHD are eligible for special services if they meet the criteria of "other health impaired"(defined as any acute or chronic condition that results in limited alertness and thereby impairs educational performance), "learning disabled," or "emotionally disturbed." The child is eligible for special services if the ADHD has a significant impact on the child's education.

    b. Section 504 of the Rehabilitation Act of 1973 (PL 93-112) and (Gearheart, Weishahm, and Gearheart, 1996).

      (1) Provides that individuals with disabilities cannot be discriminated against in any program or activity receiving federal funds.

      (2) Allows for classroom accommodations for children whose disability is causing problems that are not specifically academic.

      (3) Children with ADHD may have accommodations such as repeating instructions, modified tests or homework, daily school-home notes, extra time to complete assignments, typed rather then handwritten assignments, or teacher-checked assignment books.

  3. Children and Adults with Attention Deficit Hyperactivity Disorder (CHADD) (http://www.chadd.org) CHADD, 8181 Professional Place, Suite 201, Landover, MD 20785, 1-800-233-4050.

    a. National organization with local chapters.

    b. Four primary objectives.

      (1) Maintain a support network for parents.

      (2) Provide a forum for continuing education.

      (3) Be a community resource for information about ADHD.

      (4) Make the best educational experience available to children.

  4. Educational consultants.

    a. Perform academic testing.

    b. Assist parents in advocating for appropriate educational interventions.

H. Telephone practice.

  1. Current concerns or problem.

  2. Current medications, review of side effects and current serum levels or compliant with serum monitoring.

     3. Other confounding factors.
       a. Substitute teacher, difficult academic work, peer conflicts.
       b. Change in home routine, change in sleep habits, recent illness.
     4. What interventions have been tried thus far and results.
     5. Recommendations for discussion with counselor.
I. Communication/documentation.
     1. Current medication dose, effects, side effects, and serum monitoring.
     2. Presenting problem and what parents have tried to improve symptoms.
     3. Current involvement in counseling.
     4. In addition to documenting in chart, verbally communicate with physician.
J. Outcome management.
     1. Parent and child report of progress.
     2. Report cards and comments on behavior.
     3. Rating scales, which are scored and can be compared to document progress.
     4. Teacher feedback during parent conferences.
K. Protocol development/usage.
     1. Treatment protocols are developed based on review of literature.
     2. There are ongoing studies comparing medication effectiveness and counseling treatment strategies.

REFERENCES

AAP Task Force on Infant Sleep Position and Sudden Infant Death Syndrome (2000): Changing concepts of sudden infant death syndrome: implications for infant sleeping environment and sleep position. *Pediatrics* 105(3):650-656.

AAP Task Force on Newborn and Infant Hearing (1999): Newborn and infant hearing loss: Detection and intervention. *Pediatrics* 103(2):527-530.

American Academy of Pediatrics (1997): *Guidelines for health and supervision III,* ed 3. Elk Grove Village, IL: The Association.

Adams RJ (1994): Neurologic complications. In Embury S H, Hebbel R P, Mohandas N, Steinberg MH, editors: *Sickle cell disease: basic principles and clinical practice.* New York: Raven Press, pp. 599-622.

Adams RJ, McKie VC, Hsu L, et al. (1998): Prevention of a first stroke by transfusions in children with sickle cell anemia and abnormal results on transcranial Doppler ultrasonography. *N Engl J Med* 339:5-11.

Al-Salem AH, Nourallah H (1997): Sequential endoscopic/laparoscopic management of cholelithiasis and choledocholithiasis in children who have sickle cell disease. *J Pediatr Surg* 10:1432-1435.

Al-Salem AH, Qaissruddin S (1998): The significance of biliary sludge in children with sickle cell disease. *Pediatr Surg Int* 13:14-16.

American Academy of Pediatrics (1997): *Guidelines for health supervision III,* ed 3. Elk Grove Village, IL: American Academy of Pediatrics.

American Academy of Pediatrics Committee on Infectious Diseases (January 2000): Recommended childhood immunization schedule—United States, January-December 2000. *Pediatrics* 105(1):148-151.

American Psychiatric Association (1994): *Diagnostic and statistical manual of mental disorders,* ed 4. Washington, DC: American Psychiatric Association.

Ander DS, Vallee PA (1997): Diagnostic evaluation for infectious etiology of sickle cell pain crisis. *Am J Emerg Med* 15:290-292.

Barness LA, editor (1993): *Pediatric nutrition handbook.* Elk Grove Village, IL: American Academy of Pediatrics.

Bickley LS, Hoekelman RA (1999): *Bate's guide to physical examination and history taking,* ed 7. Philadelphia: Lippincott Williams & Wilkins.

Biederman J, Faraone SV, Keenan K, et al. (1992): Further evidence for family-genetic risk factors in attention deficit hyperactivity disorder. *Arch Gen* 49:728-738.

Boynton RW, Dunn ES, Stephens GR (1998): *Manual of ambulatory pediatrics,* ed 4. Philadelphia: JB Lippincott.

Brown FR, Voigt RG, Elksnin N (1996): AD/HD: A neurodevelopmental perspective. *Contemporary Pediatrics* 13:25-44.

Buchanan GR (1994): Infection. In Embury SH, Hebbel RP, Mohandas N, Steinberg MH, editors: *Sickle cell disease: basic principles and clinical practice.* New York: Raven Press, pp. 567-588.

Burns CE, Barber N, Brady MA, Dunn AM (1996): *Pediatric primary care: a handbook for nurse practitioners.* Philadelphia: WB Saunders.

Colson ER, Dworkin PH (1997): Toddler development. *Pediatr Rev* 18(8)255-259.

Day SW, Brunson GE, Wang WC (1997): Successful newborn sickle cell trait counseling program using health department nurses. *Pediatr Nurs* 23(6):557-561.

Eckman JR (1996): Leg ulcers in sickle cell disease. *Hematol Oncol Clin North Am* 10(6):1333-1344.

Embury SH, Hebbel RP, Mohandas N, Steinberg MH, editors (1994): *Sickle cell disease: basic principles and clinical practice.* New York: Raven Press.

Ferber R (1985): *Solve your child's sleep problems.* New York: Simon & Schuster.

Fox JA, editor (1997): *Primary health care of children.* St. Louis: Mosby.

Garganta C, Seashore MR (2000): Universal screening for congenital hearing loss. *Pediatr Ann* 29(5):302-308.

Gearheart B, Weishahn M, Gearheart C (1996): *The exceptional student in the regular classroom.* Englewood Cliffs, NJ: Prentice Hall.

Green M, Palfrey JS, editors(2000): *Bright futures: guidelines for health supervision of infants, children, and adolescents,* ed 2. Arlington, Va: National Center for Education in Maternal and Child Health.

Gribbons D, Zahr LK, Opas SR (1995) Nursing management of children with sickle cell disease: an update. *J Pediatr Nurs* 10(4):232-242.

Hakim LS, Hashmat AE, Macchia RJ (1994): Priapism. In Embury SH, Hebbel RP, Mohandas N, Steinberg MH, editors: *Sickle cell disease: basic principles and clinical practice.* New York: Raven Press, pp. 633-644.

Jackson PL, Vessey JA (1996): *Primary care of the child with a chronic condition.* St. Louis: Mosby.

Johnson CP, Blasco PA (1997): Infant growth and development. *Pediatr Rev* 18(7):224-242.

Lane PA (1996): Sickle cell disease. *Pedatr Clin North Am* 43(3):639-664.

Lieh-Lai M, Asi-Bautista M, Ling-McGeorge K (1995): *The pediatric acute care handbook.* Boston: Little, Brown.

Lowenberg ME (1993): Development of food patterns in young children. In Pipes P, editor: *Nutrition in infancy and childhood,* ed 5. St. Louis: Mosby.

McVie VC (1998): Sickle cell anemia in children: Practical issues for the pediatrician. *Pediatr Ann* 27(8):521-524.

Mercugliano M, Power T, Blum N (1999): *The clinician's practical guide to attention-deficit/ hyperactivity disorder.* Baltimore: Brooks.

Morris SE (1992): Eating readiness cues: introducing supplemental foods. *Pediatr Basics* 61:2-7.

National Asthma Education and Prevention Program (1997): *Expert panel report 2: guidelines for the diagnosis and management of asthma.* National Institutes of Health, Pub. No. 97-4051. Bethesda, MD: Author.

National Heart, Lung, and Blood Institute (1998): *Global initiative for asthma: pocket guide for asthma management and prevention.* National Institutes of Health, Pub. No. 96-3659B. Bethesda, MD: Author.

National Heart, Lung, and Blood Institute (1995): *Management and therapy of sickle cell disease,* ed 3, National Institutes of Health Pub. No. 95-2117. Bethesda, MD: Author.

National Heart, Lung, and Blood Institute (1995): *Nurses: partners in asthma care.* National Institutes of Health, Pub. No. 95-3308. Bethesda, MD: Author.

National High Blood Pressure Education Program Working Group on Hypertension Control in Children and Adolescents (1996): Update on the 1987 Task Force report on high blood pressure in children and adolescents: A working group report from the Mation High Blood Pressure Education Program. *Pediatrics* 98(4):649-658.

Needlman RD (2000): Growth and development. In Behrman RE, Kliegman RM, Jenson HB, editors: *Nelson textbook of pediatrics,* ed 16. Philadelphia: WB Saunders, pp. 61-65.

Platt OS (1997): The febrile child with sickle cell disease: a pediatrician's quandary. *J Pediatrics* 130(5):693-694.

Platt OS, Brambilla DH, Rosse WF, et al. (1994): Mortality in sickle cell disease: life expectancy and risk factors for early death. *N Engl J Med* 330:1639-1644.

Schmitt BD (1999): *Pediatric telephone advice,* ed 2. Philadelphia: Lippincott-Raven.

Steinberg MH (1999): Management of sickle cell disease. *N Engl J Med* 340(13):1021-1030.

Sturner RA, Howard BJ (1997a): Preschool development 1: Communicative and motor aspects. *Pediatr Rev* 18(9):291-301.

Sturner RA, Howard BJ (1997a): Preschool development part 2: psychosocial/behavioral development. *Pediatr Rev* 18(10):327-336.

US Department of Agriculture: Food pyramid for young children. [On-line]. Available: www.usda.gov/cnpp/KidsPyra/index.htm

US Department of Health and Human Services Office of Disease Prevention: Health Promotion Office of Public Health and Science (1998): *Clinician's handbook of preventive services: put prevention into practice,* ed 2. McLean, Va: International Medical Publishing.

US Department of Health and Human Services Public Health Services (1993a): Sickle cell disease in newborns and infants: a guide for parents (Vol. #AHCPR 93-0564).

US Department of Health and Human Services Public Health Services (1993b): Sickle cell disease: Comprehensive screening and management in newborns and infants. *Quick reference guide for clinicians: No. 6* (Vol. #AHCPR 93-0563).

US Department of Health and Human Services Public Health Services (1993c): Sickle cell disease: screening, diagnosis, management and counseling in newborns and infants. *Clinical practice guideline: No. 6* (Vol. #AHCPR 93-0562).

Vichinsky EP, Styles LA, Colangelo LH, Wright EC, Castro O, Nickerson B, and The Cooperative Study of Sickle Cell Disease (1997): Acute chest syndrome in sickle cell disease: clinical presentation and course. *Blood* 89(5):1787-1792.

Whaley LF, Wong DL (1997): *Essentials of pediatric nursing,* ed 5. St Louis: Mosby.

Wong DL (1999): *Whaley & Wong's nursing care of infants and children,* ed 6. St. Louis: Mosby.

13 Women's Health/ Gynecology

SUZANNE NELSON, MS, RN, C, CNA
MARGARET B. HOUGH, MHSA, BSN, RN
LINDA S. PASKIEWICZ, PhD, CNM, RN

PATIENT PROTOTYPES

Normal Prenatal and Postpartum Care ■ High-Risk Obstetrics ■ Perimenopause and Menopause ■ Sexually Transmitted Infections

OBJECTIVES

Study of the information presented in this chapter will enable the learner to:

1. Understand the care provided for the normal prenatal female.
2. Be able to differentiate care of the normal from the high-risk prenatal patient.
3. Describe the care provided for the menopausal female.
4. Describe the prevention and treatment of sexually transmitted infections.

■■ This chapter is designed to give an overview of ambulatory women's care, specifically related to the care of the normal and high-risk prenatal female, the menopausal female, and prevention and treatment of sexually transmitted infections. The scope of ambulatory women's health care offers opportunities to provide individualized, comprehensive nursing care to women of all ages from the onset of menses through the completion of menopause. Many women see only their obstetrics and gynecology provider for health care during their childbearing years. However, women also need information about cancer warning signs, adult immunizations, Pap smears, blood pressure, sexually transmitted infection (STI) prevention, and additional health promotion information. Professional nurses in women's health care provide many facets of nursing care, including patient assessment, education, counseling, prevention of diseases and complications, diagnosis, treatment, and evaluation of care.

NORMAL PRENATAL AND POSTPARTUM CARE

Initial assessment and care should occur within a family-centered focus and may take place before or during pregnancy. Family-focused care provides patients and families with resources and information that promotes informed decision making and active participation in their plan of care. Professional nurses assist individuals and families to:

- Identify, determine, and meet individualized health goals.
- Understand and cope with the impact of pregnancy and parenthood.
- Increase feelings of confidence and self worth.

A. Assess/screen/triage: It is recommended that the initial assessment take place before conception, but not later than the 12th week of pregnancy.

  1. Preconception care is the care provided to the nonpregnant female who is trying to conceive. Assessment and interventions will focus on achieving optimal maternal health before pregnancy and evaluating risk factors associated with maternal health status and genetic risk factors in maternal and paternal families.

  2. Prenatal care is the care provided to the pregnant female before childbirth.

  3. Perinatal care is the care provided to a woman and her family during pregnancy, delivery, and the postpartum period, up to 6 weeks after the delivery.

  4. Postpartum care is provided after delivery.

  5. Initial assessment for preconception or prenatal care includes:

    a. Genetic history incorporates assessment of the patient, her partner, and their biologic families for any history of having a child with a genetic anomaly. Maternal age over 35 increases the risk for some genetic anomalies (DiDona and Marks, 1996). Ethnic background may increase risks of some inherited diseases.

      (1) Italian, Greek, or Mediterranean background increases risk for beta thalassemia.

      (2) Alpha thalassemia is found most often in African Americans and Southeast Asians.

      (3) Sickle cell disease or trait is found primarily in African American families.

      (4) Tay-Sach's disease is primarily found in families of Jewish descent.

      (5) Hemophilia.

      (6) Muscular dystrophy.

      (7) Cystic fibrosis.

      (8) Huntington's chorea.

      (9) Mental retardation (if yes, was person tested for fragile X factor).

      (10) Other inherited or chromosomal disorder.

      (11) Neural tube defects, such as spina bifida.

      (12) Down syndrome.

    (13) More than three first trimester pregnancy losses, any second or third trimester pregnancy losses, including stillbirths.

    (14) Medication or street drugs used since last menstrual period (if yes, specific drugs and dosages).

  b. Family medical histories of patient, partner, and their biologic families (if positive, which family member affected). This assessment is used to predict relative risks of diseases and complications for the pregnant patient and her fetus (American Academy of Pediatrics [AAP] and American College of Obstetricians and Gynecologists [ACOG], 1997).

    (1) Diabetes.

    (2) Hypertension.

    (3) Heart disease.

    (4) Rheumatic fever (in patient).

    (5) Kidney disease/urinary tract infection.

    (6) Nervous or mental disorders.

    (7) Seizure disorder (date of most recent seizure, if present in patient).

    (8) Liver disease/hepatitis.

  c. Personal medical history.

    (1) Blood type and Rh. A woman who is Rh negative may form antibodies to Rh positive blood if her fetus is Rh positive.

    (2) Thyroid dysfunction.

    (3) Major accidents/trauma.

    (4) Blood transfusions may have exposed the patient to serious bloodborne diseases, such as hepatitis or HIV.

    (5) Environmental exposures.

    (6) Tuberculosis.

    (7) Asthma.

    (8) Allergies (especially to medications).

    (9) Surgeries (include history of complications).

    (10) Abnormal Pap smears. Abnormal cells in the cervix may be stimulated by pregnancy hormones to increase their growth rate.

    (11) Uterine abnormality.

    (12) Infertility.

    (13) Diethylstilbestrol (DES) exposure. This drug was used to prevent preterm labor and miscarriage in the past. Women born to mothers who took this drug in pregnancy have increased risks of cervical and uterine abnormalities. There is some evidence of increased rates of infertility in both men and women exposed to this drug in utero. The drug is currently used to treat menopausal symptoms and as palliative treatment in metastatic breast and prostate cancer (Niebyl and Kochenour, 1999).

    (14) Tobacco/smoking. Smoking cigarettes is a risk factor for intrauterine growth retardation (Novak and Broom, 1999).

(15) Alcohol use has a negative effect on the fetus. Heavy alcohol use may result in fetal alcohol syndrome (Novak and Broom, 1999).

(16) Recreational or street drugs. Cocaine use can restrict small blood vessels in the placenta and is associated with placental abruption, premature labor, and fetal death. Intravenous drug use increases risks of infections such as hepatitis and HIV (Novak and Broom, 1999).

(17) History of infections such as hepatitis, tuberculosis, HIV, viral infections since last menstrual period, previous child born with Group B streptococcal infection (Novak and Broom, 1999).

(18) Sexually transmitted infections (STIs), including human papilloma virus (HPV), gonorrhea (GC), chlamydia, syphilis, and genital herpes.

(19) Immunizations. Rubella and varicella in the pregnant mother often produce life-threatening risks to the developing fetus. Immunizations can prevent these risks.

d. Obstetric history.

(1) Number of past pregnancies (gravidity).

(2) Pregnancy outcome (parity) includes children born, premature births, abortions, and living children.

(3) History of pregnancy complications such as pregnancy-induced hypertension, premature labor and delivery.

(4) Birth outcomes including birth weight, gestational age at birth, health of newborn, labor, and postpartum complications.

(5) History of postpartum depression.

e. Social history is assessed to determine how pregnancy and child rearing may be affected by the following factors:

(1) Career/job.

(2) School.

(3) Family responsibilities.

(4) Cultural background.

(5) Expectations (i.e., childbearing).

(6) Acceptable family size.

(7) Domestic violence/abuse.

f. Family planning assessment will include:

(1) Birth control. What has the patient used in the past and what are her plans for the future?

(2) Ovulation/menstrual cycle.

(3) Previous pregnancies/outcomes.

g. Prenatal screening.

(1) ABO and Rh blood type. A woman who is Rh negative may form antibodies to Rh positive blood if her fetus is Rh positive. Antibody screens are performed during pregnancy and at delivery.

(2) Triple screen testing, including alpha fetal protein. This test, done at 15 to 19 weeks gestation, assesses relative risk for some

birth defects including Down syndrome and neural tube defects.

    (3) Ultrasound scans assess normal structural development of the fetus.

    (4) Fetal heart tones are assessed for rate and regularity.

    (5) Uterine height measurement is an indicator of fetal growth.

    (6) Measurement of maternal weight gain/loss.

    (7) Urine screening. Glucose in the urine may be an indicator of developing gestational diabetes. Protein in the urine may be an indicator of developing pregnancy-induced hypertension or infection.

    (8) Blood pressure monitoring.

    (9) Other screening based on risk assessment (TB, HIV).

B. Primary/secondary/tertiary prevention.

  1. Primary prevention for women who are newly pregnant or considering pregnancy includes:

    a. Early diagnosis of pregnancy allows interventions that can promote a healthier pregnancy outcome.

    b. Early and continuous prenatal care to improve pregnancy outcomes. Problems can be identified, and behavioral changes initiated to decrease risk factors.

    c. Nutrition during pregnancy—directly affects birth weight and developing fetus (ACOG, 1997; Newton, 1999).

      (1) Prepregnancy weight obtained.

      (2) Weight gain at each visit is measured with the goal of gaining an appropriate amount of weight to support the growing fetus and placenta.

    d. Poor nutrition, with resulting low birth weight correlates to related birth incidence of:

      (1) Perinatal mortality.

      (2) Childhood learning problems.

      (3) Neural tube and other neurologic defects (related to folic acid deficiency).

      (4) Hearing and visual defects.

      (5) Mental retardation.

      (6) Small head circumference.

    e. General nutritional needs during pregnancy (must be based on the individual). Increased caloric and protein intake emphasized.

      (1) 2500 calories/day is the minimal recommendation (to include 60 g of protein, 10 g more than the nonpregnant woman).

      (2) Vitamin D and calcium needs are increased during pregnancy.

      (3) Iron supplement.

      (4) Vitamin supplement.

      (5) Folic acid supplement.

  2. Secondary prevention during pregnancy includes:

    a. Concurrent screening for complications.

b. Gestational diabetes. Urine dipstick at all encounters.

c. Hypertensive disorders. Screen for proteinuria, elevated blood pressure at all encounters.

d. Miscarriage is the spontaneous loss of a pregnancy before the fetus can survive outside the uterus (viability). Approximately 20% of all women who become pregnant will experience a miscarriage during a pregnancy. Abortion is defined as any fetal loss, spontaneous or induced, prior to viability (Novak and Broom, 1999).

e. Threatened abortion symptoms include cramping and bleeding.

f. Inevitable abortion is fetal loss that will occur regardless of medical interventions.

g. Missed abortion occurs when an intrauterine fetal demise is identified without the expulsion of the products of conception from the uterus.

h. Incompetent cervix and possible treatment with cerclage.

i. Hydatidiform mole.

j. Ectopic pregnancy includes any pregnancy occurring outside the uterus, whether it is in the fallopian tube, the abdominal cavity, or elsewhere (Novak and Broom, 1999). Symptoms include abdominal and shoulder pain, cramping, and possible bleeding. Ectopic pregnancy can be a life-threatening emergency and may be treated with laparoscopic surgery to remove the embryo from the fallopian tube. In some cases ectopic pregnancies are treated using methotrexate, a drug mainly used for treatment of certain types of cancer.

k. Hyperemesis gravidarum. Inability to retain food or fluids for 24 hours necessitates medical intervention.

l. Infections.
   (1) Urinary tract infections (UTIs) are common during pregnancy and should be treated rapidly to prevent cramping which can cause early labor.
   (2) Pyelonephritis can occur as a complication of urinary tract infection and require hospitalization.

m. Communicable diseases should be avoided, especially during pregnancy.
   (1) Cold, flu.
   (2) Tuberculosis.
   (3) Hepatitis.
   (4) HIV.
   (5) STIs.
   (6) Rubella.
   (7) Varicella.
   (8) Cytomegalovirus.
   (9) Toxoplasmosis.

n. Anemia can result is inadequate nutrition for the fetus and possible serious health problems for the patient.

        o. Amniotic fluid abnormalities, both oligohydramnios and polyhydramnios may indicate fetal health problems.

        p. Decreased fetal movement. Nurses provide education about fetal movement monitoring.

        q. Multiple pregnancy.

            (1) Referral to resources such as Mothers of Twins Clubs or dietitians for assuring adequate nutrition may be indicated.

            (2) Moderating activity levels may increase length of gestation, increase fetal weights, and decrease premature birth complications.

        r. Eclampsia.

        s. Placenta previa.

        t. Abruptio placentae.

        u. Other antepartal bleeding.

        v. Size-dates discrepancy.

        w. Premature/postdates pregnancy.

   3. Tertiary prevention (chronic health problems compounded by pregnancy).

        a. Eating disorders.

        b. Tobacco use.

        c. Cardiac disease.

        d. Hypothyroid.

        e. Diabetes.

        f. Chronic hypertension.

        g. Neurologic disorders (multiple sclerosis).

        h. Sickle cell disease.

        i. HIV disease.

C. Clinical procedures during pregnancy may include:

   1. Ultrasound.

        a. Detects differences in tissue density by directing high frequency sound waves into tissue and measuring reflected echoes, resulting in an image of the fetus and intrauterine environment (Novak and Bloom, 1999).

        b. May be provided routinely at identified times during pregnancy.

   2. Chorionic villus sampling.

        a. Performed between 9 to 12 weeks gestation and involves the removal of chorionic cells from the placenta using a catheter through the cervix.

        b. Tests on these cells can identify the presence or absence of abnormal conditions, such as Down syndrome or spina bifida.

   3. Amniocentesis is performed during the second trimester.

        a. Amniotic fluid is removed using a thin needle placed through the abdomen into the uterus.

        b. The cells in the fluid are then tested for the presence of abnormal conditions as above.

   4. Tests that are indicators of fetal well being include:

        a. Assessment of fetal movement.

    b. Estimated fetal weight, using an ultrasound scan to measure the fetus around the head, across the head, around the abdomen, and the length of the femur.

    c. Non-stress testing, using a fetal monitor to assess fetal heart rate for acceleration with movement.

    d. Amniotic fluid index, using an ultrasound scan to estimate the amount of amniotic fluid present in the uterus in relation to the size and gestation of the fetus (Novak and Broom, 1999).

    e. Biophysical profile, using an ultrasound scan to observe fetal body movement, movement of the arms and legs, breathing movement (observing movement of the diaphragm) and the amount of amniotic fluid (APP and ACOG, 1997).

D. Care management coordination for women and their families who are at higher than normal risks due to physical or sociologic needs. Maternal support services are often provided to low-income women and their families, with or without additional pregnancy risk factors.

    1. Provider.

        a. Information shared with hospital/birthing center of choice.

        b. Utilization of specialty providers.

        c. Is home health involvement indicated?

    2. Insurance—what is covered by patient's insurance and what is not. What will out of pocket costs be to patient?

    3. Telephone triage for assessment and management of questions/problems outside scheduled visits.

    4. Case management.

        a. Assure that prenatal care meets standards set by provider and insurer.

        b. Provide education and referral to additional resources, such as social workers or dietitians, as needed.

E. Patient education for health maintenance before or during pregnancy.

    1. Nutrition.

    2. Exercise. What is the patient's normal exercise level? How could it be modified in pregnancy?

    3. Menstrual/ovulation cycle, regular or irregular.

    4. Additional patient education.

        a. Seat belt use in pregnancy.

        b. Medications that are safe to use during pregnancy.

        c. Avoid hot tubs and saunas during pregnancy.

        d. Exercise.

        e. Childbirth preparation.

        f. Selection of a physician for the new baby.

        g. Patient expectations.

            (1) Normal pregnancy.

            (2) Healthy infant.

            (3) Lifestyle changes.

            (4) Emotional changes/mood changes.

            (5) Sibling preparation for the new baby.

5. Assist patient in identification of resources/help for protecting her physical and emotional safety as needed.
6. Identification of problems and how to contact a provider 24 hours/day.
   a. Burning, pain, or bleeding with urination.
   b. Vaginal bleeding with or without pain.
   c. Persistent severe headache.
   d. Persistent severe vomiting lasting over 24 hours.
   e. Temperature above 100.6° F.
   f. Abdominal pain or painful and persistent cramping.
   g. Changes in eyesight such as blurred vision or seeing spots.
   h. Consistent persistent heartburn-like pain.
   i. Sudden swelling of face and hands.
   j. Change or decrease in fetal movement.
7. Signs and symptoms of labor. Education about contacting provider and the hospital where labor and delivery are planned.
8. Infant care/nutrition. Choose breastfeeding, bottle feeding, or plan to use combination of methods.
9. Building emotional attachments.
10. Alcohol, tobacco, recreational drugs, over-the-counter medications.
11. Birthing options, including discussion with care provider about pain relief options in labor.
12. Postpartum care and education includes:
    a. Breastfeeding/infant nutrition: resources for feeding questions may be needed.
    b. Maternal nutrition: breastfeeding requires higher nutritional intake.
    c. Exercise/rest.
    d. Infant care resources for new mothers.
    e. Birth control methods made available to patient.
    f. Postpartum checkup: emphasize the importance of assessing for return to prepregnancy state.
    g. Sexual relations: emotional and physical aspects.
    h. Plan for return to work.
    i. Plan for child care. Identification of resources in neighborhood or community.
    j. Infant vehicle safety (car seat, placement).
    k. Normal infant growth and development. Teaching resources may include books, videos, and community education classes.
    l. Family adjustments include changes for parents and siblings.
13. Maternal resources.
    a. Provider.
       (1) Physician.
       (2) Nurse midwife.
       (3) Nurse practitioner.
       (4) Staff nurse.
    b. Health educators in hospital or health center affiliated with the provider practice.
14. Family/social resources.

      a. Community-specific, such as churches, schools, and independent voluntary agencies providing services to families, such as March of Dimes, which provides resources to families of children with birth defects.

      b. Workplace-specific, such as employee health centers, exercise, stress reduction, or child care resources.

      c. Government agencies, such as local and state public health departments, that provide food, education, transportation, and linkages to local resources.

  15. Lamaze associations provide childbirth preparation classes. Many also provide support groups and classes for women returning to the workplace, breastfeeding classes, and sibling preparation classes.

  16. La Leche League provides instruction and support for breastfeeding mothers.

  17. Specialty groups and associations, especially for parents of infants with birth defects, such as cerebral palsy, or for parents with multiple births.

F. Advocacy.

  1. Provide resources when necessary: utilize community and government resources.

      a. Abuse/domestic violence often escalates during pregnancy (Novak and Broom, 1999). Caregivers should be alert to the signs and symptoms of violence and continue to ask their patients whether they are exposed to, or are at risk for violence in any of their relationships. It often takes considerable time to gain the trust of women who are abused and trust must be built before women are likely to share such personal information about themselves. Local organizations such as Safe House may provide education and resources for women and their children.

      b. Government programs, such as WIC and Maternal Support Services that identify resources for food, shelter, clothing, and transportation.

      c. March of Dimes provides resources for children with birth defects and also provides educational materials on prevention of birth defects.

      d. Home deliveries.

         (1) Help the patient to understand various risk/benefit factors to consider when choosing the appropriate place to give birth.

         (2) A care provider should be chosen carefully.

         (3) Planning/readiness for home birth: what resources will the patient and her family have available?

         (4) What factors, during labor, would indicate that hospital birth should occur?

         (5) Review birth plan with patient and family.

G. Telephone practice.

      a. Triage: are you gathering all the information you need to make an assessment?

b. Must determine if a woman needs immediate attention based on her complaints.

c. Are protocols or standards available to use in your practice site?

d. Many phone calls are related to questions about symptom management, colds, coughs, exercise, appropriate levels of activity at work and home, travel, environmental concerns (such as chemical exposures, using hair products, cat litter questions, etc.), and use of prescription medications on the developing fetus.

e. Much time is spent on allaying fears and increasing patient confidence about self-care including breastfeeding and infant feeding.

f. Information resource: the nurse is an excellent resource for information and may provide referrals to additional resources, including providers, community agencies, books, computer web sites, etc.

g. Provide reassurance. Sometimes just listening and giving reinforcing feedback may be the care the patient needs.

H. Communication/documentation.

1. Prenatal record: make available to the hospital by fax, telephone, or computer.

2. Information requirements for birth certificate: if possible, give the patient a list of information that will be asked for when she is in the hospital.

3. Hospital registration: can this be completed before admission for labor and delivery?

I. Outcome management, often kept as birth/complication studies.

1. Infant morbidity/mortality.

2. Maternal morbidity/mortality.

3. Surgical delivery: indications.

4. Perinatal/postnatal complications.

5. Patient satisfaction.

J. Patient care protocols/guidelines using algorithms for care in your practice site may include:

1. UTI. Urine culture before treatment? Antibiotics prescribed?

2. Fetal diagnostic testing. Which indicators for which type of testing?

3. Morning sickness: may include nontraditional remedies including acupressure/acupuncture.

4. When to call provider. Make sure that patients have written information about when and how to call.

5. When to go to hospital. Make sure patients have written information about when to go to the hospital and how to get there.

6. Preterm labor management.

HIGH-RISK OBSTETRICS

High-risk obstetrics is defined as the identification and care for women with an increased risk for complications of childbearing; any pregnancy in which there is a maternal or fetal factor that may adversely affect the outcome (Newton, 1999).

Women with high-risk pregnancies will have complex physiologic as well as psychosocial and cultural needs. Therefore an individualized plan of care for a high-risk woman and her family is needed.

A. Assess/screen/triage.

　　1. Risk factors identified during preconception or early prenatal care during routine assessment. Acute conditions may develop at any time regardless of identified risk status.

　　　　a. Prenatal screening includes all routine screening with additional assessment focused on specific maternal/fetal risks such as maternal age, parity, and fetal growth.

　　　　b. History of obstetric complications.

　　　　c. Preexisting medical problems (cardiac disease, diabetes).

　　　　d. Domestic violence issues.

　　2. Referral of woman to appropriate provider and level of care.

　　3. Risk assessment ongoing throughout pregnancy, labor, delivery, and postpartum.

B. Primary, secondary, tertiary prevention.

　　1. Primary prevention.

　　　　a. Educational programs on nutrition and wellness, avoidance of tobacco, substance abuse.

　　　　b. Identification of high-risk women before conception.

　　　　c. Easy access to health care including prenatal care services.

　　2. Secondary prevention.

　　　　a. Nutrition needs generally the same as uncomplicated prenatal patients, except for multiple gestation pregnancies, which require additional calories and nutrients.

　　　　b. Early identification of risk factors that affect pregnancy outcome such as maternal age, number of fetuses.

　　　　c. Concurrent screening for complications—high-risk women may be at greater risk for complications. Provision of specialty high-risk care may be provided in a high-risk practice by a perinatologist, specializing in maternal fetal medicine. Additional referral providers may include pediatric surgeons, endocrinologists, or infectious disease specialists, depending on the nature of the risk factors such as:

　　　　　　(1) Congenital defects, including genetic, such as spina bifida, and fetal heart defects.

　　　　　　(2) Fetal loss/miscarriage/abortion at various stages of pregnancy. Incompetent cervix, threatened or inevitable abortion require treatment. Additional resources include social work, psychiatric mental health services, and community support groups. Genetic counseling should be considered.

　　　　　　(3) Hypertension.

　　　　　　(4) Juvenile onset diabetes/gestational diabetes.

　　　　　　(5) Hyperemesis gravidarum.

　　　　　　(6) Premature/postdate pregnancy.

　　　　　　(7) Size-dates discrepancy.

(8) Antepartal bleeding.

(9) Other risk factors including domestic violence.

d. Signs and symptoms of complications will vary for different high-risk conditions so individualized patient education is required.

e. Planning for potential hospitalization of patient and/or infant before delivery and/or after delivery should be done with help from inpatient staff whenever possible.

3. Tertiary prevention.

a. Follow-up medical care for chronic health problems such as diabetes, hypertension.

b. Referral to social work services, substance abuse, smoking cessation programs.

c. Family planning services.

d. Postpartum follow-up, home visits.

e. Individual patient education about high-risk factors and future pregnancies.

C. Clinical procedures.

1. Procedures for high-risk women must be done at institution providing level 3 care.

2. Tests for fetal well being, (such as NSTs, biophysical profiles, etc.), as discussed under normal pregnancy, are performed more often in pregnancies identified as high risk.

3. Procedures may include intrauterine transfusion, fetal surgery, percutaneous fetal blood sampling.

D. Care management coordination involves bringing together information about all resources and care providers and sharing it with all involved parties to help all involved make informed decisions and to plan for next steps in the care of the high-risk patient and family.

1. Assures that high-risk care occurs within a level 3 institution.

2. Goals include ensuring appropriate prenatal care, education, and preparation for all services within the continuum of care.

3. Resources and care providers may include:

a. Perinatologist.

b. Other providers, including medical specialists and primary care providers and pediatric surgeons.

c. Insurance company/payer source.

d. Telephone triage.

E. Patient education: must include information specific to maternal/fetal risk factors; modification may be necessary.

1. Exercise may be modified.

2. Bed rest may be indicated.

3. Maternal expectations: are they different from normal risk women? How?

4. Indications for when to call provider or hospital may include additional signs and symptoms to watch for.

   5. Signs and symptoms of problems may include additional factors to watch for specific to the patient's high-risk condition.
   6. Infant care/nutrition: parents with anticipated feeding problems for their infant may benefit from consultation with lactation specialist and/or their pediatrician.
      a. Postpartum check up: importance of assessing for problems. Emphasize importance of follow-up visit with patient.
      b. Rest needs.
      c. Sexual relations/birth control/family planning choices.
      d. Infant care, including expectations for growth and development.
      e. Infant safety, including the choice and use of infant car seat, crib, nonflammable clothing and age-appropriate toys.
F. Advocacy.
   1. Includes for routine prenatal and postpartum care.
   2. High-risk care occurs at tertiary perinatal care center.
   3. Promote use of maternal resources.
      a. Provider.
         (1) Physician/perinatologist.
         (2) Nurse midwife/practitioner (usually transfers care to physician, but may co-manage care in some practice settings).
         (3) Staff nurses, inpatient and outpatient.
         (4) Home health, visiting nurse.
         (5) Health educators.
      b. Family/social resources.
      c. Local support/specialty groups.
      d. Genetic counseling services.
      e. Library resources.
      f. Internet resources.
G. Telephone practice.
   1. Information resource.
   2. Provide reassurance.
   3. Telemetry.
H. Communication/documentation.
   1. Outpatient medical record.
   2. Prenatal record.
   3. Hospital registration.
I. Outcome management: often kept as birth/neonatal statistics.
   1. Infant morbidity/mortality.
   2. Maternal morbidity/mortality.
   3. Perinatal/postnatal complications.
   4. Length of hospitalization, mother and infant.
   5. Birth weight of infant.
   6. Breastfeeding success.
   7. Patient satisfaction.
J. Protocol development.

    1. Algorithm for defining risk factors.
    2. Other protocols used for normal pregnancy.

PERIMENOPAUSE AND MENOPAUSE

Menopause is defined as the cessation of menses. Perimenopause is that period of time encompassing the changes leading up to and following the cessation of menstruation (Hendrix, 1997). Menopause occurs most commonly around 45 to 51 years of age. The age of menopause is genetically determined and is not related to the number of ovulations. Menopause is the result of cessation of ovulation, a normal part of aging. As the follicles age, elevation of hormones from the pituitary gland (FSH, LH) suppress ovulation. Absence of ovulation results in decreased production of gonadotropic hormones, estrogen and progesterone, by the ovary. Over time, menstrual cycles cease. Estrogen protects against several health threats, most notably heart disease and osteoporosis. Loss of these hormones, especially estrogen, causes hot flashes and other symptoms associated with menopause for most women. Menopause before age 40 is considered premature menopause. Possible causes include genetics or autoimmune disorders, and a medical evaluation is needed. Induced menopause occurs at any age after surgical removal of the ovaries or damage to ovaries after therapy such as radiation or chemotherapy. Much of the work of professional nurses working with patients in this population will consist of providing education, resources, referrals, and support for decisions made by the informed patient. Also, family life changes that occur during the perimenopause years may lead to feelings of depression. Counseling resources are often needed.

  A. Assess/screen/triage.
    1. Cause.
      a. Natural, occurring with age.
      b. Surgical.
    2. End or decreasing frequency of menstruation—length and duration of cycles, amount of bleeding.
    3. Age of onset of perimenopause, duration of symptoms.
    4. Signs and symptoms.
      a. Hot flashes/flushes.
      b. Mood swings.
      c. Sleep disorders.
      d. Vaginal dryness/itching.
      e. Decreasing hormone levels.
      f. Changes in bleeding—cycle, duration, and amount.
      g. Memory changes/difficulty concentrating.
    5. Family stability, intergenerational issues.
    6. Presence of domestic violence issues.
  B. Primary, secondary, tertiary prevention (Landwehr and Leonardi, 1997; American College of Obstetricians and Gynecologists, 1996).
    1. Primary prevention.
      a. Annual health checks.

     b. Pelvic exam.

     c. Mammogram.*

        (1) Baseline at age 35.

        (2) Every 1 to 2 years until age 50.

        (3) Annually after age 50.

        (4) Frequency based on risk factors and discussion between provider and patient.

     d. Pap smears.

     e. Cholesterol/lipid profile.

     f. Immunizations.

     g. Blood pressure check, height and weight.

     h. Kegel exercises to increase support of pelvic floor muscles.

     i. Hemoccult testing.

2. Secondary prevention: diagnostic testing for early detection and prevention of cancer, osteoporosis, heart disease, and complementary therapy.

     a. Diagnostic testing for diagnosis of menopause and early detection and prevention of diseases includes Pap smears, mammograms, blood tests, and additional procedures including:

        (1) FSH , LH (measures ovarian function).

        (2) Estradiol level.

        (3) Ultrasound: abdominal, vaginal, other.

        (4) Electrocardiograms and stress tests.

        (5) Measurement of bone density.

        (6) Endometrial biopsy.

        (7) Lipid profile.

        (8) Colonoscopy.

     b. Diet and weight management.

        (1) Dietary habits culturally and emotionally mediated.

        (2) Nutritional counseling.

        (3) Eating disorders.

     c. Complementary therapy for symptoms. Hormone replacement therapy (HRT, ERT) has varied responses by individual women and several treatment regimens may be tried before finding one that works with minimal side effects.

        (1) Estrogen replacement is used to alleviate the symptoms of perimenopause.

        (2) Estrogen is often prescribed for benefits in preventing heart disease and osteoporosis. This is becoming increasingly controversial, as the exact benefits of HRT are unclear at this time. Coronary artery disease is the number one cause of death in postmenopausal women (Hendrix, 1997). Osteoporosis ("porous bones"), is a condition which bones become weak, brittle,

*While there is a consistent agreement that screening mammograms should be done, the frequency for routine screening in a healthy population of women at various ages may vary.

and more likely to break, is a major cause of disability in older women.

(3) Progesterone is necessary for a woman who has not had her uterus removed and is given in combination with estrogen. Progesterone protects the uterus from the risk of uterine cancer caused by the effects of unopposed estrogen.

(4) Possible adverse effects from estrogen (Hendrix, 1997) include:

   (a) Endometrial hyperplasia and uterine cancer have been associated with unopposed estrogen use.

   (b) Association of estrogen to breast cancer is under investigation.

   (c) Estrogen effect is dose and duration dependent.

   (d) The addition of progesterone to estrogen has shown to decrease the occurrence of endometrial hyperplasia and cancer.

   (e) Medical history is used to determine if absolute contraindications to estrogen therapy are present.

(5) Vitamins and herbs may be used to treat perimenopausal symptoms. Educate the patient about how these substances may interact with medications (Gardner, 1999; Weed, 1999). Women must be informed of the lack of scientific evidence to support use of herb therapy.

   (a) Estrogenic herbs: anise, black cohosh, chasteberry, don quai, fennel, ginseng, red raspberry leaf, sage.

   (b) Progestogenic herbs: Mexican wild yam root, sarsaparilla.

   (c) Phytoestrogens: alfalfa, almonds, apples, cashew nuts, corn, flaxseed, lentils, licorice root, miso, oats, papaya, peanuts, peas, seaweed, soybeans, tofu, wheat.

   (d) Vitamin E (400 IU/day).

   (e) Vitamin B complex (200 mg/day).

   (f) Calcium with vitamin D (1500 mg/day) through diet or supplement.

(6) Nutrition/diet: possible referral to dietitian.

(7) Stress that weight-bearing exercise is valuable in helping to prevent osteoporosis and preventing disability.

(8) Vaginal creams: estrogen, herbal, moisturizing. Many women find painful intercourse relieved through use of these creams.

(9) Oatmeal baths (ease vaginal itching).

3. Tertiary prevention.

   a. Annual well woman physical exams including breast and pelvic exams.

   b. Annual health screening procedures as needed such as mammography.

   c. Attendance at exercise programs.

   d. Patient education programs, including nutrition and weight control, domestic violence awareness available at the community level.

      e. Support groups for intergenerational caregivers, parenting.
C. Care management.
    1. Provider.
    2. Other caregivers, as listed previously.
    3. Insurance/payer source.
    4. Telephone triage.
D. Patient education.
    1. Care options and choices to be made.
    2. Symptom management.
        a. Optimizing health, preventing disease and complications.
        b. Managing lifestyle expectations.
    3. Use of appropriate resources.
        a. Provider, which includes physician, nurse midwife, nurse practitioner, staff nurses, home health and visiting nurse, health educator.
        b. Family/social resources.
        c. Local support/specialty groups.
        d. Library resources.
        e. Internet resources.
        f. Dietitian.
        g. Counseling/psychiatry.
        h. Social work.
E. Telephone practice.
        a. Determine need for immediate care. For example, identify women who need immediate attention, such as postmenopausal bleeding.
        b. Adjust dosages of prescription and nonprescription medications, vitamins, and food supplements according to protocols.
        c. Advise about testing and treatment options.
        d. Answer questions about general health, mental health, exercise, fitness, and symptom management.
        e. Discuss test results.
        f. Serve as an information resource.
        g. Provide referrals.
        h. Provide reassurance.
F. Advocacy.
    1. Promote awareness of risk/benefit of available therapy.
    2. Provide resources when necessary.
        a. Abuse/domestic violence.
        b. Depression.
        c. Counseling.
    3. Make referrals when needed.
    4. Encourage patient participation in education to promote informed consent about treatment options.
G. Communication/documentation.
    1. Patient medical record.
    2. Telephone/advice documentation.
    3. Written notification to patient of test results such as mammograms.

    H. Outcome measurement.

        1. Early detection rate of cancer, osteoporosis, heart disease.

        2. Risk reduction of cancer, osteoporosis, and heart disease.

        3. Symptom management.

            a. Reported patient satisfaction.

            b. Number of return visits.

            c. Continued use of ERT/HRT.

  I. Protocol development.

        1. Relief of menopausal symptoms/HRT and nonmedical interventions.

        2. Components and frequency of well woman screening.

        3. Other signs/symptoms of disease.

            a. Heart disease.

            b. Cancer.

            c. Hypertension.

            d. Mental health.

            e. Osteoporosis.

SEXUALLY TRANSMITTED INFECTIONS

Sexually transmitted infections (STIs) are very common, affecting one in four adults in the United States. STIs affect women of all social and income levels. Women are at greater risk of being infected than men, and younger women are at greater risk than older. Women may develop health problems associated with STIs, such as infections spreading to the uterus and fallopian tubes leading to pelvic inflammatory disease (PID), a major cause of female infertility and ectopic pregnancy. Human papillomavirus (HPV) infections increase the risk of cervical cancer. HIV can be sexually transmitted and upon progression to AIDS, may cause numerous debilitating symptoms and lead to death (Centers for Disease Control and Prevention [CDC], 1998). Prevention of STIs is a major nursing focus when caring for any sexually active female. Communication between a woman and her sexual partner about sexual history and STIs is of primary importance. Counseling about testing for HIV and other STIs is one way that a professional nurse can make a difference in the long-term health status of their patients. Providing reassurance about the confidential nature of the patient's treatment/testing is critical in gaining the trust of your patient and allowing her to share information necessary to develop a plan of care to meet her needs.

  A. Assess/screen/triage.

        1. Determine the level of sexual risk.

            a. Number of sexual partners.

            b. Partner history of STIs.

            c. Personal history of STIs.

            d. History of abnormal Pap smears.

            e. Condom use.

        2. Determine presence of partner violence.

        3. Signs and symptoms of STIs. (Many STIs have no symptoms.)

            a. Vaginal burning, itching.

       b. Unusual vaginal discharge.

       c. Chancre or vaginal, perianal lesions.

       d. Rash.

       e. Acute discomfort/pain.

       f. Foul smelling discharge.

4. Diagnosis.

       a. Vaginal/pelvic exam.

       b. Culture.

       c. Slide prep.

       d. Pap smear.

       e. Colposcopy.

       f. Biopsy.

       g. Blood tests.

5. Treatment depends on the causative agent. Bacterial infections, such as gonorrhea, chlamydia, and syphilis, can be cured with antibiotics. Viral infections, such as HPV, herpes, and HIV, cannot be cured. Medications can be taken to control the symptoms, but there is no way to completely remove the virus from the body.

       a. Appropriate antibiotic(s).

       b. Antivirals.

       c. Antifungals.

       d. Ensure partner treatment.

B. Primary/secondary/tertiary prevention.

   1. Primary prevention.

       a. Annual health checks.

          (1) Pelvic exam.

          (2) Pap smear.

          (3) Other tests as indicated.

       b. Patient education.

          (1) Communication with sexual partner.

          (2) Abstinence.

          (3) Barrier protection using condoms, female condoms, spermicides, diaphragm.

          (4) Signs and symptoms (and prevalence of infections with no symptoms).

   2. Secondary prevention.

       a. Education.

          (1) Individualized teaching, tailored to the patient.

          (2) Include specific actions the patient can take.

          (3) Use effective communication skills.

          (4) Use all opportunities for proactive interviewing.

       b. Detection of asymptomatically infected persons.

       c. Detection of symptomatic persons unlikely to seek diagnosis and treatment.

       d. Effective diagnosis and treatment, counseling to complete treatment.

       e. Evaluation, testing, treatment, and counseling of sex partners.

  f. Preexposure vaccination if at risk for:
   (1) Hepatitis B.
   (2) Hepatitis A.
  g. Reporting requirements.
   (1) According to state law.
   (2) Reports are maintained in strictest confidentiality.
   (3) Most states require public health officials to verify diagnosis and treatment.
 3. Tertiary prevention.
  a. Assisted life style changes.
  b. Reinfection prevention education.
  c. Long-term effects.
   (1) Infertility.
   (2) Fetal risk.
   (3) Death.
  d. Support groups for women with herpes, HIV.
C. Clinical procedures.
 1. Pelvic/penile exam for patient and partner.
 2. Blood tests.
 3. Biopsy.
 4. Microscopy, including wet prep for Trichomonas, yeast, and WBCs.
D. Care management.
 1. Providers.
 2. Health clinics.
 3. Insurance/payer source.
 4. Telephone triage.
E. Patient education: see under Primary/secondary/tertiary prevention section B on page 235.
F. Advocacy.
 1. Provide resources and referrals when appropriate.
  a. Personal provider.
   (1) Physician.
   (2) Nurse practitioner.
   (3) Certified nurse midwife.
   (4) Staff nurse.
  b. Planned Parenthood clinics and public health clinics.
  c. Family/social services/community services.
  d. Specialty groups.
  e. Library and Internet information resources.
 2. Provide education.
 3. Support patient decision-making.
G. Telephone practice.
 1. Information resource.
 2. Triage/referrals.
 3. Provide reassurance when indicated.
 4. Maintain confidentiality.

H. Communication/documentation.
   1. Patient record.
   2. Telephone advice documentation.
   3. Number system (for confidentiality purposes) vs. names, often used for STI/HIV testing.
I. Outcome measurement.
   1. Early detection and treatment rate.
   2. Risk-reducing behavior changes.
   3. Improvement in health status.
   4. Patient satisfaction.
J. Protocol development.
   1. Centers for Disease Control is a resource for protocol development. Available at: *www.cdc.gov*
   2. Areas for protocol development include:
      a. Contact mechanisms for informing patients of test results.
      b. Reporting of positive STI test protocols (usually based on government requirements). Partner identification may also be required.
      c. Diagnosis/treatment protocols for patients and partners.
      d. Domestic violence, substance abuse screening.

REFERENCES

American Academy of Pediatrics and American College of Obstetricians and Gynecologists (1997): *Guidelines for perinatal care,* ed 4. Elk Grove Village, IL: American Pediatric Association.

American College of Obstetricians and Gynecologists (1996): *Guidelines for women's health care.* Washington, DC: ACOG.

American College of Obstetricians and Gynecologists (1997): *Planning for pregnancy, birth and beyond.* New York: Signet.

Centers for Disease Control and Prevention (1998): Guidelines for treatment of sexually transmitted diseases. *MMWR* 47 (RR-1):1-118.

DiDona NA, Marks MG (1996): *Introductory maternal newborn nursing.* Philadelphia: JB Lippincott.

Gardner C (1999). Ease through menopause with homeopathic and herbal medications. *J PeriAnesthesia Nurs* 14(3):139-143.

Hendrix S (1997): Menopause. In Random S, McNeeley SG Jr, editors: *Gynecology for the primary care provider.* Philadelphia: WB Saunders, pp. 183-199.

Landwehr J, Leonardi M (1997): Preventive gynecology care. In Random S, McNeeley SG Jr, editors: *Gynecology for the primary care provider.* Philadelphia: WB Saunders, pp. 17-20.

Newton E (1999): Maternal nutrition. In Queenan JT, editor: *Management of high-risk pregnancy,* ed 4. Malden, MA: Blackwell Science, pp. 3-19.

Niebyl J, Kochenour N (1999): Medications in pregnancy and lactation. In Queenan JT, editor: *Management of high-risk pregnancy,* ed 4 Malden, MA: Blackwell Science, pp. 43-51.

Novak J, Broom B (1999): *Ingalls and Salerno's maternal and child health nursing,* ed 9. St. Louis: Mosby.

Weed S (May/June 1999). Menopause and beyond: The Wise woman way. *J Nurs Midwifery* 44 (3):267-278.

Internet Resources

American College of Obstetricians and Gynecologists—www.acog.org

Healthfinder—www.healthfinder.gov

National Mental Health Association—www.nmha.org

Centers for Disease Control—www.cdc.org

National Cancer Institute—www.cancernet.nci.nih.gov

National Domestic Violence Hotline—www.ndvh.org

National Institutes of Health—www.nih.gov

National Osteoporosis Foundation—www.nof.gov

National Women's Health Information Center—www.4woman.gov

Office of Consumer Affairs, Food and Drug Administration—www.4woman.gov

Planned Parenthood—www.plannedparenthood.org

Smart Moms, Healthy Babies—www.smartmoms.org

Resolve, Inc (Impaired fertility)—www.resolve.org

La Leche League—www.lalecheleague.org

Special Supplemental Nutrition Program for Women, Infants, and Children (WIC)—www.usda.gov/fns/wic.html

14 Male Health

DOROTHY A. CALABRESE, MSN, RN, CURN, CNP

PATIENT PROTOTYPES

Benign Prostatic Hyperplasia ▪ Prostate Cancer ▪ Impotence ▪ Testicular Cancer

OBJECTIVES

Study of the information presented in this chapter will enable the learner to:

1. Discuss common symptoms of benign prostatic hyperplasia (BPH).
2. Explain the value of the prostate specific antigen (PSA) in the diagnosis of prostate cancer.
3. Discuss the importance of testicular self-examination (TSE).
4. Describe two common treatment options for the man experiencing impotence.

Men experiencing urologic problems might be seen originally in primary care. As the symptoms change or worsen, the patient will be referred to a urologist for management or treatment of the problem. The age range for men experiencing urologic problems varies; it can include men in their teens or twenties (testicular cancer), men ranging in age from 40 to 90 (with prostate problems), or men of any age experiencing erection difficulties. Men with urologic problems rarely experience a medical emergency (acute urinary retention, priapism, and torsion of the testicle being exceptions); often their symptoms are chronic and bothersome, and the patients are seen regularly for ongoing medical evaluation of the condition. Men diagnosed with prostate cancer can be healthy men who are going through diagnosis and treatment (localized disease) or men living with the chronic problem of metastatic disease. Each of these patient types is seen at regular intervals for evaluation of their disease status, and they are evaluated when medical issues arise or changes in their condition occur.

The goal of this chapter is to discuss men's common urologic problems (benign prostatic hyperplasia [BPH], prostate cancer, impotence, and testicular cancer) and to describe the common symptoms and treatments available for each condition. Nursing interventions and educational needs of patients and families will also be addressed.

BENIGN PROSTATIC HYPERPLASIA

Benign prostatic hyperplasia (BPH) is a noncancerous enlargement of the prostate gland, which is a walnut-shaped gland located at the base of the bladder, in front of the rectum, and surrounding the urethra. The gland produces the fluid for transport of sperm during ejaculation.

A. Assess/screen/triage.
  1. The prostate is composed of muscular and glandular tissues that tighten with BPH, leading to urinary symptoms.
     a. Dysuria: painful urination as a result of enlarged prostate pushing on bladder.
     b. Weak urinary stream.
     c. Straining: difficulty starting urinary stream.
     d. Nocturia: awakening at night to urinate.
     e. Frequency: frequent urination
     f. Double voiding: sense of incomplete bladder emptying and needing to urinate soon after voiding (< 30 minutes).
     g. Terminal dribbling: involuntary postvoid dripping of urine.
     h. Urgency: difficulty postponing urination.
     i. Intermittency: interruption of stream.
     j. Urinary tract infections.
     k. Hematuria: blood in the urine.
     l. Acute urinary retention.
  2. Diagnosis of BPH.
     a. History of urinary symptoms, change/worsening of urinary symptoms.
     b. Physical examination including a digital rectal examination (DRE) to estimate the size of the prostate and determine any areas of abnormal texture or nodules (may feel larger and harder than normal prostate and may feel rubbery; may also feel normal, a rounded structure with no nodules or irregularities).
  3. Screening/triage.
     a. Assess the baseline status of patient symptoms.
     b. Evaluate the change in severity of symptoms, effect on lifestyle.
     c. If symptoms indicate that patient might be developing urinary retention, arrange for immediate appointment for catheter insertion.
B. Primary, secondary, tertiary prevention.
  1. Primary prevention: none.
  2. Secondary prevention (to maintain the integrity of the bladder and preserve function of the kidneys and ureters).
     a. Appointment for evaluation of a change in urinary symptoms.
     b. Take prescribed medications as directed.
     c. If medication not controlling symptoms, appointment to discuss surgical options.
     d. Surgery (if indicated).
  3. Tertiary prevention: none.
C. Clinical procedures.

1. Urinalysis.
   a. Detect presence of infection in the urine (white cells, + nitrites).
   b. Detect presence of blood or red cells in the urine.
2. Bladder pressure flow studies: measure urinary flow and help determine the extent of urinary blockage.
3. Residual urinary volume: measures the amount of urine left in the bladder following urination by catheterization or use of bladder scanner (noninvasive).
4. Other tests may include an intravenous pyelogram (IVP) (detect kidney damage) and a cystoscopy (directly visualize the bladder).

D. Care management.
   1. Not all patients with BPH need medical intervention.
   2. Treatment should begin when symptoms become bothersome or when the integrity of the urinary tract (kidney or bladder function) can be compromised.
   3. Treatments include:
      a. Watchful waiting.
         (1) Used with patients with mild symptoms.
         (2) Patients seen at predetermined interval (usually annually) for evaluation of symptoms.
         (3) Lifestyle changes may help decrease symptoms.
      b. Medications: generally the first line of therapy.
         (1) Alpha-blocker drugs (Minipress, Hytrin, Cardura, Flomax) relax the muscles in the prostate and may relieve part of the urinary blockage.
         (2) Proscar (finasteride) can cause the prostate to shrink.
      c. Surgery: provides relief of symptoms but is not a cure. Transurethral resection of the prostate (TURP)—the most common surgery performed on American men. Transurethral incision of the prostate (TUIP)—often used when the prostate is small to moderately enlarged.
         (1) Laser surgery to destroy prostate tissue (long-term effects not known).
         (2) Thermal therapy (Prostatron)—use of microwave energy to destroy prostate tissue (long-term effects not known).

E. Patient education.
   1. Symptoms or change of BPH symptoms that necessitate follow-up appointment (e.g., an increase in nocturia from 1x to 2x per night).
   2. Lifestyle changes that may help decrease urinary symptoms.
      a. Limit alcohol, table salt, caffeine, and spicy foods.
      b. Limit the amount of fluids taken after dinner.
      c. Taking time to empty the bladder completely.
      d. Not allowing long intervals to pass without voiding. Recognizing medications that might affect the prostate: cough and cold medications, selected tranquilizers, antidepressants, antihypertensive medications.

3. Alpha-blocker medications (Minipress, Hytrin, Cardura, Flomax) are to be taken as directed (daily or twice each day).
   a. The medications work fairly quickly if they are going to work (generally within 2 to 6 weeks) and their effects can last for several years.
   b. Side effects include: dizziness or lightheadedness, low blood pressure, headache, weakness, fatigue, retrograde ejaculation, rhinitis, and headache (Presti, 2000).
4. Proscar is to be taken daily; symptoms return if medication stopped.
   a. Benefit of medication occurs slowly (may take 3 to 6 months) and long-term administration is generally necessary.
   b. Decreases the PSA value by 50% after 6 months of treatment.
   c. Side effects include: impotence; decreased libido; decreased amount of semen ejaculated; tenderness or swelling of the breasts.
5. Surgery: provides relief of symptoms but is not a cure.
   a. With most surgeries, patient will need to have a Foley catheter for a period of time following surgery.
   b. Symptoms usually improve quickly.
   c. Surgical procedure may need to be repeated in the future.
   d. Long-term effects of laser surgery, thermal therapy not known.

F. Advocacy.
   1. Patients should be aware that a change in urinary symptoms is not necessarily a normal part of aging and changes must be evaluated.

G. Telephone practice.
   1. Triage phone calls related to changes in symptoms (reassurance, scheduling appointment for follow-up evaluation) and discuss with physician.
   2. Explanation of medications: effects and side effects, how and when to take medication.

H. Communication/documentation.
   1. Ongoing communication with physician regarding changes in patient condition.
   2. Relaying information from physician to patient, from patient to physician.
   3. Document pertinent information (change in symptoms, change in medication, or effect of medication).

I. Outcome management.
   1. Patient will have an understanding of cause of BPH and importance of notifying health care provider of significant changes in symptoms.
   2. Patient will have an understanding of treatment options available to treat BPH, the expectations of each treatment, and the side effects of the treatment.

PROSTATE CANCER

Prostate cancer is a malignant tumor of the prostate gland (which lies under the bladder neck and in front of the rectum). It is the most commonly diagnosed male cancer and is the second most common cause of male cancer deaths in the United States (ACS, 2000). Prostate cancer is often considered a disease of aging, but the advent of the PSA blood test has changed the face of prostate cancer, allowing diagnosis at an earlier curable stage in many younger men.

A. Assess/screen/triage.

1. The American Cancer Society (ACS) estimates that 180,400 men (29% of male cancers) will be diagnosed with prostate cancer and 31,900 men will die from prostate cancer (11% of male cancer deaths) in 2000 (ACS, 2000).

2. The natural history of the disease is unknown.

3. Biologic behavior and metastatic potential vary widely, leading to controversy regarding management of the disease.

4. The natural progression of the disease is unknown.

5. Risk factors include:

   a. Increasing age.

   b. Race (more common in African-American men).

   c. Familial tendency (increased risk with increased number of relatives with the disease).

   d. Environmental factors might play a part.

   e. Hormonal factors might play a part.

   f. Dietary factors appear to influence the growth of cancer (e.g., high fat diet may accelerate growth; tomatoes may inhibit growth).

   g. Vasectomy (conflicting data).

6. Symptoms.

   a. Localized disease (cancer that is contained in the prostate): none.

   b. Locally advanced disease (cancer that has spread to the structures adjacent to the prostate).

      (1) Urinary symptoms: hesitancy, dribbling, straining, dysuria (painful urination), hematuria.

      (2) Bladder outlet obstruction: acute urinary retention.

      (3) Bone pain.

   c. Metastatic disease (cancer that has spread to distant lymph nodes, bones, or other organs).

      (1) Bone pain.

      (2) Anemia.

      (3) Urinary obstruction.

7. Diagnosis: a prostate biopsy provides the only definitive diagnosis.

8. Treatment depends upon:

   a. Stage of the disease.

   b. Grade of the cancer.

   c. Patient preference.

   d. General health of the patient.

B. Primary, secondary, and tertiary prevention.

1. Primary prevention: none (although current studies are ongoing to determine if Proscar may prevent the development of prostate cancer; a clinical trial regarding the use of Vitamin E and selenium to prevent

prostate cancer may soon be started. Results of these won't be known for 5 to 7 years).

2. Secondary prevention.
   a. The American Cancer Society and the American Urologic Association recommend that men should begin regular screening for prostate cancer at age 50 (African American men and men with a family history of prostate cancer should begin screening at age 40) (Houde, 1999).
      (1) Yearly digital rectal examination (DRE).
      (2) Yearly prostate-specific antigen (PSA).
   b. An elevated PSA (> 4 ng/ml) or an abnormality on DRE will dictate need for a prostate biopsy.
   c. Positive prostate biopsy will necessitate treatment based on stage of the cancer, grade of the cancer, and preference of the patient.
3. Tertiary prevention.
   a. Management of symptoms following treatment for localized disease (surgery or radiation therapy). These might include incontinence and impotence.
   b. Management of symptoms of hormone therapy for patients with metastatic disease (including hot flashes, lethargy, decrease in libido).
   c. Routine, regularly scheduled follow-up appointments with DRE and PSA to evaluate for recurrence of cancer.
C. Clinical procedures.
   1. Diagnosis.
      a. The normal range for the PSA is 0 to 4 ng/ml.
         (1) A glycoprotein produced by the prostate gland.
         (2) While the PSA value is usually elevated in prostate cancer, it can be elevated as a result of prostatitis or BPH.
      b. DRE used to determine any abnormalities of the prostate gland.
      c. Transrectal ultrasound (TRUS) to evaluate prostate, any areas of abnormality.
      d. Prostate biopsy: identifies cancer and defines the tumor grade (aggressiveness of the tumor).
         (1) Lower the score, the less aggressive the cancer.
         (2) Higher the score, the more aggressive the cancer.
   2. Other tests might include: bone scan, CAT scan of abdomen and pelvis, or Prostascint scan to evaluate the extent of the disease.
D. Collaboration/resource identification and referral.
   1. Resources might include reading material (books and pamphlets), the Internet, other patients who have undergone treatment, support groups.
   2. Referrals might include radiation oncologist or medical oncologist.
E. Care management.
   1. Treatment options for localized prostate cancer include:
      a. Watchful waiting.
         (1) Indicated in elderly men or men with low-grade prostate cancer.

(2) Patient reevaluated at regular intervals (3 or 6 months) by PSA and DRE.
   b. Surgery: radical retropubic prostatectomy or perineal prostatectomy.
      (1) Removal of the prostate and seminal vesicles.
      (2) Postoperative incontinence and impotence occur (length of time varies) and may be temporary or permanent.
   c. Radiation therapy: external beam or seed implants.
      (1) External beam: radiation to the prostate; treatment occurs over 6 to 7 weeks.
      (2) Seed implants: radioactive seeds (e.g., ^{131}I) are implanted into the prostate under ultrasound and remain there permanently (occasionally the seeds can be expelled spontaneously via the urethra).
   d. Cryosurgery: freezing of prostate tissue to kill cancer cells.
      (1) Tissue sloughing, hematuria, inability to urinate are common effects immediately following treatment.
      (2) Incontinence and impotence are potential problems.
      (3) Long-term effects not known; patients who do not wish to undergo radiation therapy or surgical removal of prostate may consider this treatment. Cost may not be covered by insurance.

2. Treatment options for metastatic prostate cancer (rationale is to decrease the amount of testosterone produced by the body or utilized by the cancer cells) include:
   a. LHRH agonists: Lupron depot (leuprolide acetate) or Zoladex (goserelin acetate) (medical castration).
   b. Diethylstilbestrol (DES, [rarely used due to cardiovascular side effects], medical castration) decrease the production of testosterone by the testicles.
   c. Antiandrogen medications: Eulixin (flutamide), Casodex (bicaluta-mide), or Nilandron (nilutamide)—block the prostate cancer cells from utilizing circulating testosterone.
   d. Complete androgen deprivation: LHRH agonist or bilateral orchiectomy plus antiandrogen.
   e. Bilateral orchiectomy: surgical castration. Surgical removal of source of testosterone (testicles).
   f. Chemotherapy: variety of new chemotherapy options are available through clinical trials.

F. Patient education: explanation of procedures from diagnosis through treatment.
   1. Prostate biopsy.
      a. No aspirin/aspirin-containing products or anticoagulants for 7 to 10 days before procedure.
      b. May experience hematuria or blood in semen following biopsy.
      c. Restrict heavy lifting for approximately 24 hours following procedure.

2. Surgery for radical retropubic prostatectomy or perineal prostatectomy (these are general guidelines; individual urologist preferences will dictate specifics).
   a. Generally, patients can return to presurgical diet following discharge from hospital (usual stay is 2 to 5 days); liquids are encouraged, but carbonated beverages should be avoided until bowel function returns.
   b. Activity: no heavy lifting or driving the car for approximately 4 weeks after surgery; walking is strongly encouraged. Patient may need frequent rests for 2 to 4 weeks following surgery. Return to work is per physician protocol.
   c. Patient should avoid use of enemas or suppositories for approximately 4 weeks following surgery because the surgery is near the rectum; use of stool softeners and/or laxatives may be necessary.
   d. Catheter care is per routine; catheter will remain in for approximately 8 to 21 days following surgery. Following removal of the Foley catheter, pelvic muscle exercises (Kegel exercises) are often recommended to help the patient regain urine control.
3. Radiation therapy: treatment is daily for 6 to 7 weeks on Monday through Friday.
   a. Patients may experience fatigue; frequent rest may be indicated and patients will need to plan the rest periods into their day.
   b. Urinary symptoms: urgency, frequency, and painful urination.
      (1) Increase fluid intake to 8 + glasses per day.
      (2) Antibiotics as ordered if patient has a urinary tract infection.
      (3) Antispasmodic medications to relax the bladder (as indicated).
   c. Gastrointestinal symptoms: diarrhea, rectal spasms (usually resolve following completion of treatment).
      (1) Use of over-the-counter antidiarrheal medications (for example, Kaopectate or Imodium).
      (2) Use of antispasmodic medications as ordered.
      (3) Use of symptomatic treatment as necessary (e.g., sitz baths, topical creams, or ointments).
   d. Hormone therapy (Lupron depot or Zoladex).
      (1) Importance of adhering to medication schedule (every 3 to 4 months, depending on preparation used).
      (2) Side effects of medication include: hot flashes, decreased libido, gynecomastia, nausea.
      (3) Vitamin E 800 mg per day or Megace (prescription needed) may decrease intensity of hot flashes.
      (4) Report any problems or changes in condition to nurse or MD: any increase in or new bone pain (metastasis to bone), any change in urination (increased frequency, inability to start stream, decrease in urinary stream, increase in nocturia, feeling of not emptying bladder—obstruction of bladder outlet).
      (5) A patient who has metastasis to the spine and experiences

urinary incontinence or urinary retention or reports an increase in back pain and an inability to walk up or down stairs, *must* be evaluated for spinal cord compression (a medical emergency).

G. Advocacy.
   1. Individuals: importance of annual screening with DRE and PSA (age 40 for African American men or men with a family history of prostate cancer; age 50 for other men) to detect prostate cancer at early, potentially curable stage.
H. Telephone practice.
   1. Answer questions, re-explanation of information that health care provider had discussed with patient. Specific questions may include questions about treatment options, side effects of treatment options, incontinence, impotence.
   2. Triage phone calls related to side effects of treatment, change in patient condition; reinforce Kegel exercises to help regain urinary control.
   3. Assess patient understanding of "red flag" symptoms (symptoms of potentially serious problems) and what to do if these occur.
      a. Increased pain, especially back pain (think bone metastasis, spinal cord compression).
      b. Change in urination, difficulty starting stream (think bladder outlet obstruction, spinal cord compression, especially if patient is experiencing bowel symptoms along with urinary symptoms).
I. Communication/documentation.
   1. Ongoing communication with physician regarding changes in patient condition.
   2. Relaying information from physician to patient, from patient to physician.
   3. Documentation of pertinent information (change in symptoms, medications changes).
J. Outcome management.
   1. Patient will have an understanding of side effects of the treatment option and/or medication and common ways to manage those side effects.
   2. Patient will know and understand red flag symptoms (those that can have serious complications if ignored) and will know whom to contact (day or night) to report those symptoms.

ERECTILE DYSFUNCTION

Erectile dysfunction (ED) is a problem with gaining or sustaining erections sufficient for intercourse. The causes of ED can be physical, psychologic, or a combination of both. In the 1970s and 1980s, impotence was thought to be primarily a psychologic problem, but it is now known that 50% of the cases of impotence have an organic cause (Leu, 2000).

A. Assess/screen/triage.
   1. Sexuality/sexual functioning is an important part of life at all ages. When it is absent, people can feel that an important part of their life is missing.

2. The pathogenesis of ED can involve psychologic, neurologic, hormonal, arterial, or cavernosal factors.
3. Many conditions are called ED; each of these is treated differently. Some of these are:
    a. Impotence (ED): inability to achieve and maintain a firm erection.
    b. Premature ejaculation: uncontrolled ejaculation before or shortly after the vagina is entered.
    c. Retarded ejaculation: an unusually delayed ejaculation.
    d. Retrograde ejaculation: backflow of semen into the bladder during ejaculation because of incompetent bladder neck mechanics.
4. Causes of ED.
    a. Psychologic: normal erections during sleep; normal physical examination; good general health.
        (1) Causes may include anxiety, depression, anger, poor body image, stress, concern over aging, misinformation regarding sexuality.
        (2) Performance anxiety: a man may feel tremendous burden to be able to achieve erection and perform sexually.
        (3) Treatment may include sex therapy, a short-term form of counseling (5 to 20 sessions); may include reading material, exercises (such as touching exercises, practicing better sexual communication). The partner is usually a part of the treatment.
    b. Physical.
        (1) Medication-induced: most common treatable cause of erection problems. Common medications involved include sedatives, antihypertensive medications, weight control drugs, peptic ulcer medications, alcohol, nicotine, and opiates.
        (2) Blood flow abnormalities: reduce the blood flow to the penis. Causes include: hardening of the arteries, high blood pressure, diabetes, Peyronie's disease (scar tissue in the penis).
        (3) Nerve impulse abnormalities include: diabetes, strokes, spinal cord injuries, pelvic surgery, alcoholism.
        (4) Hormonal abnormalities include: kidney disease (and dialysis), liver disease, alcoholism.
5. Diagnosis.
    a. Physical examination: helpful in determining if the cause is physical.
        (1) Special attention paid to sex organs to be sure that blood vessels, nerves, and tissues of the penis are functioning normally.
        (2) Penile nerves may be evaluated to ensure adequate sensation in and around penis.
        (3) Digital rectal examination to assess for prostatitis, an inflammation of the prostate gland (can disrupt blood flow or nerve sensation in the penis).
        (4) Observation for genital abnormalities (e.g., Peyronie's disease).
    b. Laboratory tests: may be needed (for example, hormone levels, cholesterol, triglycerides, liver, kidney function, glucose).

6. Screening/triage.
   a. Ask questions in calm, matter of fact manner; recognize that many people have a difficult time discussing intimate details with health care providers.
   b. May need to ask questions in very specific, nonmedical terms.
B. Primary, secondary, tertiary prevention.
   1. Primary prevention: related to nutrition, management of general health to delay onset of medical conditions that affect erections (e.g., diabetes, hypertension).
   2. Secondary prevention.
      a. Take prescribed medication to manage underlying medical condition.
      b. Medical management of underlying medical problem to prevent further sequelae.
   3. Tertiary prevention: none.
C. Clinical procedures: tests that may be used to evaluate sexual function.
   1. Penile blood flow studies.
      a. Vasodilation: a drug to increase penile blood flow is injected into the shaft of the penis, bypassing the penile nerves (checks if the blood vessels of the penis are healthy).
      b. Cavernosography: dye is injected into the penis and an x-ray study is done to identify leaking veins that may make erection impossible.
      c. Ultrasound: an imaging test that uses painless, high-frequency sound waves to measure the rate of blood flow through the penile arteries. It is often done before and after vasodilation.
      d. Sleep monitoring: a test to monitor whether the patient has erections during sleep. If the person does not have nighttime erections, it may indicate that the nerve or blood supply to penis is inadequate for erections. Types of test are Snap-Gauge, stamp test, RigiScan, or strain gauge.
D. Care management: a variety of treatment options is available to the patient.
   1. Viagra: an oral therapy for ED.
      a. Effect of medication takes 30 to 90 minutes.
      b. Medication not effective unless sexual stimulation occurs.
      c. Dosage is 25 mg, 50 mg, or 100 mg.
      d. Absolute contraindication is use of nitrate medications (nitroglycerin, Isordil, isosorbide, or Sorbitrate).
      e. Side effects include headache, flushing, nasal congestion, blue tinge to objects (disappear with excretion of medication from the body).
   2. Muse: a transurethral drug delivery system of alprostadil (prostaglandin E).
      a. Patient inserts a small applicator into the urethra and pushes the applicator button to deliver the medication. The medication is then absorbed by the mucosa.
      b. Dosage is titrated under medical supervision.
      c. Side effects: priapism (rigid erection lasting >6 hours), penile pain, vaginal burning/itching.

  d. Contraindicated in men with hypersensitivity to alprostadil, men with abnormal penile anatomy. It should not be used for intercourse with a pregnant woman unless the couple uses a condom barrier.

 3. Vacuum constriction device.

  a. Used primarily when the cause of ED is related to blood flow (poor blood flow into the penis or excessive blood flow out of the penis during erections) or when there is damage to the nerves that control erection reflex.

  b. Safe to use; few side effects.

  c. Process: An external pump is placed over the penis when a man wants to have an erection. The air is pumped out (by hand or by a battery-operated device) creating a vacuum, which causes the blood to be drawn into the shaft of the penis. A retaining band (a plastic or rubber ring) is placed onto the penis to keep the blood in the penis (can be left in place for 30 minutes).

  d. Cost is $300 to $500, part may be covered by Medicare/private insurance.

 4. Injection therapy.

  a. Used for medically caused erection problems resulting from poor circulation or nerve damage.

  b. The medication is injected into the shaft of the penis. The drugs relax the smooth muscle in the penis, promoting blood flow.

  c. Caverject (alprostadil), prostaglandin E are main medications used.

  d. Concerns: prolonged erection (over 3 hours)—a medical emergency and the patient should be seen by MD or in ER for treatment; men often feel squeamish about injecting their penis.

  e. Cost: for supplies and medication varies, about $40 per month; insurance may pay part of cost.

 5. Penile prosthesis.

  a. A surgical system that is implanted in the penis, allowing the man to have erections whenever he chooses.

  b. Used when there is a clear medical reason for ED and natural erections unlikely to improve.

  c. Cylinders are placed in the penis; the reservoir is implanted under the groin muscle; the pump is placed in the scrotum. Following a healing period, usually about 6 weeks, the patient inflates the prosthesis by activating the pump.

  d. A surgical procedure, insurance may cover if medical indication documented.

TESTICULAR CANCER

Testicular cancer is a rare type of cancer (accounts for less than 1% of all cancers) that is the most common malignancy in the 15 to 34 year age group for male cancers (Presti, 1995).

 A. Assess/screen/triage.

  1. A potentially curable form of cancer even at advanced stages.

   2. Average age at diagnosis is 25 years (range is 15 to 44 years).
   3. The striking incidence.
      a. Peak incidence is in young men.
      b. Rising incidence over the past 20 years in young Caucasian men.
      c. Low incidence in young African American males.
   4. Cause is unknown.
   5. Risk factors.
      a. Cryptorchidism.
      b. Cancer of the alternate testicle.
      c. Race: more common in Caucasians.
      d. Socioeconomic status: more common in higher economic status.
      e. Infertility.
      f. Exposure to DES in utero.
   6. Signs and symptoms.
      a. Painless swelling of the testicle.
         (1) Often described as heaviness.
         (2) Occurs more often on the right.
         (3) Pain is rare (but can occur).
      b. Gynecomastia.
      c. No symptoms in 10% (Presti, 2000).
   7. Diagnosis.
      a. History: describe lump in scrotum, feeling of heaviness.
      b. Physical examination (examines and compares testicle to alternate testicle).
      c. Laboratory values: testis profile (tumor markers): alpha fetoprotein (AFP), beta human chorionic gonadotropin (HCG), LDH.
      d. Patients often delay 3 to 6 months after noting symptoms to see physician (Presti, 2000).
   8. Screening/triage.
      a. Patients should be seen and examined as soon as possible (because of metastatic potential of tumor).
      b. Patient and parents are usually very anxious.
B. Primary/secondary/tertiary prevention.
   1. Primary: If born with undescended testicle, surgery should be done before age 6, returning the testicle to the scrotum. Young men should be taught testicular self-examination.
   2. Secondary: If a mass is present, an inguinal orchiectomy would be done; based on the pathology, observation, radiation therapy, retroperitoneal lymph node dissection, or chemotherapy might be recommended.
   3. Tertiary: none.
C. Clinical procedures: x-rays to further define patient status.
   1. Testicular ultrasound: to evaluate cystic vs. solid mass in testicle.
   2. Chest x-ray: to evaluate the lungs for metastatic disease.
   3. CAT of abdomen and pelvis: to evaluate for enlarged lymph nodes.
D. Care management.
   1. First step is an inguinal orchiectomy.
   2. Additional treatment depends on type of tumor.

    a. Tumor types.
      (1) Seminomas (35% to 40%).
      (2) Nonseminomas (60% to 65%): teratoma, embryonal, mixed or teratocarcinoma, and choriocarcinoma.
    b. Pure seminoma tumors: respond to radiation therapy to the retroperitoneal lymph nodes.
    c. Nomseminoma tumors.
      (1) Chemotherapy: cisplatin, vinblastine, bleomycin, and VP 16.
      (2) Retroperitoneal lymph node dissection.
      (3) Low stage nonseminomas may be observed (every month to every 3 months) as a treatment option.

E. Patient education.
  1. Awareness of the potential seriousness of a testicular mass.
  2. Testicular self-examination monthly.
  3. For patients with testicular cancer, sperm banking as a possible option prior to treatment.
  4. Importance of follow-up care; testicular cancer is highly curable even with metastatic disease.

F. Advocacy.
  1. Men/boys need to be aware of the importance of monthly testicular self-examination.
  2. Testicular cancer can be cured even when it has metastasized; because of the age of the patients when diagnosed, the impact of early detection and treatment will affect many years of the patient's life.

G. Telephone practice.
  1. Patient with complaint of testicular mass should be evaluated as soon as possible.
  2. The importance of follow-up cannot be overemphasized.

H. Outcome management.
  1. Patient and parents will understand the treatment options, effects of treatment, and the importance of follow-up tests, examinations.
  2. The patient will be able to cope with changes in body image and will be able to verbalize fears and feelings about sexual functioning, fertility.
  3. The patient will be able to correctly perform testicular self-examination.

REFERENCES

American Cancer Society (2000): *CA: A cancer journal for clinicians.* New York: Lippincott Williams and Wilkins, pp. 12-13.

Houde SC (1999): Prostate disorders. In Buttaro TM, Trybulski J, Bailey PP, Sandberg-Cook J, editors: *Primary care: a collaborative practice.* St. Louis: Mosby, pp. 595-602.

Leu TF (2000): Male sexual dysfunction. In Tanagho EA, McAninch JW, editors: *Smith's general urology,* ed 15. Norwalk, CT: Appleton & Lange, pp. 788-810.

Presti JC, Herr HW (2000): Neoplasms of the prostate gland. In Tanagho EA, McAninch JW, editors: *Smith's general urology,* ed 15. Norwalk, CT: Appleton & Lange, pp. 399-421.

15 Adult Health

Compiled by JOANN APPLEYARD, PhD, RN

PATIENT PROTOTYPES

Hypertension ■ Diabetes Mellitus ■ Congestive Heart Failure ■ Chronic Obstructive Pulmonary Disease

OBJECTIVES

Study of the information presented in this chapter will enable the learner to:

1. Describe the symptoms, physical signs, and laboratory and radiologic findings of patients with hypertension (HTN), diabetes, congestive heart failure (CHF), and chronic obstructive pulmonary disease (COPD).

2. Discuss the risk factors and elements of primary, secondary, and tertiary prevention for the chronic diseases of HTN, diabetes, CHF, and COPD.

3. Describe the essential treatment plans for HTN, diabetes, CHF, and COPD.

4. Discuss the educational elements necessary to improve the disease outcomes and quality of life for patients with HTN, diabetes, CHF, and COPD.

5. Identify resources available to medical professionals and patients to enhance their knowledge about HTN, diabetes, CHF, and COPD.

■
■■ Ambulatory nursing roles in adult health are numerous and varied. Adult health services are provided to people with a wide range of ages from 18 years on. At some point, geriatric health services may be needed for most clients, but adult health encompasses a large portion of the lifespan. During adulthood people progress through many life stages, and their health needs include the maintenance and/or achievement of wellness, the prevention of injury and illness, and the diagnosis and management of chronic conditions. This chapter focuses on the ambulatory nurse's role in managing four chronic diseases: hypertension (HTN), diabetes, congestive heart failure (CHF), and chronic obstructive pulmonary disease (COPD).

Ambulatory nurses who work in settings focusing on wellness and prevention should have knowledge of effective clinical preventive measures and skills and competencies essential to implementing these measures, including individual and group teaching skills (United States Public Health Services [USPHS], 1998). Nurses who work in more disease-focused ambulatory settings need knowledge and skills related to common, serious chronic conditions, including those cited in this chapter.

■ TABLE 15-1
■ ■ **Classification of Blood Pressure for Adults Aged 18 Years and Older***

	Blood Pressure (mm Hg)		
Category	Systolic		Diastolic
Optimal	< 120	and	< 80
Normal	< 130	and	< 85
High-normal	130-139	or	85-89
Hypertension			
Stage 1	140-159	or	90-99
Stage 2	160-179	or	100-109
Stage 3	≥ 180	or	N ≥110

From National Heart, Lung, and Blood Institute (1997): *The sixth report of the joint national committee on prevention, detection, evaluation, and treatment of high blood pressure.* NIH Publication No. 98-4080. Bethesda, MD: National Institutes of Health.
* Not taking antihypertensive drugs and not acutely ill.

HYPERTENSION

Pamela S. Del Monte, MS, RN
Mary G. Daymont, MSN, RN

Hypertension is present in approximately 50 million Americans and may be diagnosed at any age. It is a significant risk factor for adverse neurologic and cardiac events. The complications of hypertension are preventable with screening, early detection, and adequate blood pressure control. The role of the ambulatory care nurse is paramount in all these areas, as these patients often have no obvious symptoms.

A. Assessment/screen/triage (National Heart, Lung and Blood Institute, 1997).
1. Risk factors.
   a. Family history of hypertension, cardiovascular disease, coronary artery disease.
   b. Patient history of smoking, elevated lipid levels, renal disease, medication history to include prescription and over-the-counter drugs.
   c. Patient demographics: age, race, gender. African Americans are more likely to have hypertension than other ethnic and racial groups. Men are more likely than women to have hypertension.
2. Physical assessment.
   a. Blood pressure reading in both arms lying, seated, standing (Table 15-1). Measurement taken after a minimum of 5 minutes of rest. Cuff size appropriate to circumference of arm. Mercury sphygmomanometer preferred. Record systolic blood pressure and diastolic blood pressure. Two or more readings spaced 2 minutes apart, then averaged. If there is a greater than 5 mm Hg difference, take average of additional readings.

     b. Previous blood pressure readings.

     c. Height and weight.

     d. Heart sounds.

     e. Associated signs and symptoms of elevated blood pressure. These can include: headache, palpitations, dizziness, fatigue, chest discomfort.

   3. Lifestyle assessment.

     a. Smoking history.

     b. Level of activity.

     c. Nutrition history to include consumption of salt, saturated fats, cholesterol, alcohol, caffeine.

     d. Stress and stress management.

     e. Psychosocial history, family situation, employment status, working conditions, educational level.

B. Primary, secondary, and tertiary prevention (National Heart, Lung and Blood Institute, 1997).

   1. Primary prevention.

     a. Identify those at risk and educate to risk factors and nonpharmacologic interventions to include lifestyle modifications and watchful blood pressure monitoring.

     b. Home blood pressure screening. Have patient demonstrate technique. Readings from home screening should be validated by the clinician.

     c. Weight appropriate to body mass index (BMI).

     d. Physical conditioning.

     e. Medical nutrition therapy: decrease sodium, decrease saturated fat.

   2. Secondary prevention.

     a. Identify patient in whom nonpharmacologic interventions have not suitably controlled blood pressure. Add medication therapy and agreed-upon next steps. Create an action plan with patient participation.

     b. Adequate potassium and calcium intake as appropriate to medication regime and any target organ dysfunction. Including foods high in potassium (approximately 4700 mg per day) may protect against the development of hypertension and improve blood pressure control in those diagnosed with hypertension. Also, foods high in calcium (approximately 1240 mg per day) may lower blood pressure in some patients with hypertension. An inverse relationship has been reported between dietary magnesium (500 mg) and blood pressure. Supplements are not recommended (Mahan and Escott-Stump, 2000).

   3. Tertiary prevention.

     a. Minimize target organ damage (heart, brain, eyes, kidneys) with thorough and ongoing history and physical examination.

     b. Additional laboratory monitors to monitor therapy and target organ function.

C. Clinical procedures (National Heart, Lung and Blood Institute, 1997).

   1. Monitoring.

  a. Blood pressure measurements should be obtained at each encounter.
  b. Frequency of blood pressure re-checks is determined by the degree and severity of elevation. For example:
    (1) Immediate evaluation: systolic ≥ 180 or diastolic ≥ 110.
    (2) Reevaluation within 1 month: systolic 160 to 179 and/or diastolic 100 to 109.
    (3) Reevaluation within 2 months: systolic 140 to 159 and/or diastolic 90 to 99.
    (4) Reevaluation within 1 year: systolic 130 to 139 and/or diastolic 85 to 90.
    (5) Reevaluation within 2 years: systolic < 130 and/or diastolic < 85 (National Heart, Lung and Blood Institute, 1997, p. 11).

2. Lifestyle management.
  a. Smoking cessation.
  b. Physical conditioning and activity. Aerobic physical activity 30 to 45 minutes most days of the week.
  c. Stress management and stress reduction.
  d. Relaxation and biofeedback.
  e. Dietary modifications: cholesterol, saturated fat, salt, alcohol. Healthy weight, sodium, and alcohol are going to have a direct impact. Cholesterol and saturated fat have an indirect impact. Caffeine has been shown to cause a transient increase in blood pressure.
  f. Avoid over-the-counter medications such as nasal decongestants, cold remedies, diet medications, herbal remedies.

3. Pharmacologic management.
  a. Diuretics lower blood pressure primarily by reducing extracellular fluid volume.
  b. Beta-blockers block the effect of catecholamines.
  c. ACE inhibitors prevent angiotensin II formation.
  d. Calcium channel blockers produce vasodilation and reduced vascular resistance.

4. Hypertensive emergencies.
  a. Hypertensive crisis is an acute life-threatening rise in blood pressure that if left untreated can result in severe target organ damage. Diastolic blood pressure may exceed 140 mm Hg.
    (1) Goals of therapy include:
      (a) Immediate blood pressure reduction by 25% within 2 to 6 hours.
      (b) Minimization and prevention of target organ damage.
      (c) Prevention of organ and tissue damage from too rapid and too vast a decrease in blood pressure.
      (d) Seek out organic and treatable cause of elevated blood pressure (Smeltzer and Bore, 2000).
    (2) Pharmacologic intervention with parenteral medications (e.g., vasodilators [sodium nitroprusside, nitroglycerine, hydralazine hydrochloride, nicardipine hydrochloride] and adrenergic inhibitors [labetalol hydrochloride]).

   b. Hypertensive urgencies are associated with rapid vascular changes and the potential sequela of a hypertensive crisis. Diastolic blood pressure may exceed 120 mm Hg.

   (1) Goal of therapy includes blood pressure reduction within a few hours.

   (2) Pharmacologic intervention with fast-acting oral medications (e.g., loop diuretics, beta-blockers, ACE inhibitors, alpha$_2$-agonists, calcium antagonists) (Smeltzer and Bore, 2000).

D. Collaboration (National Heart, Lung and Blood Institute, 1997).

   1. Utilization of ancillary services such as pharmacy, nutrition, health education.

   2. Reinforce patient education with patient and significant other(s). Note factors such as educational level, socioeconomic status, employment status, which influence understanding and potential for lifestyle changes.

   3. Utilization of specialty services as needed.

E. Care management (National Heart, Lung and Blood Institute, 1997).

   1. Regular evaluation of blood pressure control.

   2. Referrals as necessary.

   a. Nutrition.

   b. Cardiology.

   c. Nephrology.

   d. Ophthalmology.

   e. Neurology.

F. Patient education (National Heart, Lung and Blood Institute, 1997).

   1. Risk factor modification.

   a. Smoking cessation.

   b. Stress and stress management.

   2. Dietary modifications.

   a. Weight management. Weight appropriate to BMI.

   b. Limit cholesterol and saturated fat intake. Calories from dietary fat intake to be < 30% of total daily calories decreasing to < 20% to 25% for weight control.

   c. Limit sodium intake to 2400 mg per day or less.

   d. Limit alcohol intake to (for men) 1 oz ethanol, 24 oz beer, 10 oz wine, or 2 oz 100-proof whiskey. Half amounts for women and lightweight people.

   e. Intake of potassium to 4700 mg per day, with normal renal function.

   3. Activity modifications.

   a. Increasing activity safely, slowly, and progressively.

   b. Stress and stress management.

   4. Medication administration.

   a. Compliance with prescription.

   b. Side effects.

   5. Lack of overt symptoms.

   6. When to access health care.

   a. Routine access for blood pressure screening and monitoring of blood pressure control.

  b. Emergency access for signs and symptoms of untoward event. Call 911. These can include:

   (1) Onset of severe headache.

   (2) New onset of mental status changes.

   (3) New onset of vision changes, numbness, and weakness.

   (4) Chest pain.

   (5) Palpitations.

   (6) Shortness of breath.

   (7) Dizziness and facial drooping.

  c. Urgent access for fluid retention, edema, rapid weight gain, confusion.

 7. Self-monitoring of blood pressure. Bring BP record to each visit. Patient demonstrates BP technique during visit. Compare home machine readings with a mercury manometer.

G. Advocacy.

 1. Health care resources such as American Heart Association, American Dietetic Association, National Center for Nutrition and Dietetics, National Institutes for Health, National Heart, Lung and Blood Institute, local and community programs.

 2. Routes to access health care.

 3. Health education classes such as nutrition classes, disease-specific classes, relaxation and meditation programs, stress management programs.

H. Telephone practice.

 1. Assessment, triage, and management, usually by protocol.

  a. Onset of symptoms.

  b. Pertinent history.

  c. Current blood pressure readings.

  d. Associated symptoms: severe headache, visual changes, weakness, numbness, chest pain, diaphoresis, shortness of breath, radiation of chest pain, dizziness or lightheadedness.

  e. Severity of symptoms.

I. Communication/documentation.

 1. Self-documentation of at-home blood pressure readings.

 2. Documentation of all encounters.

 3. Documentation and evaluation of teaching plan.

J. Outcome management (National Heart, Lung and Blood Institute, 1997).

 1. Medication compliance.

 2. Blood pressure readings to optimal/normal.

 3. Minimize target organ damage.

 4. Weight control.

 5. Increased activity level.

 6. Decreased sodium intake.

 7. Decreased saturated fat and cholesterol intake.

 8. Smoking cessation.

K. Protocol development/usage (National Heart, Lung and Blood Institute, 1997).

1. Teaching plans.
2. Medication dosage and side effects.
3. Lifestyle modifications.
4. Dietary modifications.
5. Hypertensive crisis.
6. Blood pressure monitoring and when to report variations.
7. National Guideline Clearinghouse.
   http://www.guideline.gov
8. Agency for Healthcare Research and Quality.
   http://www.ahrq.gov
9. National Heart, Lung and Blood Institute.
   http://www.nhlbi.nih.gov/

DIABETES MELLITUS

Chris Schaefer, MSN, RN, CDE
Linda Edwards, MHS, RN, CDE

Diabetes mellitus, a serious chronic disease, affects more than 16 million people in the United States, consuming 1 in 7 health care dollars spent. Diabetes is the seventh leading cause of death in the United States. People with diabetes are at increased risk for heart disease, strokes, blindness, kidney disease, and amputations (Centers for Disease Control and Prevention, 1997). Approximately 90% of all people with diabetes receive their medical care in the primary care setting. The nurse who works in an ambulatory setting, especially in primary care, can significantly and positively affect quality of care for people with diabetes by coordinating, paying attention to the continuum of care, and facilitating communications between the patient and the provider (Hiss and Greenfield, 1996). Diabetes care and management knowledge, tools, and strategies change frequently with the continual inclusion of new research evidence. It may be difficult for the staff nurse working in an ambulatory setting to remain current in all diabetes management issues in addition to other areas of practice. Many organizations are implementing basic competencies for nurses in those areas of practice that include high-volume and high-risk patient groups. The ambulatory nurse does not need to demonstrate knowledge and skill in *all* areas of diabetes care and education; however, it is recommended that the nurse demonstrate basic diabetes competencies, including the knowledge and skill necessary to support, assess, and teach basic *patient* competencies (Edwards, 1999). A full-spectrum diabetes program is coordinated by a certified diabetes educator (CDE).

A. Assess, screen, triage.
   1. Risk factors.
      a. Obesity.
      b. First-degree relative with diabetes.
      c. High-risk populations: African American, Hispanic, Native American, and Asian.
      d. Previous gestational diabetes, baby over 9 lbs, history of glucose intolerance.

2. Diagnosis.
   a. Type 1 diabetes (previously called insulin-dependent diabetes): lack of insulin production, must take insulin injections (American Diabetes Association [ADA], 1994a).
   b. Type 2 diabetes (previously called non–insulin-dependent diabetes): treated by diet, exercise, oral medications and/or insulin (ADA, 1994b).
   c. Fasting glucose 126 mg/dl or higher; random glucose over 200 mg/dl.
3. Diabetes history.
   a. Diabetes: when diagnosed, success of previous treatment(s).
   b. Current status: blood glucose (bg) patterns, acute complications, presenting problem(s), symptoms.
   c. Hypertension, other diagnoses, comorbidities.
   d. Presence of diabetes complications, foot infections, delayed wound healing.
4. Lifestyle.
   a. Current weight, weight changes.
   b. Eating patterns: usual foods, meal/snack times, portion sizes.
   c. Exercise/activity patterns.
   d. Smoking, alcohol usage.
   e. Stress levels, coping skills, stress management patterns.
   f. Social/family support systems.
5. Laboratory parameters.
   a. Blood glucose control: fasting glucose, hemoglobin A1c.
   b. Fasting lipid panel.
   c. Kidney function: urine microalbumin, serum creatinine.
B. Primary, secondary, tertiary prevention (ADA, 1999).
   1. Primary prevention: No primary prevention strategy is known to prevent the development of diabetes. A large NIH-sponsored study, the Diabetes Prevention Program, is currently underway to determine if education and lifestyle intervention can prevent or delay the onset of Type 2 diabetes in first-degree relatives of people with Type 2 diabetes.
   2. Secondary prevention: Preventing/delaying the onset of diabetes-related long-term complications through the achievement of appropriate blood glucose control, blood pressure, lipid management through time.
   3. Tertiary prevention: management of the complications of diabetes: retinopathy, neuropathy, nephropathy, cardiovascular complications to reduce the morbidity and mortality associated with these problems.
C. Clinical procedures (ADA, 1999).
   1. Blood glucose monitoring.
      a. Observe patient perform bg test using own meter.
      b. Evaluate patient bg patterns/record.
   2. Foot exam.
      a. Annual comprehensive foot exam including evaluation of skin integrity, circulation status, sensitivity (using monofilament), deformities.
      b. Visual inspection of feet at each visit for signs of infection.

■ TABLE 15-2
■ ■ **Oral Diabetes Medications**

Generic Name	Brand Name	Dosage Range	Comments
SULFONYLUREAS			
Glipizide	Glucatrol	2.5-40 mg	Once or twice daily dosing.
	GlucatrolXL	5-20 mg once daily	Stimulates increased insulin production.
Glyburide	Diabeta	1.23-20 mg	May be used alone or in combination
	Micronase		with metformin, acarbose, or insulin.
	Glynase	0.75-12 mg	*Can cause hypoglycemia.*
	PresTab		
Glimepiride	Amaryl	1-8 mgonce/day	
OTHER ORAL ANTIDIABETICS			
Metformin	Glucophage	500-2550 mg	May be used alone or in combination with sulfonylurea and/or insulin. Decreased liver glucose output. Twice daily dosing. Does not cause hypoglycemia when used alone. *Contraindicated if serum creatinine elevated. Use with caution in patients with history of CHF.*
Acarbose	Precose	75-300 mg	Taken 3/day with meals. Delays carbohydrate digestion and glucose absorption. Used alone or in combination with other orals/insulin.
Troglitazone	Rezulin	200-600 mg	Taken once daily at breakfast in combination with insulin. Increases insulin sensitivity and decreases insulin resistance. *See recommendations for monthly liver function studies.*
Repaglinide	Prandin	0.5-4 mg with meals	Taken 30 minutes before eating. Skip dose if meal is skipped. Dosing is titrated to number and quantity of meals. Used alone or in combination with metformin.

Data from Stone MS, Swenson K (1997): *Managing diabetes and its complications: a guide for health care providers.* Milpitas, CA: LifeScan.

   3. Treatment plan.
     a. Nutrition: individualized meal plan facilitated by a registered dietitian (RD), who is a CDE when possible, which addresses bg goals, patient goals, family/work schedule, cultural traditions, and timing according to medications/insulin being used.
     b. Medication.
        (1) Oral diabetes medications (Table 15-2).

■ TABLE 15-3
■ ■ **Insulin Action Times**

Insulin	Starts	Peaks	Ends	Low bg* Likely at	When to Check bg for Effect
Lispro (Humalog)	10 min	1.5 hr	3 hr	2-4 hr	2-4 hrs after injection
R (Regular)	20 min	3-4 hr	8 hr	3-7 hr	Before next meal
N (NPH)	1.5 hr	4-12 hr	22 hr	6-12 hr	AM dose: ac dinner
					PM dose: ac breakfast
L (Lente)	2.5 hr	7-15 hr	24 hr	7-13 hr	Same as above
UL (Ultralente)	4 hr	10-24 hr	36 hr	12-28 hr	Before breakfast
70/30	0-1 hr	3-4 hr	12-20 hr	3-12 hr	Before meals and
70% N		and			at bedtime
30% R		4-12 hr			
50/50		Same as above			
50% N					
50% R					

Data from Stone MS, Swenson K (1997): *Managing diabetes and its complications: a guide for health care providers.* Milpitas, CA: LifeScan.
**bg*, Blood glucose.

      (a) Sulfonylureas increase insulin production (can cause hypoglycemia).
      (b) Biguanides, thiazolidinediones improve effectiveness of insulin.
      (c) Alpha-glucosidase inhibitor, delay glucose absorption.
      (d) Repaglinide (Prandin), useful for patients with postprandial hyperglycemia; stimulates insulin secretion.
    (2) Insulin or insulin mixtures (Table 15-3).
      (a) Very fast-acting.
      (b) Fast-acting.
      (c) Intermediate-acting.
      (d) Long-acting.
  c. Physical activity: negotiated level of activity including type of exercise, intensity, frequency, and timing in relation to meals and medications.
  d. Blood glucose monitoring: frequency of routine testing, additional testing to determine causes of bg problems, such as hypoglycemia.
  e. Follow-up plan: includes expectations for both routine follow-up and when to contact physician when bg pattern changes, problems occur.
    (1) Next contact for routine review of bg patterns.
    (2) Next physician visit.
    (3) When lab tests are due.
    (4) When next eye exam, foot exam are due.
4. Blood pressure management.
  a. Target: < 130/85.

b. ACE inhibitors, drug of choice for managing hypertension in people with diabetes, has additional renal-protective benefit.

5. Lipid management.

　　a. Nutrition management.

　　b. Lipid-lowering drugs to achieve LDL cholesterol level < 130 (under 100 in people with coronary artery disease [CAD]).

6. Management of hypoglycemia (in patients taking sulfonylureas and/or insulin).

　　a. Assess for signs and symptoms each visit/encounter.

　　b. Evaluate bg patterns for wide fluctuations, which include bg below normal.

　　c. Determine causes, whether clinical management or patient behavioral, and implement intervention to reduce possibility of future episodes.

　　d. Establish follow-up plan to be followed until bg stable.

7. Management of acute hyperglycemia, "sick days": blood glucose over 240 mg/dl or presence of infection, gastroenteritis, other acute illness including fever, nausea, diarrhea.

　　a. High risk for severe hyperglycemia, dehydration, ketoacidosis, requiring hospitalization, if treatment delayed or inadequate.

　　b. Requires immediate intervention.

　　　(1) Guidance for patient to maintain hydration.

　　　(2) Short-term, frequent advice about insulin adjustments.

　　　(3) Blood glucose/urine ketone monitoring.

　　c. Ambulatory intravenous (IV) administration if patient unable to maintain hydration.

D. Collaboration, resource identification, and referral.

1. Endocrinology consultation.

　　a. Recommended for all patients with Type 1 diabetes, those with multiple endocrinopathies, and those with other complex management issues.

　　b. Provides ongoing consultation, education to primary care providers.

2. Certified diabetes educators: RN, RD, other professionals with diabetes education experience who have passed the CDE examination (Funnell, 1998).

　　a. Provide patient education, individually or in groups to support patient progress toward self-management.

　　b. Provide education and support to primary care team and other professionals regarding standards of care, management of complex issues, and changes in current knowledge base and state-of-the-art care.

3. Resources supporting appropriate routine care.

　　a. Pharmacy.

　　b. Ophthalmology.

　　c. Podiatry.

　　d. Exercise specialist, physical therapist.

    e. Mental health professionals.

  4. Resources to manage diabetes complications/special needs.

    a. Nephrology.

    b. Cardiology.

    c. Neurology.

    d. Other as needed: GI, GU, home care.

E. Care management (Ward and Rieve, 1997).

  1. Primary care.

    a. Blood glucose management and medication management in uncomplicated cases: newly diagnosed and stable Type 2 diabetes.

    b. Facilitate patient achievement of diabetes control goals and manage episodes of blood glucose variations to regain stability.

    c. Facilitate appropriate ongoing care (see Protocol Development/ Usage) and access to appropriate resources according to patient need.

  2. Diabetes care management.

    a. RN specially trained in diabetes management/education, care management, and diabetes risk reduction strategies, such as coordination of blood pressure and lipid management, access to annual dilated eye exam, complete foot exams, and other resources as needed.

    b. Targets population segments that have dropped out of routine care, are at known risk for diabetes complications (elevated Hb A_{1c} levels), and/or those who frequently use health care resources inappropriately (frequent ED, hospital admissions).

    c. Provide diabetes management, education, access to appropriate resources and follow-up for a predetermined period of time or until patient has engaged in the process of active participation in the care and management of their own diabetes.

    d. Goals: improved clinical outcome, risk reduction, reduced cost, appropriate resource utilization.

F. Patient education.

  1. Basic skills: provided/coordinated by primary care team that focuses on immediate knowledge and skills patient and/or caregivers need to perform the treatment plan safely, without supervision in their own environment (Edwards, 1999).

    a. Describes type of diabetes, treatment plan elements, blood glucose targets.

    b. Eats reasonably appropriate meals at consistently spaced times (does not skip meals).

    c. Performs blood glucose monitoring accurately.

    d. Takes medication(s)/insulin correctly.

    e. Recognizes signs/symptoms of hypoglycemia and treats promptly.

    f. Follow-up plan: calls appropriately for bg extremes, schedules routine follow-up visits and lab tests as directed.

  2. Intermediate: referral to Diabetes Education Program, preferably ADA-recognized as meeting the standards of care for diabetes self-management education programs (ADA, 1999).

    a. Usually group education programs provided by CDEs, which include expanded diabetes management education information and behavior change strategies.

    b. Patient able to make appropriate decisions about daily bg management issues and effectively manage bg fluctuations.

    c. Patient actively participates in own care and uses health care resources appropriately.

  3. Advanced: patient has knowledge, skill, and motivation to design own treatment plan to meet individual needs.

    a. Example: Type 1 patient who proactively anticipates insulin needs based on variations in food intake and exercise.

    b. Provided by expert diabetes team, experienced in insulin intensification.

  4. Community support groups.

    a. Often provided by American Diabetes Association local chapters.

    b. May be facilitated by organizations providing care for patients with unique or similar needs: Hispanic communities, etc.

  5. Special needs: additional education may be needed for individuals experiencing unique problems (i.e., visual impairment, renal dialysis, stroke rehabilitation, etc).

G. Advocacy.

  1. Facilitate appropriate communication between patient and physician.

  2. Facilitate access to appropriate resources (see Collaboration and Patient Education pp. 263-264).

  3. Assist with insurance interface for durable medical equipment needs and referrals.

  4. Provide patient-focused, flexible support and interventions.

  5. Promote positive, proactive expectations with patient, physician, and other providers.

H. Telephone practice.

  1. Supports day-to-day blood glucose management.

  2. Provides timely patient access for acute situations.

  3. Reminds patients of annual lab tests and examinations.

I. Communication/documentation.

  1. Baseline.

    a. General health status.

    b. Current diabetes control.

    c. Patient competencies.

  2. Patient goals, relating to:

    a. Blood glucose, Hb A_{1c} targets.

    b. Lipid, blood pressure targets.

    c. Weight.

    d. Lifestyle changes.

    e. Comorbidities.

  3. Progress.

    a. Clinical targets.

    b. Accomplishment/readjustment of patient goals through time.

J. Outcome management.

1. Individual outcomes.
   a. Demonstrated competencies.
   b. Quality of life, such as perceived sense of well being, personal/job productivity, loss of work/school time because of diabetes-related problems.
2. Clinical.
   a. Process criteria.
      (1) Documented performance of recommended annual lab tests.
      (2) Documented performance of annual dilated eye and complete foot exams.
   b. Outcome criteria.
      (1) Lab values in target ranges.
      (2) Eye, foot exams with normal results.
      (3) BP managed within target range.
   c. Resource utilization/cost outcomes.
      (1) Fewer ED visits, hospitalizations, demonstrating reduced use of the highest cost resources.
      (2) Appropriate primary care provider visits for recommended routine care, according to the recommended standards for proactive care.
K. Protocol development/usage. ADA Standards: criteria by which regulatory bodies evaluate quality of care provided by health care organizations and managed care organizations.
   1. Diabetes treatment algorithms.
      a. Promote consistent level of care throughout an organization.
      b. Guide provider through steps to advance therapy in order to help patient achieve diabetes control goals in an efficient and appropriate manner.
   2. Nursing care pathways: useful to promote consistent level of care, timely patient access to appropriate care and education, and continuity of care within the resources and systems of each organization (Zander, 1997), such as:
      a. Newly diagnosed Type 1 or Type 2 diabetes.
      b. Diabetes "out-of-control," "sick day" management competencies (see C7 on p. 263).
   3. Include CDEs in pathways for both patient education and staff nurse access to information that exceeds basic parameters.
   4. If CDE resources are not available within the organizations, consider collaborating/contracting with other local CDEs or contact the American Association of Diabetes Educators for other CDE resources.

CONGESTIVE HEART FAILURE

Nancy M. Albert, MSN, RN, CCRN, CNA

Heart failure is an acute or chronic syndrome in which the cardiac myocytes or contractile apparatus of the heart does not pump enough blood to meet the needs of the tissues (Committee on Evaluation and Management of Heart Failure, 1995; Albert, 1998; Packer and Cohn, 1999). Peripheral bed perfusion is altered, leading to subsequent mechanical, neuroendocrine, and inflammatory responses in an attempt to improve systemic organ flow. Compensatory mechanisms fail to improve contractility over time and lead to a maladaptive state characterized by ventricular remodeling (myocyte hypertrophy, cardiac dilation and reshaping of the left ventricle from an elliptical to a spherical or globular shape) and hemodynamic alterations (systemic and venous vasoconstriction, increased afterload and preload, and low cardiac output). Chronic myocyte dysfunction may be a result of systolic (ejection fraction below 40%) and/or diastolic (normal ejection fraction) changes in regional myocyte workload and/or passive tension, respectively (Albert, 1998; Albert, 1999a). Heart failure patients are evaluated based on New York Heart Association (Criteria Committee of NYHA, 1973; Packer and Cohn, 1999) functional status assessment or classification. Class I reflects the ability to carry out ordinary exercise *without physical activity limitation* resulting from symptoms of fatigue, dyspnea, chest pain, or palpitations. Class II is designated when the patient is comfortable at rest but has symptoms with ordinary exercise, which causes a *slight limitation of physical activity.* In class III heart failure, less than ordinary activity results in symptoms, therefore, the patient has a *marked limitation of physical activity.* When the patient develops *discomfort with any physical activity or has symptoms at rest,* functional class IV is designated. The ultimate goal of therapy is to cause reversal or prevent progression of left ventricular remodeling.

A. Assessment, screening, and triage (Konstam, et al., 1994; Packer and Cohn, 1999).

   1. History.

     a. History of chronic coronary artery disease, myocardial infarction, hypertension, diabetes, valve or thyroid disease, or anemia.

     b. Prevalence increases with age.

     c. Type of cardiac dysfunction (systolic versus diastolic, right versus left heart failure) and stage syndrome severity (NYHA functional class).

     d. Precipitating disease processes that can lead to reversal of heart failure with proper surgical intervention (i.e., cardiac revascularization or valve repair).

     e. Lifestyle issues.

       (1) Alcohol/drug abuse.

       (2) Tobacco use.

       (3) Excessive fluid intake.

       (4) Diet (sodium and fat content).

       (5) Activity/exercise level.

       (6) Stress management.

       (7) Medication noncompliance.

     f. Potentially detrimental medications (Mills and Young, 1998; Packer and Cohn, 1999).

       (1) Chronic nonsteroidal antiinflammatory drugs.

       (2) High dose (> 325 mg/day), chronic aspirin.

       (3) Decongestants.

       (4) Calcium channel blockers *except* amlodipine or felodipine.

      (5) 1st generation beta-blockers with intrinsic sympathomimetic activity in the heart: propranolol or timolol.

      (6) Class 1a and 1c antiarrhythmic agents.

      (7) Antacids (sodium-containing).

2. Assess medication drug and dose history (including therapy compliance) related to core pharmacologic therapies for heart failure (Packer and Cohn, 1999).

    a. ACE inhibitors.

    b. 2nd or 3rd generation beta-adrenergic blockers.

    c. Diuretics if signs of volume overload.

    d. Digoxin in systolic heart failure.

    e. Angiotensin II receptor blockers, hydralazine/nitrate combination or other systemic vasodilators.

    f. Aldosterone inhibitor (spironolactone) if in NYHA functional class III or IV.

3. Assess signs and symptoms of volume overload. Note: only 35% of patients have congestive symptoms; therefore, must assess for subclinical volume overload (Packer and Cohn, 1999).

    a. Dyspnea, orthopnea, paroxysmal nocturnal dyspnea.

    b. Edema, ascites, anasarca, acute pulmonary edema.

    c. Worsening cough, rales, weight gain.

    d. S_3 gallop, neck vein distention, or elevated jugular venous pressure (> 10 cm H_2O pressure); positive abdominojugular reflux test.

4. Assess for signs and symptoms of resting hypoperfusion.

    a. Fatigue, decreased exercise tolerance.

    b. Mental obtundation, dizziness, lightheadedness.

    c. Nausea, anorexia.

    d. Resting tachycardia (> 85 bpm), decreased systolic blood pressure and increased intracardiac pressures.

5. Assess for arrhythmias (palpitations, atrial fibrillation, slow or rapid heart rate, dizziness or lightheadedness).

6. Assess serum lab work for electrolyte balance (basic metabolic panel, magnesium) renal function (creatinine) and thyroid function.

7. Determine need for hospitalization (Mills and Young, 1998).

    a. Hypotension with organ hypoperfusion.

    b. Severe dyspnea.

    c. Profound volume overload, especially if not relieved with intravenous loop diuretic agent administration in the outpatient setting.

    d. Severe electrolyte imbalances.

    e. New onset atrial fibrillation, non-sustained ventricular tachycardia or other cardiac rhythm problem requiring immediate evaluation and treatment.

    f. New onset angina or refractory angina, clinical suspicion of myocardial infarction.

    g. Uncontrolled hypertension requiring immediate evaluation and treatment with intravenous agents.

      h. Acute pneumonia concomitant with heart failure.

      i. Advanced renal or hepatic disease with decompensated heart failure.

  8. Determine need for critical care hospitalization due to complex decompensation (Albert, 1999b; Mills and Young, 1998).

      a. Severe or refractory symptoms of volume overload and/or resting hypoperfusion (with metabolic sequelae) requiring intravenous preload and afterload reduction and/or intravenous inotrope therapies.

      b. Hemodynamic instability requiring right heart catheterization and continuous hemodynamic monitoring.

      c. Hypoxemia requiring respiratory support via ventilator.

      d. Recent respiratory or cardiac arrest.

      e. Shock.

      f. Complex cardiac arrhythmias requiring close electrocardiographic monitoring and medication and/or technical therapies.

B. Primary, secondary, and tertiary prevention.

  1. Major modifiable primary and secondary prevention strategies (Mills and Young, 1998; Packer and Cohn, 1999; Uretsky, et al., 1998).

  2. Hypertension control.

      a. Hyperlipidemia control.

      b. Cigarette smoking cessation.

      c. Curbing physical inactivity; promotion of aerobic exercise.

      d. Weight reduction.

      e. Hormone replacement at menopause.

      f. Prevention of glucose intolerance.

      g. Alcohol cessation; limiting caffeine intake; habitual drug withdrawal.

      h. Low sodium diet (i.e., 2000 mg/day in NYHA Class III or IV failure or 3000 mg/day in NYHA Class I or II failure).

  3. Other secondary prevention strategies (Konstam, et al., 1994; Mills and Young, 1998; Packer and Cohn, 1999).

      a. Self-management education related to fluid management (weight monitoring, fluid intake limitation, and managing thirst by sucking on ice chips or hard candy rather than drinking fluid).

      b. Compliance with pharmacologic therapies.

      c. Yearly flu vaccine; pneumococcal vaccine (every 6 to 10 years).

      d. Regular physical examinations.

      e. Social (family) support of lifestyle changes.

  4. Tertiary prevention (Konstam, et al., 1994; Mills and Young, 1998; Packer and Cohn, 1999).

      a. Prompt recognition and treatment of signs and symptoms of worsening condition (Packer and Cohn, 1999).

         (1) Obtaining lab work of renal function, electrolytes, thyroid, and complete blood count.

         (2) Chest film to detect the presence of cardiac enlargement, pulmonary congestion, or other pulmonary disease and electrocardiogram to detect evidence of prior myocardial infarction, left

ventricular hypertrophy, cardiac arrhythmia, or diffuse myocardial disease, as necessary.

    (3) Pulmonary function test and 24- to 48-hour Holter monitor, as necessary for pulmonary dysfunction and cardiac electrophysiology issues, respectively.

  b. Identification and treatment of exacerbating factors (Mills and Young, 1998).

    (1) See Primary and Secondary Prevention.

    (2) New or worsening stress.

    (3) Atrial arrhythmias.

    (4) Infection.

    (5) Anemia.

    (6) COPD.

    (7) Pulmonary emboli.

    (8) Thyroid disease.

    (9) Environmental conditions.

    (10) Pregnancy.

C. Clinical procedures (Konstram, et al., 1994; Packer and Cohn, 1999).

  1. Two-dimensional echocardiogram (coupled with Doppler flow study when possible) or radionuclide ventriculography: to evaluate the presence and severity of left ventricular systolic dysfunction (ejection fraction). These tests can reveal segmental wall motion abnormalities.

    a. Echocardiogram: can assess chamber size, valve abnormalities, pericardial effusion, ventricular thrombus, and presence of cardiac hypertrophy.

      (1) Echocardiogram is the single, most useful diagnostic tool in the evaluation of heart failure.

      (2) Echocardiogram is less expensive and more generally available than radionuclide ventriculography; it does not require preparation.

    b. Radionuclide ventriculogram: provides a more precise measurement of ejection fraction and better assessment of right ventricular function. It provides a limited assessment of valvular abnormalities and left ventricular hypertrophy.

      (1) Radionuclide ventriculogram requires venipuncture and radiation exposure; it does not require prep.

  2. Special studies.

    a. Diagnostic right heart catheterization/hemodynamics: catheter inserted into a vein and guided to the right side of the heart to determine low cardiac output and elevated right ventricular filing pressures. Uses local anesthetics. Does not require prep.

    b. Electrophysiologic testing: heart catheterization that records electrical activity in the heart and can reveal serious rhythm disturbances after electrical stimulation.

    c. Maximal cardiopulmonary exercise testing: graded treadmill or bicycle exercise protocol to measure total duration of exercise and peak oxygen consumption. Does not require preparation except to hold medications as necessary.

   3. Routine assessment, metabolic status assessment (diabetes, lipids, weight).

D. Collaboration/resource identification and referral (Albert, 1999b; Fonarow, et al., 1997; Roglieri, et al., 1997).

   1. Ancillary services: nutrition, social work, pharmacy, cardiac or physical rehabilitation.

   2. Preventive cardiologist, heart failure specialist cardiologist; palliative care medicine.

   3. Group therapy programs (smoking cessation, stress management, relaxation); heart failure education/social support group.

E. Care management (Fonarow, et al., 1997).

   1. Medical therapies.

     a. Determine need for changes based on patient signs and symptoms.

     b. Routine medication up-titration as tolerated for ACE inhibitors, diuretics, and beta-blocker therapies.

   2. Regular evaluation of self-care practices, education needs, and symptoms.

   3. Regular surveillance monitoring via telephone or other means following an emergency department visit, inpatient hospitalization, or if history of therapy noncompliance.

   4. Assess psychosocial issues: anxiety, depression, social isolation.

F. Patient education (Albert, 1999b; Uretsky, et al., 1998).

   1. Knowledge of heart failure; signs and symptoms of worsening condition; when to access health care.

   2. Medication management; compliance with prescriptions, side effects; polypharmacy issues.

   3. 2000 to 3000 mg sodium diet; low animal fat diet; limit alcohol intake; limit caffeine intake.

   4. Fluid management: daily weight monitoring, fluid restriction/monitoring, tips to quench thirst.

   5. Activity and exercise; increasing activity level safely; prevention of overexertion.

   6. Health promotion strategies.

     a. Self-management of symptoms (dyspnea, weight gain, dizziness/lightheadedness).

     b. Risk factor modification (smoking, stress, alcohol, obesity, over-the-counter medications that may worsen heart failure).

     c. Follow-up management (flu shot, regular check-ups).

     d. Self-monitoring of blood pressure and heart rate; including when to notify provider of changes.

   7. Prognosis counseling.

G. Advocacy: There is a great need for patient advocacy in heart failure. Current heart failure research literature has led to an alteration in patient management recommendations, and past assumptions regarding care may no longer apply in today's health care environment, that is, in the past, rest was promoted; currently, exercise and activity are promoted; in the past, beta-blocker therapy was contraindicated because it has a negative inotropic effect (worsens contractility); now selective beta-blocker therapy is recommended because it favorably alters neurohormone levels and leads to regression of cardiac remodeling. Nurses are a key link to physician ordering practices, especially when the nurse initiates communication with the physician regarding patient complaints and symptoms. Nurses must be proactive in clearly communicating the patient's situation and offering ideas based on current consensus recommendations so that patient quality of life is optimized and survival is prolonged.

1. Nurse knowledge of advanced pathophysiology concepts (ventricular remodeling, neuroendocrine changes, effects on the vascular and end-organ systems).
2. Nurse knowledge of the hemodynamic goals of therapy.
    a. Optimized systolic blood pressure (Albert, 1999b).
        (1) Lowest systolic blood pressure that maintains mentation, urine output, and does not cause prolonged orthostatic response (dizziness and lightheadedness).
        (2) 80 mm Hg; 90 mm Hg in the frail elderly.
    b. Optimized afterload values and definitions if using noninvasive hemodynamic monitoring to guide therapy.
        (1) 800 to 1200 dynes/sec/cm^{-5} or uses systolic blood pressure value.
        (2) Lowest value that leads to an increase/maintenance of cardiac index and does *not* cause systolic blood pressure and/or renal perfusion to fall, even if cardiac index is increased.
    c. Optimized afterload values and definitions if using noninvasive hemodynamic monitoring to guide therapy.
        (1) Right atrial pressure of 8 mm Hg or 11 cm H_2O; right internal jugular venous pressure of 6 cm H_2O; pulmonary artery wedge pressure of 15 mm Hg.
        (2) The lowest preload value that can be maintained without a decrease in systolic blood pressure and/or cardiac index.
3. Nurse knowledge of the pharmacologic goals of therapy; steps to reach goals, and measures to minimize and/or alleviate side effects and complications.
4. Nurse understanding and communication of heart failure nonpharmacologic principles.
5. Common errors in patient management that can be overcome through advocacy (Fonarow, et al., 1997; Mills and Young, 1998; Roglieri, et al., 1997).
    a. Nonaggressive treatment in managing concomitant hypertension.
    b. Inadequate patient, family, and caregiver education.
    c. Inappropriate treatment when heart failure is not the result of systolic dysfunction.
    d. Close weight monitoring is not specifically stated and/or the patient

does not understand what to do (self-management) with slight weight changes to decrease risk of worsening symptoms.

   e. Causes of patient noncompliance are not recognized and/or acted on appropriately.

   f. In patients with chronic coronary artery disease (three vessel disease) and systolic dysfunction, myocardial metabolic function must be assessed and revascularization must be considered.

   g. In patients with severe mitral regurgitation and systolic dysfunction, mitral valve repair is often not considered.

   h. Heart transplantation referral is often delayed and severe decompensation or secondary multisystem organ failure develops.

   i. Cardiac rehabilitation program or an exercise prescription is underused.

   j. Home health care specialty program for heart failure is underused in homebound patients.

   k. Suboptimal dosing of ACE inhibitors and/or beta-blockers; in many cases it is based on concerns of possible side effects rather than on actual issues.

   l. Underdosing of diuretics when overt or subclinical signs and symptoms of volume overload persist.

   m. Failure to remove medications from the patient's pharmacologic profile that have been clearly shown to cause deleterious effects.

   n. Failure to offer self-management instructions to offset the development of symptoms of worsening condition. Assuming that telling the patient to "call your doctor" is adequate instruction when symptoms develop or worsen in severity.

   o. Not providing prompt response and early intervention to patients when they phone into the office with complaints or new symptoms.

  H. Telephone practice.

    1. Rapid response telephone practice.

     a. Priority evaluation protocols that direct the patient to an immediate emergency department visit, when necessary.

     b. Assessment of medical history and heart failure history.

     c. Cardiac medication assessment including recent changes or additions/deletions.

     d. Current symptom(s) assessment including onset and severity.

     e. Treatment plans for fluid overload, hypoperfusion, and for symptoms that reflect worsening heart failure with or without obvious volume overload. These plans must offer specific treatment options (i.e., additional dose of diuretic, hold ACE inhibitor) rather than just referring the patient to the emergency department or an office visit the following day.

    2. Surveillance or vigilance monitoring programs.

     a. Physical and psychosocial status; current symptoms.

     b. Compliance with the pharmacologic and nonpharmacologic plan of care.

 I. Communication/documentation.

1. Subjective and objective assessment and plan of care.
2. Patient's understanding of education taught and compliance monitoring with plan of care.
3. Patient and/or nurse initiated follow-up telephone calls or results from another surveillance system.
4. Ancillary program results: home health care or cardiac rehabilitation programs.

J. Outcome management.
  1. Determine standards of care utilizing one or more of the following resources:
     a. Advisory Council to Improve Outcomes Nationwide in Heart Failure (ACTION-HF) consensus recommendations for the management of chronic heart failure (Packer and Cohn, 1999).
     b. AHA/ACC task force heart failure guidelines (Committee on Evaluation and Management of Heart Failure, 1995).
     c. AHCPR clinical practice guidelines for patients with left-ventricular systolic dysfunction (Konstam, et al., 1994).
  2. Identify outcomes and benchmarks.
     a. Based on current issues (length of stay when hospitalized, mortality, readmission rates, cost).
     b. Based on issues of concern (patient knowledge base, high-risk patients, improved quality of life, self-care ability, coordination of care, promotion and/or adherence to standards).
  3. Develop interventions to meet outcomes.
     a. Multidisciplinary team.
     b. Physician champion who understands the complexity of heart failure and is an expert in this field of care.

K. Protocol development/usage.
  1. Pharmacologic therapy algorithms for ACE inhibitors, beta-blockers, diuretics, digoxin, hydralazine, nitrates, and angiotensin II receptor blockers and aldosterone inhibitors (Albert, 1999b).
     a. Initiation and up-titration schedules.
     b. Serum electrolyte, vital signs, and other monitoring information.
  2. Decision tree based on clinical severity of symptoms (mild, moderate, or severe) (Konstam, et al., 1994).
  3. How to treat persistent:
     a. Volume overload.
     b. Dyspnea.
     c. Hypertension.
     d. Concomitant angina.
     e. Concomitant atrial fibrillation.
     f. Hypotension.
  4. Nonpharmacologic expectations related to education (Uretsky, et al., 1998).
  5. Surveillance/compliance monitoring questionnaire or system (Fonarow, et al., 1997).

6. Patient-initiated communication (rapid-response program) algorithm regarding treatment options based on current symptoms.
7. Multidisciplinary consultation and support group expectations (i.e., aggressive home care heart failure program).
8. When to consult a heart failure specialist.
9. When should a patient be directly hospitalized; routine floor versus a critical care environment.
10. End-of-life issues and guidelines.

CHRONIC OBSTRUCTIVE PULMONARY DISEASE

Nancy Bair, MSN, RN

Chronic obstructive pulmonary disease (COPD) was defined in 1995 by the American Thoracic Society (ATS) as a group of diseases that exhibit airflow obstruction as a result of chronic bronchitis or emphysema. These diseases may be accompanied by airway hyperreactivity, are usually progressive, but somewhat reversible. Further, the ATS defined emphysema as an abnormal permanent enlargement of the airspaces distal to the terminal bronchioles with destruction of their walls and without obvious fibrosis. Chronic bronchitis is the presence of a productive cough for 3 months in each of 2 successive years when other causes of chronic cough have been excluded (ATS, 1995; Petty, 1998).

A. Assess/screen/triage.
  1. Assessment of illness (ATS, 1995; Phillips and Hnatiuk, 1998).
    a. Risk factors.
      (1) Smoking history 20 cigarettes/day for > 20 years before symptomatic.
      (2) Passive smoking/environmental tobacco smoke (ETS).
      (3) Ambient air pollution.
      (4) Hyperresponsive airways.
      (5) Occupational factors.
      (6) Sex, race, socioeconomic status.
      (7) Alpha-1 antitrypsin deficiency (A_1ATD).
    b. Presents in 5th decade with a productive cough or acute illness.
    c. Dyspnea occurs in the 6th or 7th decade.
    d. Sputum.
      (1) Initially occurs in morning.
      (2) Daily volume rarely exceeds 60 ml.
      (3) Mucoid but becomes purulent with exacerbations.
    e. Wheezing.
    f. Acute chest illness occurs intermittently and with increased frequency.
      (1) Increased cough.
      (2) Purulent sputum.
      (3) Wheezing.
      (4) Dyspnea.

(5) Fever.
g. Late stages of COPD.
   (1) Hypoxia with cyanosis.
   (2) Morning headaches suggest hypercapnia.
   (3) Hypercapnia with severe hypoxemia (end stage).
   (4) Cor pulmonale with right heart failure and edema.
2. Physical exam (ATS, 1995; Phillips and Hnatiuk, 1998).
   a. Chest auscultation.
      (1) Slowed expiration becomes more prolonged as disease progresses.
      (2) Wheezing on forced expiration.
      (3) Decreased breath sounds.
      (4) Heart sounds distant as anterior-posterior (A-P) diameter increases.
      (5) Coarse bibasilar crackles.
   b. Positioning.
      (1) Forward leaning with arms outstretched and weight supported on palms.
   c. Accessory muscles of neck and shoulders. Paradoxical indrawing of lower interspaces (Hoover's sign).
   d. Expiration through pursed lips.
   e. Cyanosis (may be present).
   f. Enlarged, tender liver with right heart failure.
   g. Asterixis with acute hypercapnia.
3. Diagnosing and monitoring COPD (ATS 1995; Phillips and Hnatiuk, 1998).
   a. Chest radiography findings.
      (1) Low, flat diaphragm.
      (2) Increased retrosternal airspace.
      (3) Long, narrow heart shadow.
      (4) Hypertransradiance and bullae.
   b. Computed tomography (CT) indications.
      (1) Not indicated for routine care.
      (2) Indicated for consideration of pulmonary resection or diagnosis of bronchiectasis.
   c. Pulmonary function testing.
      (1) Spirometry with bronchodilators.
      (2) Arterial blood gases.
B. Primary, secondary, tertiary prevention.
   1. Primary prevention (ATS, 1995; Petty and Nett, 1995; Phillips and Hnatiuk, 1998).
      a. Risk factors.
         (1) Tobacco smoke: increased morbidity/mortality for cigarette smokers. Pipe and cigar smokers have increased morbidity/mortality for COPD but not as high as cigarette smokers.
         (2) Passive smoking/ETS: children with parents who smoke have a

high rate of respiratory symptoms/disease. Relationship to development of COPD is unclear.

(3) Air pollution: high levels of urban air pollution are harmful to people with lung disease. Role in development of COPD is unclear.

(4) Hyperresponsive airways: hyperreactivity is inversely related to FEV_1 and may be predictive of an accelerated decline of lung function in smokers.

(5) Sex, race, and socioeconomic status: high prevalence of respiratory symptoms for men. Mortality higher in whites but this difference is decreasing in males. Morbidity and mortality inversely related to socioeconomic status (higher in blue-collar workers).

(6) Occupational factors: inhalation of occupational dusts (e.g., coal, grain) can cause COPD.

(7) Alpha-1 antitrypsin deficiency: genetic defect that can lead to COPD in smokers and non-smokers (later age development).

b. Education programs/resources.*

(1) National Lung Health Education Program: national health care initiative aims to promote early identification and intervention in COPD and related disease. Internet: *www.nlhep.org*

(2) American Lung Association: information on asthma, tobacco control, air quality, and lung disease. Internet: *www.lungusa.org*, *www.Coloradohealthnet.org/site/index_copd.html*

(3) Alpha$_1$ National Association and other related references: information on alpha-1 antitrypsin deficiency. Internet: *www.alpha1. org*, *www.alphalink.org*

(4) Children's Liver Disease Foundation: pamphlet on alpha-1 antitrypsin deficiency caused by a relationship between liver disease and alpha-1 antitrypsin deficiency (ATD). Internet: *www.childliverdisease.org*

2. Secondary prevention (ATS, 1995; Donado and Hill, 1998; Petty and Nett, 1995; Phillips and Hnatiuk, 1998).

a. Smoking cessation.

(1) Group therapy.

(2) Pharmacologic therapy: nicotine substitutes and antidepressants (Zyban).

(3) Hypnosis.

b. Pharmacologic therapy for COPD.

(1) Bronchodilators: beta$_2$-agonists, anticholinergics, theophylline.

(2) Antiinflammatory agents: oral, intravenous, inhaled steroids.

(3) Mucolytic agents: reducing mucus viscosity for symptomatic relief.

(4) Antibiotics: use of intermittent courses for patients with four or

---

*Note: Caution patients to discuss outside information and resources with their physician to determine accuracy and appropriateness of the information.

more exacerbations/year. Not shown to prevent exacerbations in stable patients.

(5) Psychoactive agents: for dyspnea relief.

(6) Cardiovascular therapy: for controlling the secondary pulmonary hypertension and right heart dysfunction of cor pulmonale.

(7) Immunization (influenza and Pneumovax vaccinations).

(8) Antiprotease therapy for alpha-1–antitrypsin deficiency: administered by intravenous route.

c. Surgical treatments (Deslauriers and LeBlanc, 1994; Edelman and Kotloff, 1998).

(1) Bullectomy: eliminates large bullae to allow reexpansion of functional lung tissue.

(2) Lung volume reduction surgery (LVRS): removal of 20% to 30% of most severely affected lung tissue that improves the function of the remaining lung tissue by altering the lung, chest wall, and diaphragmatic mechanics. National Emphysema Treatment Trial (NETT) is ongoing to compare LVRS with standard therapy.

(3) Lung transplantation: patients may have either a single or double lung transplant.

3. Tertiary prevention (ATS, 1995; Donado and Hill, 1995; Heffner, 1998; Petty, 1998; Petty and Nett, 1995; Phillips and Hnatiuk, 1998; Resnikoff and Ries, 1998).

a. Pulmonary rehabilitation.

(1) Exercise training that improves large muscle groups and relates to activities of daily living.

(2) Education about the disease and behavioral changes.

(3) Psychosocial support.

(4) Breathing retraining: pursed lip and diaphragmatic breathing.

(5) Nutrition/weight control and maintenance.

(6) Mobilization of secretions: hydration, postural drainage, chest percussion and vibration, directed coughing, positive expiratory pressure techniques.

b. Long-term oxygen therapy.

(1) Determination of need: long-term oxygen therapy improves survival in hypoxemic COPD patients. Need for O_2 is based on room air measurements of P_aO_2.

(2) Oxygen systems: oxygen concentrators, compressed gas cylinders, and liquid oxygen.

(3) Oxygen delivery method: nasal cannulas, masks, or transtracheal systems.

(4) Reimbursement criteria (U.S. Health Care Financing Agency for Medicare reimbursement guidelines).

(a) Continuous O_2: $PaO_2 \geq 55$ mm Hg or oxygen saturation ≤ 88 at rest; PaO_2 of 56 to 59 mm Hg or oxygen saturation of 89% at any time, in the presence of polycythemia (Hct > 56%), cor pulmonale, pulmonary hypertension.

(b) Noncontinuous O_2: $PaO_2 \leq 55$ mm Hg or oxygen saturation $\leq 88\%$ on exertion; $PaO_2 \leq 55$ mm Hg or oxygen saturation $\leq 88\%$ with sleep.

   c. Ethical issues: discussion of end-of-life treatment must occur before the crisis.

     (1) Discuss limitations of treatments and document the discussion before the patient becomes seriously ill/incompetent.

     (2) Know the state's laws concerning a living will or durable power of attorney for health care.

C. Clinical procedures.

  1. Suctioning.

  2. Assisting with initiation of transtracheal oxygen therapy. Setting up oxygen delivery systems.

  3. Using metered-dose inhalers and spacers.

  4. Measuring pulse oximetry.

  5. Drawing of arterial blood gases.

D. Collaboration/resource identification/referral.

  1. Primary care physician/nurse practitioner.

  2. Pulmonologist.

  3. Cardiologist.

  4. Otorhinolaryngologist.

  5. Respiratory therapy.

  6. Home care nurse.

E. Care management/telephone practice.

  1. Frequency of follow-up calls based on severity of disease.

  2. Assess for need of a follow-up visit/hospitalization.

    a. Response of symptoms to outpatient management.

    b. Ability to eat and sleep.

    c. Ability to walk between rooms (patient previously mobile).

    d. Family opinion of patient's ability to manage at home.

    e. High-risk comorbid condition.

    f. Prolonged, progressive symptoms.

    g. Altered mental capacity.

    h. Level of dyspnea.

    i. Sputum.

  3. Assess patient's understanding of current therapeutic regimen.

  4. Assess psychosocial issues.

  5. Maintain contact with home care providers.

  6. Assess functioning of equipment.

  7. Documentation of discussion and changes in care management.

F. Patient education.

  1. Disease process.

    a. Normal lung function vs. COPD lung function.

    b. Progression of the disease.

    c. Treatment options.

  2. Smoking cessation.

    a. Encourage patient to progress in a stepwise manner.

    b. Provide information on smoking cessation techniques and reinforce the teaching throughout.

3. Oxygen therapy.

    a. Use and care of equipment.

    b. Safety measures for use of oxygen: remind patients of potential hazards of oxygen and its ability to support combustion. Continued cigarette smoking is considered a contraindication for oxygen therapy.

    c. Adjustment of oxygen flow rates is determined by the physician. Patients are placed on low flow rates (0.5 to 2 L/min) initially with recommendation of an increase by 1 L/min for sleep.

4. Medication management.

    a. Inform patient about prescribed medications (indications, side effects, dose).

    b. Teach use and care of delivery devices (e.g., nebulizers, spacers).

5. Nutrition/weight control and maintenance.

    a. Assess nutritional status.

    b. Instruct on good dietary habits.

    c. Achieve ideal body weight.

    d. Encourage several small meals per day.

6. Breathing techniques.

    a. Pursed lip/diaphragmatic breathing: patient inhales slowly and deeply through the nose while expanding the abdomen. They exhale through slightly parted lips.

    b. Leaning forward on a table or with arms resting on the thighs can relieve breathlessness.

7. Exercising.

    a. Prescription to include mode, frequency, intensity, and duration.

    b. Incorporate large muscle groups and closely relate to daily activities (e.g., walking, cycling).

    c. Upper extremity training.

    d. Inspiratory muscle training.

8. Mobilization of secretions.

    a. Maintain adequate hydration.

    b. Postural drainage: gravity-assisted positioning to help with mucous clearance.

    c. Chest percussion and vibration: uses external vibration to loosen mucous plugs.

    d. Directed coughing: patient leans forward and inhales deeply; then coughs several times while exhaling through pursed lips.

    e. Positive expiratory pressure techniques: exhaling against a resistive device (flutter valve) to prevent airway collapse and helps to clear mucus.

9. Travel guidelines (in-flight oxygen requirements).

    a. Requires advance planning. Contact airlines on requirements for physician prescription for oxygen administration in-flight.

      b. Assess cost of oxygen in-flight and coverage by insurance.

      c. Generally increasing oxygen by 1 to 2 L/min is adequate.

  10. Ethical issues.

      a. Involve patient and family in discussions.

      b. Teach differences of living wills vs. durable power of attorney for health care. Retain a copy for the patient's record.

G. Advocacy.

  1. Assess the environment of outpatient area.

  2. Interact with caregivers in other areas.

  3. Meet with outpatient management team on a regular basis.

  4. Determine appropriate patient support/education organizations.

H. Outcome management.

  1. Improved exercise tolerance.

  2. Decreased dyspnea.

  3. Decreased anxiety/depression.

  4. Improved quality of life.

  5. Decreased health care utilization.

  6. Improved survival rate.

I. Protocols for management of COPD (ATS, 1995).

  1. Management of the COPD patient.

  2. Cessation of smoking.

  3. Pharmacologic therapy for the COPD patient.

  4. Indications for long-term oxygen therapy.

  5. Long-term oxygen therapy for the COPD patient.

  6. Correcting hypoxemia in the acutely ill COPD patient.

  7. Emergency room evaluation of COPD patients with acute exacerbation.

  8. Indications for hospitalization.

  9. Indications for ICU admission of COPD patients with acute exacerbation.

  10. Discharge criteria for COPD patients with acute exacerbation. Management of the preoperative patient with COPD.

REFERENCES

Albert NA (1998): Advanced systolic heart failure: emerging pathophysiology and current management. *Prog Cardiovasc Nurs* 13(3):14-30.

Albert NA (1999a): Heart failure: the physiologic basis for current therapeutic concepts. *Crit Care Nurse* June (Suppl.):1-13.

Albert NA (1999b): Manipulating survival and life quality outcomes in heart failure through disease state management. *Crit Care Nurs Clin North Am* 11:121-141.

American Diabetes Association (1999, January): Clinical practice recommendations 1999. *Diabetes Care* (Suppl.1).

American Diabetes Association (1994a): Medical management of insulin-dependent (Type 1). *Diabetes,* ed 2. Alexandria, VA: Author.

American Diabetes Association (1994b): Medical management of non-insulin-dependent (Type 2). *Diabetes,* ed 3. Alexandria, VA: Author.

American Thoracic Society (1995): Standards for the diagnosis and care of patients with chronic obstructive pulmonary disease. *Am J Respir Crit Care Med* 152(Suppl):S77.

Centers for Disease Control and Prevention (1997, November): *Diabetes fact sheet*. Atlanta: Author.

Committee on Evaluation and Management of Heart Failure. (1995): Guidelines for the evaluation and management of heart failure. *Circulation* 92:2764-2784.

Criteria Committee of the New York Heart Association (NYHA) (1973): *Criteria for diagnosis of disease of the heart and great vessels*, ed 7. Boston: Little, Brown.

Deslauriers J, LeBlanc P, editors (1994): Management of bullous disease. *Chest Surg Clin North Am* 4 (5):539-559.

Donado JR, Hill NS (1998): Outpatient management. In Heffner JE, Petty TL, editors: Chronic obstructive pulmonary disease. *Respir Care Clin North Am* 4(3):391-423.

Edelman JD, Kotloff RM (1998): Surgical approaches to advanced emphysema. In Heffner JE, Petty TL, editors: Chronic obstructive pulmonary disease. *Respir Care Clin North Am* 4(3):513-539.

Edwards LL (1999): Phased competency: A new model to prepare nurses for enhanced roles in diabetes disease management. *Disease Management and Health Outcomes* 5(5):253-261.

Fonarow GC, Stevenson LW, Walden JA, et al. (1997): Impact of a comprehensive heart failure management program on hospital readmission and functional status of patients with advanced heart failure. *J Am Coll Cardiol* 30:725-732.

Funnell MM, editor (1998): *A core curriculum for diabetes education*, ed 3: Chicago: American Association of Diabetes Educators.

Heffner JE (1998): End-of-life ethical issues. In Heffner JE, Petty TL, editors: Chronic obstructive pulmonary disease. *Respir Care Clin North Am* 4(3):541-559.

Hiss R, Greenfeld S (1996): Forum three: changes in the U.S. healthcare system that would facilitate improved care for non-insulin-dependent diabetes mellitus. *Ann Intern Med* 124(Pt 2):180-186.

Konstam MA, Dracup K, Baker DW, et al. (1994); Heart failure: evaluation and care of patients with left-ventricular systolic dysfunction. Clinical Practice Guideline No. 11. (AHCPR Publication No. 94-0612). Rockville, MD: Agency for Health Care Policy and Research.

Mahan LK, Escott-Stump S, editors (2000): *Krause's food, nutrition, and diet therapy*, ed 10. Philadelphia: WB Saunders.

Mills RM, Young JB, editors (1998): *Practical approaches to the treatment of heart failure*. Baltimore: Williams & Wilkins.

National Heart, Lung and Blood Institute (1997): *The sixth report of the joint national committee on prevention, detection, evaluation, and treatment of high blood pressure*. (NIH Publication No. 98-4080). Bethesda, MD: National Institutes of Health.

Packer M, Cohn J (1999): Consensus recommendations for the management of chronic heart failure. *Am J Cardiol* 83(2A):1A-38A.

Petty TL, Nett LM (1995): *Enjoying life with chronic obstructive pulmonary disease*, ed 3. Cedar Grove, NJ: Laennec Publications.

Petty TL (1998): Definitions, causes, course, and prognosis of chronic obstructive pulmonary disease. In Heffner JE, Petty TL, editors: Chronic obstructive pulmonary disease. *Respir Care Clin North Am* 4(3):371-389.

Phillips YY, Hnatiuk DW (1998): Diagnosing and monitoring the clinical course of chronic obstructive pulmonary disease. In Heffner JE, Petty TL, editors: Chronic obstructive pulmonary disease. *Respir Care Clin North Am* 4(3):371-389.

Resnikoff PM, Ries AL (1998): Maximizing functional capacity: pulmonary rehabilitation and adjunctive measures. In Heffner JE, Petty TL, editors: Chronic obstructive pulmonary disease. *Respir Care Clin North Am* 4(3):475-491.

Roglieri JL, Futterman R, McDonough KL, et al. (1997): Disease management interventions to improve outcomes in congestive heart failure. *Am J Managed Care* 3:1831-1839.

Smeltzer S, Bore B, editors (2000): *Brunner and Suddarth's textbook of medical-surgical nursing,* ed 9. Philadelphia: Lippincott.

Stone MS, & Swenson K (1997): *Managing diabetes and its complications: a guide for health care providers.* Milpitas, CA: LifeScan.

Uretsky BF, Pina I, Quigg RJ, et al. (1998): Beyond drug therapy: nonpharmacologic care of the patient with advanced heart failure. *Am Heart J* 135:S264-S284.

US Preventive Services Task Force (1996): *Guide to clinical preventive services,* ed 2. Baltimore: Williams & Wilkins.

United States Public Health Services (USPHS) (1998): *Clinician's handbook of preventive services,* ed 2. McLean, VA: International Medical Publishers.

Ward MD, Rieve JA (1997): The role of case management in disease management. In Todd WE, Nach D, editors: *Disease management: a systems approach to improving patient outcomes.* Chicago: American Hospital Publishing, pp. 235-259.

Zander K (1997): Classic nursing management skills and disease management: something old, something new. *Semin Nurse Managers* 5(2):85-90.

MARGARET ROSS KRAFT, MS, RN
JAN SHELDON, MS, RN, ANP

PATIENT PROTOTYPES

Osteoarthritis ■ Osteoporosis ■ Depression ■ Cataracts ■ Advocacy

OBJECTIVES
Study of the information presented in this chapter will enable the learner to:

1. Identify risk factors that interfere with activities of daily living in older adults.

2. List health promotion activities relevant to older adults.

3. Dispel the myths of late onset depression.

4. Describe treatment strategies for common chronic conditions of aging.

5. Recognize the importance of the nurse's role in advocacy for the elderly.

■■ Throughout the world, numbers of older persons are increasing at a rapid rate. In the United States, the number of Americans age 65 and older has tripled since 1900, and by 2030, one in every five Americans will be 65 or older. The fastest growing segment of the population is that of the "oldest old" age 80 and above; by 2002, U.S. census projections estimate that the number of adults over age 85 will triple. American life expectancy of 76 years in 1999 is expected to reach 83 by the year 2030 (American Association for World Health, 1999).

Population aging means that more people reach ages at which the risk for developing chronic debilitating diseases is very high. At least 30% of the over 85 group are impaired in one or more activities of daily living (Edelman and Mandle, 1998). Healthy aging goes beyond the prevention or treatment of disease to consider the physical, psychologic, social, and spiritual health of the whole person. The United Nations has defined healthy aging as "the interaction of factors such as maintenance of physical and mental functioning; being active, productive, and involved in society; independence in stable social environments; and involvement in meaningful personal relationships" (American Association for World Health, 1999, p 6).

The idea that aging means inevitable disease and deterioration does not have to be true if healthy lifestyles choices are made. Nurses in ambulatory care settings are well situated to influence quality of life for older persons by helping them make wise choices regarding diet, exercise, and health care, which contribute to healthy aging.

Nurses also serve in an important role as patient advocate with this population dealing with many complex factors that influence both physiologic and psychologic health.

OSTEOARTHRITIS

Osteoarthritis, also known as degenerative joint disease (DJD), is the most common type of arthritis and is generally a disease of older adults. It occurs as the result of normal "wear and tear" on joints but its presence can be hastened through repetitive joint strain, injury, and/or obesity. This disease is manifested by progressive degeneration of cartilage in joints—usually weight-bearing joints although any joint could be affected. As cartilage becomes thin, bone ends come closer together; bone spurs develop at tendon and ligament attachment sites; synovial fluid may leak; and cysts may develop on the bone (Gulanick, Klopp, Galanes, Gradishar, and Puzas, 1998). The result is impaired joint functioning. After the age of 75, some degree of osteoarthritis is found in almost all persons; osteoarthritis is the leading cause of disability for those over age 80.

   A. Assess/screen/triage.
      1. Joint assessment.
         a. Spine.
         b. Knee.
         c. Fingers.
         d. Hip.
      2. Symptom assessment.
         a. Pain.
         b. Changes in mobility: maintenance of mobility in elderly can mean the difference between living independently in the community and institutionalization.
         c. Body image changes.
      3. Risk factor screening.
         a. Repetitive joint motion. Take work history.
         b. Familial tendency.
         c. Obesity.
   B. Primary, secondary, tertiary prevention.
      1. Primary prevention: maintain ideal body weight.
      2. Secondary prevention.
         a. Treatment to reduce pain.
         b. Maintenance of joint mobility.
      3. Tertiary prevention.
         a. Referral to dietitian for weight reduction.
         b. Rehabilitation after joint surgery to promote mobility.
   C. Clinical procedures.
      1. Surgical interventions.
         a. To correct deformities.
         b. To improve function.
         c. To relieve pain.

        d. To prevent deformity (Harkness and Dincher, 1996).

    2. Common surgical interventions.

        a. Tendon transplants.

        b. Synovectomy.

        c. Total joint replacement.

D. Care management.

    1. Treatment is aimed at relieving pain, which tends to be worse in the morning or after any extended period of inactivity (Ebersole and Hess, 1998).

        a. Maintenance of optimal joint function.

        b. Position changes.

        c. Joint support.

        d. Medication for control of pain and inflammation.

        e. Hot or cold packs.

            (1) Moist heat (i.e., pads, soaks, paraffin baths).

            (2) Ice packs for a duration of no more than 20 minutes.

        f. Adequate regular and intermittent rest periods.

        g. Use of adaptive equipment as necessary.

        h. Elimination of stressors.

    2. Prevention of progressive disability.

E. Patient education.

    1. Medication management.

        a. Use of salicylates.

            (1) Teach side effects.

            (2) Toxicity of sustained use of large doses.

            (3) Teach precautions/contraindications.

        b. Use of nonsteroidal antiinflammatory drugs (NSAIDs) and COX2-inhibitors (i.e., celecoxib [Celebrex], rofecoxib [Vioxx]).

            (1) Evaluate for GI upset, which is a major risk for the elderly.

            (2) Monitor for increased bruising.

        c. Use of corticosteroids; preferred for short-term therapy for acute exacerbations.

            (1) Avoid use with uncontrolled diabetes.

            (2) Monitor for extension of existing cataracts.

            (3) Rule out osteoporosis.

        d. Muscle relaxants.

            (1) May be used for painful muscle spasms.

            (2) Caution about drowsiness and driving.

        e. Topical application of capsaicin cream for pain relief.

            (1) Wear cotton gloves if applied to hands.

            (2) Wash hands thoroughly to avoid irritation to nonmedicated body areas.

    2. Weight control: excess weight stresses involved joints.

    3. Exercise program stressing the importance of exercise to maintain joint mobility.

        a. Maintain range of motion (ROM) of all joints.

        b. Encourage rest between activities.

        c. Evaluate pain during exercise.

        d. Discuss environmental barriers to mobility.

        e. OT/PT/RT/KT consult as indicated.

    4. Teach relaxation and stress reduction techniques.

    5. Teach ADL adaptations.

    6. Orthopedic consultation regarding possible joint replacement.

F. Telephone practice.

    1. Evaluate for exacerbation of symptoms.

    2. Assess compliance with medication regimen.

G. Documentation.

    1. Be sure subjective and objective data are documented along with the nursing assessment and treatment plan.

H. Outcomes management.

    1. Pain reduction.

    2. Increased mobility and functional status.

    3. Increased quality of life.

OSTEOPOROSIS

Osteoporosis is a disease characterized by low bone mass, demineralization, and structural deterioration of bone tissue, which leads to bone fragility, brittleness, and increased susceptibility to fractures. Bone loss affects both men and women in middle to late life but is accelerated rapidly in women after menopause. Among adults over age 50, 50% of women and 12% of men can expect to have an osteoporosis-related fracture. Osteoporosis is so prevalent that it is considered to have reached epidemic proportions in the older age group. Treatment costs for hip fractures alone are estimated at between $10 and $20 billion annually (Ebersole and Hess, 1998) with an estimated 1.5 million fractures per year (Burke and Walsh, 1997). The most common fractures associated with osteoporosis are compression fractures of the vertebrae, hip fractures, and fractures of the femur and forearm. Unfortunately, the disease may go unnoticed until a fracture occurs. The key to management of osteoporosis is prevention as well as health promotion. Prevention really begins by ensuring that children and teenagers have an adequate calcium intake.

    A. Assess/screen/triage.

        1. Risk factor assessment.

            a. Menopause: Type I osteoporosis is associated with estrogen deficiency in women between 50 and 75. Women lose approximately 25% of bone mass compared to a loss of approximately 12% of bone mass in men (Edelman and Mandel, 1998).

            b. Specific medication usage may alter bone mass.

                (1) Prolonged use of corticosteroids.

                (2) Diuretics such as furosemide.

                (3) Anticonvulsants such as phenytoin.

                (4) Tetracycline.

                (5) Heparin.

(6) Methotrexate.
   c. Physical build: presence of small thin frame, fair skin, and light hair and eyes.
   d. Caucasian or Asian ancestry.
   e. Use of alcohol and tobacco.
   f. Inadequate calcium intake. Average daily intake should be approximately 1 g.
   g. Decreased physical activity, especially weight-bearing activity.
2. Assessment of loss of height with deformity of the spine.
3. Screening.
   a. Bone density testing (Dexascan). Test is positive if bone density is 2.5 standard deviations below the mean for a normal young (age 30 to 40) adult.
   b. Biochemical assessment.
      (1) Decreased alkaline phosphatase.
      (2) Increased serum calcium.
      (3) Increased thyroid stimulating hormone (TSH).
      (4) Calcium oxalate in urine.
      (5) Testosterone screen for men.
B. Primary, secondary, tertiary prevention.
   1. Primary prevention.
      a. Ensure that the diet has adequate levels of calcium and vitamin D across the entire life span.
      b. Promotion of weight-bearing exercise and regular physical activity is effective for both primary and secondary prevention. Recommend 50 minutes of jogging or walking three times per week.
         (1) Resistance and weight training improve strength and functional mobility.
         (2) Weight-bearing and muscle building exercise helps to maintain skeletal integrity and improve muscle mass and strength and flexibility (Edelman and Mandle, 1998).
   2. Secondary prevention.
      a. Regular exercise may actually reverse the demineralization process.
      b. Intake of vitamin D.
         (1) 400 to 800 I.U. daily. Can be found in a multivitamin.
         (2) Urge 10 to 15 minutes of daily exposure to sunlight with appropriate sun block.
      c. Estrogen replacement for menopausal women if indicated.
      d. Improved nutrition (Figure 16-1).
      e. Calcium supplements.
         (1) Should be maintained at 1 to 2 g daily for women not getting estrogen or men who are testosterone-deficient. Women on estrogen replacement therapy and men with normal testosterone levels need 1 g daily.
         (2) Age-related changes in vitamin C synthesis negatively affect calcium absorption resulting in Type II osteoporosis. Most

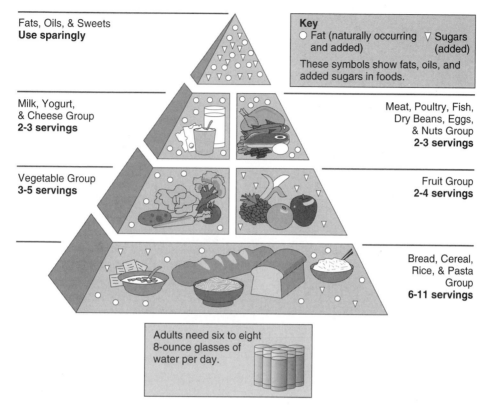

Fats, Oils, & Sweets
Use sparingly

Key
○ Fat (naturally occurring   ▽ Sugars
    and added)   (added)
These symbols show fats, oils, and
added sugars in foods.

Milk, Yogurt,
& Cheese Group
2-3 servings

Meat, Poultry, Fish,
Dry Beans, Eggs,
& Nuts Group
2-3 servings

Vegetable Group
3-5 servings

Fruit Group
2-4 servings

Bread, Cereal,
Rice, & Pasta
Group
6-11 servings

Adults need six to eight
8-ounce glasses of
water per day.

FIGURE 16-1 ■ Food Guide Pyramid for Persons 50 Plus (Courtesy U.S. Department of Agriculture, Washington, D.C.)

commonly seen in persons over 75. Frequent result is hip fracture.

(3) Avoid foods that reduce calcium absorption such as coffee and caffeinated soft drinks, high fat foods, and alcohol.

(4) The average diet usually does not supply adequate calcium so supplements are often essential.

f. Smoking cessation.

g. Avoidance of excessive use of alcohol.

h. Fall prevention.

(1) Home environment modifications.

(a) Removal of tripping hazards.

(b) Installation of grab bars.

(c) Appropriate lighting and elimination of glare.

(d) Appropriate footwear.

(2) Vision and hearing assessment.

(3) Work environment modifications as appropriate.

i. Medication review.

(1) Discuss medication side effects.

(2) Explain expected therapeutic effects of medications.
C. Clinical procedures.
  1. Rule out bone-thinning diseases.
     a. Osteomalacia.
     b. Multiple myeloma.
  2. Treat secondary causes.
     a. Hyperparathyroidism.
     b. Hyperthyroidism.
     c. Diabetes.
     d. Alcoholism.
     e. Hypotestosterone-hypogonadism.
     f. Prolonged use of corticosteroids. Often see in patients with COPD.
D. Referrals.
  1. Dietary referral for weight control.
  2. Specialty practice referral for treatment of secondary conditions.
     a. Endocrine consult.
     b. Pain management consult.
     c. Therapy (OT and PT) consults.
     d. Substance abuse treatment.
E. Documentation.
  1. Be sure subjective and objective data are documented along with the nursing assessment and treatment plan.
F. Outcomes management.
  1. Prevention of fractures.
  2. Annual assessment for vertebral fractures determined by measurement of height and single lateral thoracolumbar x-ray (Kassirer and Greene, 1997).
  3. Treatment follow up with Dexascan (bone density testing).
     a. Some sources recommend repeat Dexascan 1 year after initial treatment and every other year after that (Goroll, May, and Mulley, 1998).
     b. Other sources feel that treatment is 95% effective in postmenopausal women and the cost of additional Dexascan is not justified (Kassirer and Greene, 1997).
  4. Improved quality of life as defined by the client.

DEPRESSION

Mental health problems in older adults may be hidden or unrecognized even though as many as one of every eight community-based older adults may suffer from a psychiatric disorder, most commonly late-life onset depression. Depression is not part of normal aging but the rate of occurrence does increase with age (Ebersole and Hess, 1998). Events like retirement, illness, the loss of family and friends can all contribute to depression. By reducing the quality of life, depression can seriously affect a person's health and ability to function. Depression is an affective disorder characterized by feelings of unworthiness, sadness, apathy, and hopelessness.

Everyone gets the "blues" now and then. When the mood lasts longer than a couple of weeks, the ambulatory care clinician needs to tune into symptoms of depression.

For the older adult, depression is more prevalent in patients who have a medical illness. The greater the severity of illness, the greater the chance of developing depression. Diseases that may increase the risk of late-life depression include coronary artery disease, hypertension, diabetes, and hyperthyroidism (Hance, Carney, Freedland, and Skala, 1996). Vascular changes are particularly interesting in that lesions in the left frontal lobe and the left basal ganglia are more likely to be associated with late-onset depression (Greenwald, Kramer-Ginsberg, and Krishnan, 1997). Older patients can develop a number of risk factors for vascular disease, including diabetes, hypertension, and hyperlipidemia. Studies have suggested that persons developing late onset depression are at increased risk for developing dementia (Alexopoulos, Meyers, and Young, 1993). Persons with vascular depression may not respond to standard treatment for depression but therapy to prevent the progression of vascular changes in the brain, including aspirin daily, lipid-lowering medications, and estrogen for postmenopausal women may be the treatments of choice.

A. Assess/screen/triage.
  1. Health history.
   a. Physical domain.
    (1) Weight gain or loss.
    (2) Pallor, weakness, posture, eye contact.
    (3) Fatigue, constipation, incontinence, sense of "not feeling good."
    (4) Dependent edema.
    (5) Nutritional status including 24-hour dietary review.
    (6) Mobility and activities of daily living (ADLs).
   b. Affective appearance/mentation.
    (1) Suicidal and/or homicidal ideation and means to carry out intentions.
    (2) Slow responses.
    (3) Vague responses to direct questions.
    (4) Changes in usual behavior.
    (5) Confusion.
    (6) Disengaged from usual activities or patterns of normal behavior.
    (7) Well dressed/groomed vs. unkempt.
   c. Prior laboratory findings.
    (1) Anemia or decreasing trend in RBCs, HCT, Hgb, and B_{12} level.
    (2) Hyperlipidemia or increasing trend in lipid profile.
    (3) Hypothyroidism or increasing TSH.
    (4) Electrolyte imbalance.
   d. Medications.
    (1) New medications since last visit.
    (2) Dosing and/or frequency modified by patient.
    (3) Method for self-administration of medications.
   e. Social support.
    (1) Recent losses of family members.

       (2) Changes in living situation.

  B. Primary, secondary, tertiary prevention.

     1. Primary prevention: Primary care practitioners must identify those at risk and work with them to develop a successful prevention program. Ambulatory care nurses have an important role in screening for risk factors and symptoms.

       a. Assist the elder to prepare for major life changes such as retirement, death of a spouse, or friend.

       b. Assess prior responses to life changes and coping patterns.

       c. Encourage the older adult to maintain friendships over the years.

       d. Initiate conversation about the development of hobbies or interests.

       e. Develop a plan to keep the mind and body active.

       f. Listen to the family/significant others to assess whether the patient exhibits signs and symptoms of depression.

       g. Screen as appropriate using the 15 to 30 item Geriatric Depression Scale (GDS) and compare scores when life stress situations change (Figure 16-2).

       h. Identify ways to maintain physical fitness.

       i. Encourage eating a balanced diet.

       j. Screen for signs of metabolic disease, illness, atherosclerosis, neurologic changes every visit.

       k. Monitor for constipation and incontinence and develop prevention program if necessary.

     2. Secondary prevention.

       a. Assist the older adult to accept help when help is needed.

       b. Assess response to medical treatment for other conditions that may have contributed to the depression (metabolic disorders, infection, atherosclerosis, neurologic changes).

       c. Identify misconceptions that the elder or family/significant other may have about depression including:

         (1) Depression is a sign of weakness.

         (2) A depressed person can quickly snap out of it.

         (3) An older adult is too old for help.

         (4) Treatment options are too expensive.

         (5) Treatment is not covered by insurance for the elder seeking care.

         (6) Medications will cure depression immediately.

       d. Identify with the older person or family/significant other referral sources for the care of depression.

       e. Assess with the GDS pre- and posttreatment and compare scores over time.

     3. Tertiary prevention.

       a. Assess response to intervention each visit.

       b. Support the older adult by showing interest in treatment response.

       c. Assess suicidal/homicidal ideation each encounter.

       d. Report suicidal/homicidal ideations to appropriate person or facility.

       e. Consider direct observed therapy (DOT) for patients not compliant

Thirty (30) item mood assessment scale with fifteen (15) item scale indicated by an asterisk (*).
Response indicating depression is typed in all capital letters.
Scoring indicative of depression is described below.

*	Are you basically satisfied with your life?	yes/NO
*	Have you dropped many of your activities and interests?	YES/no
*	Do you feel that your life is empty?	YES/no
*	Do you often get bored?	YES/no
	Are you hopeful about the future?	yes/NO
	Are you bothered by thoughts you can't get out of your head?	YES/no
*	Are you in good spirits most of the time?	yes/NO
*	Are you afraid that something bad is going to happen to you?	YES/no
*	Do you feel happy most of the time?	yes/NO
*	Do you often feel helpless?	YES/no
	Do you often get restless and fidgety?	YES/no
*	Do you prefer to stay at home, rather than going out and doing new things?	YES/no
	Do you frequently worry about the future?	YES/no
*	Do you feel that you have more problems with memory than most?	YES/no
*	Do you think it is wonderful to be alive now?	yes/NO
	Do you often feel downhearted and blue?	YES/no
*	Do you feel pretty worthless the way you are now?	YES/no
	Do you worry a lot about the past?	YES/no
	Do you find life very exciting?	yes/NO
	Is it hard for you to get started on new projects?	YES/no
*	Do you feel full of energy?	yes/NO
*	Do you feel that your situation is hopeless?	YES/no
*	Do you think that most people are better off than you are?	YES/no
	Do you frequently get upset over little things?	YES/no
	Do you frequently feel like crying?	YES/no
	Do you have trouble concentrating?	YES/no
	Do you enjoy getting up in the morning?	yes/NO
	Do you prefer to avoid social gatherings?	YES/no
	Is it easy for you to make decisions?	yes/NO
	Is your mind as clear as it used to be?	yes/NO

30 Item scoring: Normal 0-9; Mild depressive 10-19; Severe depressive 20-30.
15 Item scoring: For clinical purposes a score greater than five (5) is suggestive of depression
and should warrant a follow-up interview. Scores greater than ten (10) indicate depression.

FIGURE 16-2 ■ The Geriatric Depression Scale (From Yesavage J, Brink T, Rose T, et al. [1983]: Development and validation of a geriatric depression scale. *J Psychiatric Res* 17:37-49.)

with medications. Clients in a DOT program receive medications at the clinic to ensure compliance.

C. Clinical procedures.
  1. Acute management.
    a. Psychotherapies.
      (1) Individual therapy.
      (2) Family therapy.
    b. Pharmacologic agents.
      (1) Serotonin reuptake inhibitors (SSRIs).

(a) Examples: sertraline (Zoloft), fluoxetine (Prozac), paroxetine (Paxil), citalopram (Celexa).
(b) Considerations.
   (i) Decrease dosing for the elderly. Start with the lowest recommended dose.
   (ii) Transitory GI effects should disappear within the first 2 weeks.
(2) Tricyclic antidepressants (TCA) in lower doses.
   (a) Nortriptyline and desipramine are preferred because of lower anticholinergic effects, less sedation, and less orthostatic hypotension.
   (b) Avoid amitriptyline (Elavil) and imipramine (Trofinil).
(3) Monoamine oxidase inhibitors (MAOI).
   (a) Examples: phenelzine (Nardil) and tranylcypromine (Parnate).
   (b) Avoid using with the elderly because of food-drug and drug-drug interactions.
c. Adjunctive therapy: electroconvulsive therapy (ECT) is reserved for psychotic depression or for when antidepressants are contraindicated.
D. Referral to a specialist if no improvement after a month of medical treatment. Specialists include:
   1. Geriatric psychologist.
   2. Geriatric social worker.
   3. Geriatric psychiatrist.
   4. Geriatrician.
E. Care management.
   1. DSM-IV (1994) criteria for diagnosis of major depression: at least five of the following symptoms have been present during the same 2-week period and represent a change; at least one of the symptoms is depressed mood or loss of interest or loss of pleasure.
      a. Depressed mood most of the day.
      b. Diminished interest or pleasure in all, or almost all, activities most of the day.
      c. Significant weight loss or weight gain or a decrease or increase in appetite.
      d. Insomnia or hypersomnia.
      e. Psychomotor agitation or retardation.
      f. Fatigue or loss of energy.
      g. Feelings of worthlessness, excessive or inappropriate guilt.
      h. Diminished ability to think or concentrate.
      i. Recurrent thoughts of death, recurrent suicidal ideation without a specific plan, or a suicide attempt, or a specific plan for committing suicide.
   2. GDS score indicative of depression.
   3. Physiologic and/or substance use causes for behavior have been ruled out.

4. Symptoms cause significant distress or impairment in social, occupational, or other important areas of functioning.
5. Symptoms are not accounted for by bereavement.
6. All patients suspected of new late-onset depression will be screened for physiologic causes for the depression.
   a. CBC to rule out anemia and infections.
   b. TSH to rule out hypothyroidism.
   c. Lipid panel to assess atherosclerosis.
   d. Nutrition screen to assess intake of a balanced diet.
   e. Presence/progression of chronic disease such as CHF.
   f. Medication assessment.
F. Patient/caregiver education.
   1. The most common signs and symptoms of depression in the older adult include:
      a. An empty feeling, ongoing sadness, and anxiety.
      b. Tiredness, lack of energy.
      c. Loss of interest or pleasure in everyday activities, including sex.
      d. Sleep problems including very early morning waking.
      e. Problems with eating and weight (gain or loss).
      f. A lot of crying.
      g. Aches and pains that just won't go away.
      h. A hard time focusing, remembering, or making decisions.
      i. Feeling that the future looks grim; feeling guilty, helpless, or worthless.
      j. Being irritable.
      k. Thoughts of death or suicide; a suicide attempt.
   2. Medication teaching.
      a. Intended action.
      b. Side effects.
      c. Adverse reactions.
      d. Possible drug/drug interactions.
      e. Drug/food interactions.
      f. Anticipated duration of treatment.
      g. Anticipated onset of action.
   3. Treatment options.
      a. Electroconvulsive therapy.
      b. Group therapy.
      c. Individual therapy.
G. Advocacy: many senior centers have lists of organizations that can help the depressed elder and/or family with problems of depression.
   1. The National Depressive and Manic Depressive Association
      730 N. Franklin Street, Suite 501
      Chicago, Il., 60610-3256
      1-800-826-3632
      http://www.ndmda.org
   2. The National Alliance for the Mentally Ill
      200 North Glebe Road, Suite 1015

Arlington, Va., 22203-3754

1-800-950-NAMI

http://www.nami.org

3. The National Mental Health Association

1021 Prince Street

Alexandria, Va., 22314-2971

1-800-969-6642

http://www.nmha.org

4. The American Association for Geriatric Psychiatry

7610 Woodmont Avenue, Suite 1350

Bethesda, Md., 20814-3004

http://www.aagpga.org

5. The American Psychological Association

750 First Street NE

Washington, D.C. 20002-4242

1-800-374-3120

http://www.apa.org

6. The National Institute on Aging

P.O. Box 8057

Gaithersburg, Md., 20898-8057

1-800-222-2225

http://www.nig.gov.nia

H. Telephone practice: the GDS is used because it has been validated for use in telephone screening (Burke, Roccaforte, Wengel, Conley, and Potter, 1995).

1. Assessment of initial diagnosis.

2. Assessment of response to treatment. The GDS is also used here and offers a feasible way to do telephone assessments. Both the long (30 questions) and the short form (15 questions) are considered valid and reliable (D'Arth, Katona, Mullan, Evans, and Katona, 1994).

3. Assessment of suicidal ideation. Evaluate presence of support or notify authorities for intervention if suicidal thoughts and plan are expressed.

I. Documentation.

1. Subjective and objective data is documented along with the nursing assessment and treatment plan.

2. Failure to keep appointments is documented.

3. Telephone follow-up should be part of the plan.

J. Care management.

1. All patients with a diagnosis of late-onset depression will be treated with an appropriate antidepressant medication.

2. All patients receiving treatment for depression will have follow-up appointments at 2 months, 6 months, and 1 year.

K. Protocol development/usage: the Agency for Health Care Policy Research (AHCPR) Guidelines (http://www.ahcpr.gov, 1999) recommend treatment through recovery.

1. Phase one: acute treatment phase (6 to 12 weeks) characterized by deterioration from normalcy to depression with the initiation of therapy.

    2. Phase two: continuation of treatment phase (4 to 9 months) characterized by remission and recovery.

    3. Phase three: maintenance of treatment phase (1 or more years) characterized by continuation of treatment and return to normalcy.

L. Outcome management.

    1. Decrease in symptoms of depression.

    2. No suicidal/homicidal ideation.

    3. Compliance with treatment.

    4. Return to normal activities of daily living.

CATARACTS

Many older people have good eyesight but some type of visual impairment affects many others. There are many causes of visual loss including age-related macular degeneration, glaucoma, and diabetic retinopathy. Often, however, the cause of visual deficits in the elderly is the presence of cataracts. Cataracts are the result of increased density and opacity in the lens of the eye and are a common eye problem with aging. Forty percent of cataracts occur between the ages of 75 and 85 (Ebersole and Hess, 1998). The loss of visual acuity with cataracts may result in a loss of ability to function independently. When loss of eyesight as a result of cataracts has a negative impact on daily living and reduces quality of life, surgical removal is the treatment of choice.

A. Assess/screen/triage.

    1. Symptoms of cataract formation.

        a. Difficulty in reading.

        b. Difficulty with night driving.

        c. Increased sensitivity to glare.

        d. Decreased color vision.

        e. Presence of double vision.

        f. Halos of light around objects.

    2. Medical conditions contributing to cataract formation. Severity of illness is a factor.

        a. Diabetes.

        b. Hypertension.

        c. Renal disease.

        d. Eye trauma.

        e. Long-term use of prednisone.

B. Primary, secondary prevention.

    1. Primary prevention.

        a. Eye exam including pupil dilation every other year after age 60.

        b. Use of appropriate sunglasses to avoid ultraviolet light.

        c. Brimmed hats when in sun.

    2. Secondary prevention: nonsurgical interventions.

        a. Diabetes screening and treatment if appropriate.

        b. Use of visual aids like stronger eyeglasses.

        c. Use of magnification devices.

      d. Better illumination.
C. Clinical procedures: surgical interventions.
    1. Cataract extraction.
        a. Outpatient surgery with local anesthesia except when preexisting medical conditions exist (i.e., mental disturbances, physical disability; need for extended nursing) observation.
        b. Lens replacement.
           (1) Interocular lens implant.
           (2) Glasses.
           (3) Contact lenses.
D. Care management is aimed at keeping the elderly person functional and active.
E. Patient education.
    1. Preoperative teaching.
        a. Proper administrative of eye drops or ointments; return demonstration by patient and/or caregiver.
        b. Use of patch and shield and eventually glasses after surgery.
        c. Postoperative expectations and restrictions.
        d. Determine whether help in the home environment will be needed.
    2. Postoperative teaching.
        a. Stress necessity for temporary activity restrictions.
           (1) Avoid deep bending, driving.
           (2) Avoid heavy lifting.
        b. Avoidance of strain during elimination.
           (1) Increase intake of fiber and fluids.
           (2) Use a mild laxative if necessary.
        c. Medication compliance.
           (1) Use a mild analgesic for discomfort.
           (2) Use eye drops appropriately.
        d. Necessity for postsurgery follow-up.
        e. Resumption of driving based on physician recommendation.
        f. Use of visual aids as appropriate: large print books, magnifying glass.
F. Telephone practice.
    1. Do phone follow-up first day postoperatively and as determined by facility policy.
    2. Practice active listening.
    3. Verify patient understanding of information.
    4. Be sure speech is slow and at a low pitch.
G. Documentation.
    1. Subjective and objective data as well as interventions and outcomes are included in the documentation of care.
H. Outcome management.
    1. Maintenance and improvement of vision.
    2. Follow up with physician for at least 6 weeks after surgery. Total rehabilitation after surgery takes from 6 to 12 weeks.
    3. Improved quality of life.

    I. Advocacy: senior centers may have a list of local resources that assist persons with vision loss. National organizations provide information and educational material about vision loss.

       1. National Eye Institute
       2020 Vision Place
       Bethesda, Md., 20892-3655
       http://www.nei.nih.gov

       2. American Society of Cataract and Refractive Surgery
       4000 Legato Road, Suite 850
       Fairfax, Va., 22033
       703-591-2220
       http://www.ascrs.org

ADVOCACY

Nurses advocate for the elderly by acting in their behalf. This is especially important for those who cannot act for and protect themselves. Advocacy may address the assurance of adequate care and service, the provision of necessary referrals, ethical protection of research subjects, and the prevention of abuse.

Abuse of the vulnerable elderly has seemed to increase as the general violence level in society has increased. The National Center on Elder Abuse estimates from 820,000 to 1,860,000 cases of elder abuse annually (Ebersole and Hess, 1998, p. 562). Abuse experienced by the elderly may include physical and verbal abuse, financial exploitation, forced confinement, and denial of rights. The abuser is often an adult child or spouse and is often the caregiver of the elderly victim. Nurses must be aware of the definitions of abuse, the symptoms of abuse, and the reporting policies in their practice areas.

    A. Ambulatory care nurses must be aware of the complexity of factors that influence the lives of the elderly, which include:

       1. Economic status.

       2. Health status.

         a. Expected normal aging changes.

         b. Presence of chronic diseases.

         c. Personal definition of health, which determines personal perception of wellness, a state that can be achieved and maintained.

       3. Support systems.

       4. Relationships with family and significant others.

       5. Spiritual beliefs.

       6. Cultural and value differences.

       7. Issues of grief, death, and dying.

    B. Resource identification and referral: ambulatory care nurses need to know about resources available for seniors.

       1. Community resource identification.

         a. Area Agency on Aging (AAoA) administers Older American Act funds.

           (1) Meals on Wheels and congregate meal programs.

        (2) Information and referral programs.

        (3) Case coordination services.

        (4) Chore housekeeping/homemaker services.

        (5) Transportation.

        (6) Protective Services.

    b. American Association of Retired People (AARP).

        (1) Educational resources.

        (2) Senior driving programs.

        (3) Political action.

        (4) Prescription benefits.

        (5) Insurance.

    c. Self-help/peer support groups: many of these groups are for persons with specific disease conditions (e.g., Alzheimer's, stroke, arthritis, etc.). Local senior centers should have listings.

    d. YMCA or church-sponsored exercise programs.

    e. Senior citizen centers.

        (1) Older adult day care.

        (2) Socialization activities.

        (3) Congregate meal programs.

        (4) Volunteer programs.

  2. Medicare A & B. 98% of Americans over 65 have some kind of Medicare benefits.

    a. Medicare Part A provides coverage for acute care and limited skilled nursing care.

    b. Medicare Part B provides for lab tests, outpatient visits, and durable medical equipment.

C. Prevention of elder abuse: the elderly are particularly vulnerable to abuse.

  1. Abuse is willful infliction of physical or emotional pain, injury, or debilitating mental anguish; unreasonable confinement or deprivation of services necessary to maintain physical and mental health.

  2. Ambulatory care nurses have the opportunity to assess for signs of abuse including:

    a. Physical abuse: bruises, sprains, lacerations, fractures, malnutrition.

    b. Mental abuse: isolation, fear, verbal assault/name-calling by caregivers.

    c. Material abuse: misuse or theft of money or other assets.

    d. Medical abuse: withholding of medications or other treatments.

    e. Active or passive neglect: refusal or failure to provide care; abandonment.

  3. Ambulatory care nurses should assess whether a patient should be interviewed alone if abuse is suspected.

  4. Ambulatory care nurses should know about the legal requirements for reporting suspected abuse.

    a. Many states mandate reporting of suspected abuse.

    b. Nurses must be aware of facility policy when acting as an agent of the facility in the reporting of abuse.

    c. Protective service agencies are available to assist the abused elder.
D. Goals for improving the health status of aging adults.
    1. Decrease suicide among older white males.
    2. Decrease deaths of the elderly from motor vehicle accidents and falls.
    3. Decrease hip fractures in the elderly.
    4. Decrease the numbers of elderly with significant visual impairment.
    5. Encourage elderly participation in light to moderate activity 30 minutes per day.
    6. Increase elder participation in health promotion activities.
    7. Increase the number of medication reviews for elderly clients. Remember that polypharmacy creates major health problems in this population.
    8. Increase participation in health screening exams such as breast and prostate exams.

REFERENCES

Agency for Health Care Policy and Research (1993): *Depression in primary care. vol. 2: treatment of major depression.* Clinical Practice Guideline #5. Publication #93-0551. Available at: http://www.ahcpr.gov

Alexopoulos G, Meyers B, and Young R (1993): The course of geriatric depression with "reversible dementia:" a controlled study. *Am J Psychiatry* 150 (11):1693-1699.

American Association for World Health (1999): *Healthy aging, healthy living—start now.* Washington, DC: Author.

American Psychiatric Association (1994): *Diagnostic statistical manual of mental disorders (DSM-IV).* Washington, DC: Author.

Burke M, Walsh M (1997): *Gerontological nursing: wholistic care of the older adult,* ed 2. St. Louis: Mosby.

Burke W, Roccaforte W, Wengel S, et al. (1995): The reliability and validity of the Geriatric Depression Rating Scale administered by telephone. *J Am Geriatr Soc* 43(6):574-579.

D'Arth P, Katona P, Mullan E, et al. (1994): Screening, detection and management of depression in elderly primary care attenders. *Family Practice* 11(3):260-266.

Ebersole P, Hess P (1998): *Toward healthy aging: human needs and nursing response,* ed 5. St. Louis: Mosby.

Edelman C, Mandle C (1998): *Health promotion throughout the lifespan,* ed 4. St Louis: Mosby.

Goroll A, May L, Mulley A (1998): *Primary care medicine* (on CD). Philadelphia: Lippincott-Raven.

Greenwald B, Kramer-Ginsberg E, Krishnan K (1997): Neuroanatomical localization of MR hyperintensities in geriatric depression. Abstract. Presentation at Annual Meeting, American Psychiatric Association. San Diego.

Gulanick M, Klopp A, Galanes S, et al. (1998): *Nursing care plans: nursing diagnosis and intervention,* ed 4. St. Louis: Mosby.

Hance M, Carney R, Freedland K, Skala J (1996): Depression in patients with coronary heart disease. *Gen Hosp Psychiatry* 18(1):61-65.

Harkness G, Dincher J (1996): *Medical-surgical nursing: total patient care,* ed 9. St. Louis: Mosby.

Kassirer J, Greene H (1997): *Current therapy in adult medicine,* ed 4. St. Louis: Mosby.

Yesavage J, Brink T, Rose T, et al. (1982): Screening tests for geriatric depression. *Clin Gerontologist* 1:37-44.

17 Oncology Pain Management

MARY SZYSZKA, MSN, RN, AOCN
PATRICIA JASSAK, MS, RN, AOCN

OBJECTIVES

Study of the information presented in this chapter will enable the learner to:

1. List appropriate pain assessment strategies to assess cancer pain.

2. Identify appropriate pain prevention for acute, chronic, and terminal pain.

3. List four pain relief procedures.

4. Identify three professional resources for pain management.

5. Identify pain protocols for telephone triage.

6. Identify patient self-assessment strategies for the management of cancer pain.

7. Identify two barriers to effective pain management.

8. List four pain management outcomes.

■■ "Two thirds of cancer patients experience pain at some point during the disease process" (Goldstein, 1999, p. 531). The International Association for the Study of Pain and the American Pain Society have accepted the following definition, "pain is an unpleasant sensory and emotional experience associated with actual or potential tissue damage, or described in terms of such damage" (Merskey, 1986, p. 217). In 1968, Margo McCaffery defined pain as "whatever the experiencing person says it is, existing whenever he/she says it does" (McCaffery and Portenoy, 1999, p. 17). Pain is a subjective experience, requiring consistent assessment for optimal clinical management. Pain is to be treated as an emergency with appropriate and immediate intervention.

    A. Pain assessment/screening/triage. Pain assessment is aimed at preventing pain if possible, identifying pain as soon as it occurs, and monitoring interventions (McGuire, Yarbro, and Ferrell, 1995).

        1. Patient is primary source of pain assessment.

        2. Ask patient/family about pain experience.

        3. Include pain as the fifth vital sign assessment.

4. Initial pain assessment should include:
  a. History.
      (1) Onset of pain.
      (2) Duration of pain.
      (3) Location of pain.
      (4) Alleviating/aggravating characteristics of pain.
      (5) Pain intensity and character.
      (6) Current pain alleviating measures, pharmacologic and nonphar-macologic.
      (7) Side effects to pain alleviating measures if any.
  b. Physical examination.
      (1) Clinical examination.
      (2) Appropriate scans and tests.
      (3) Emphasize neurologic examination.
  c. Psychosocial assessment.
      (1) Emotional response (depression, anxiety, mood responses).
      (2) Ability to perform ADLs.
      (3) Meaning of pain to patient and family.
      (4) Past pain experiences.
      (5) Patient's knowledge of pain and pain treatment.
      (6) Patient resources (social, financial, etc.).
  d. Pain intensity tools. Several tools are available to help a patient objectively rate the pain experience.
      (1) Numeric rating scale, 1 to 10.
      (2) Visual analogue scales.
      (3) Pain faces.
      (4) Pain intensity scales (Figure 17-1).
5. Pain classifications.
  a. Nociceptive pain: normal processing of stimuli that damages normal tissues or has the potential for damage if prolonged.
      (1) Somatic pain: arises from bone, joint, muscle, skin, or connective tissue. Usually described as aching or throbbing. It is localized pain.
      (2) Visceral pain: arises from visceral organs such as GI tract.
          (a) Tumor involvement of the organ capsule causing aching and fairly well localized pain.
          (b) Obstruction of hollow viscus, causing intermittent cramping and poorly localized pain (McCaffery and Pasero, 1999, p. 19).
  b. Neuropathic pain: an abnormal processing or sensory input by the peripheral or central nervous system and is described as burning, tingling, or shock-like.
6. Temporal relationships.
  a. Acute pain: recent onset associated with overt pain behavior such as moaning, grimacing, splinting with diaphoresis, hypertension, and tachycardia.

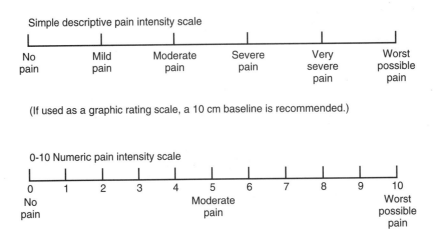

FIGURE 17-1 ■ Pain Intensity Scales. (Jacox A, Carr D, Payne R, et al. (1994): *Management of cancer pain*. Clinical Practice Guideline, No. 9, AHCPR Publication No. 94-0592. Rockville, MD: US Department of Health and Human Services, Agency for Health Care Policy Research.)

 b. Chronic pain: persistence of pain for 3 months or more beyond the usual course of an acute illness or injury. Overt pain behaviors and vital sign changes are often absent.

 c. Chronic pain with acute exacerbations (e.g., sickle cell anemia).

 d. Breakthrough pain: common in both acute and chronic pain states. May be precipitated by an action or without an identifiable cause.

 e. Idiopathic pain: perceived as excessive for the extent of identifiable organic pathology.

7. Special populations: assessment and treatment of special populations should be given extra attention and individual intervention.

 a. Infants/children.

  (1) Develop awareness of developmental age of child.

  (2) Assess nonverbal behavior (i.e., facial expression, movements, responses to cuddling, crying, lack of crying, staring into space).

  (3) Assess past procedural related pain experience.

  (4) Develop trust with child and parents.

  (5) Tailor interventions to specific child's needs and anxieties.

  (6) Use topical analgesics for invasive procedures including peripheral blood draws.

  (7) Instruct parents to use topical analgesia prior to coming to outpatient setting for an invasive procedure.

(8) Use music, games, and other forms of distraction with children.

8. Elderly population.

    a. Assess chronic nonmalignant pain as well as cancer pain (e.g., arthritis).

    b. Complete a full medication history to assess for possible drug interactions. Include all over-the-counter medications.

    c. Individualize opioid doses and titration as the elderly may experience a higher peak effect and longer duration of pain relief (Jacox, et al., 1994).

    d. Continuous reassessment and management are necessary to achieve optimal pain control in the elderly.

9. Cognitively impaired elderly.

    a. Believe patient self-report of pain when available.

    b. When self-report is not available, the presence of painful stimuli such as a wound or incision should prompt medication administration.

    c. Attempt to use a visual pain-rating scale.

    d. Observe overt signs and symptoms of acute or chronic pain.

10. Patients with a history of substance abuse. Fears, misconceptions, and lack of knowledge about addiction affect prescribing of opioid analgesics to persons experiencing pain (Compton, 1999).

    a. It is important to understand the terms related to substance abuse.

        (1) Addiction is characterized by a persistent pattern of dysfunctional drug use.

        (2) Opioid addiction is a pattern of compulsive drug use with a craving for the opioid for reasons other than pain relief.

        (3) Chemical dependence is physical dependence on a drug or medication.

        (4) Physical dependence is an expected physiologic occurrence with continuous use of particular drugs such as opioid analgesics. Physical dependence does not imply or cause addiction.

        (5) Substance abuse is a term that describes a less severe form of addiction, which is often a predecessor to addiction.

        (6) Tolerance is the decreased drug effect that results from chronic drug administration requiring increases in the dose of drug to reach the same analgesic effect. Tolerance is an expected physiologic effect (Compton, 1999).

    b. The nurse should be aware of his/her own personal biases related to addiction and consciously put these biases aside to meet patient needs.

    c. Assess the current and past history of drug use.

    d. At each patient visit assess and chart:

        (1) Pain severity and quality.

        (2) Level of function.

        (3) Opiate analgesic use.

        (4) Evidence of opiate misuse.

        (5) Evaluation and plan (Compton, 1999).

e. Use opioid agents with less street value, such as codeine, controlled release morphine, oxycodone, transdermal patch.

f. Educate patient on dose, time drug should be taken, route, and side effects.

g. Opioid treatment should be a part of the recovery plan and should be shared with a recovery counselor if the patient is in active recovery treatment.

11. Patient with psychiatric history.
    a. Patient may not be able to verbalize the pain experienced.
    b. Observe for obvious causes of pain.
    c. Observe for acute or chronic pain behaviors.

B. Primary, secondary, tertiary prevention. Pain prevention or control requires an interdisciplinary approach to pain management utilizing continuous quality improvement intended to identify pain presence, location, classification, treatment, and outcome.

1. Primary prevention activities are actions taken to prevent pain in an identifiable situation where pain is likely to occur (acute pain).
   a. Administer appropriate premedication with procedures.
   b. Treat cause of pain.
   c. Provide padding on exam and treatment tables to add to comfort during procedures.
   d. Educate patient and family.
      (1) Take analgesics early when pain is mild or when pain starts.
      (2) Prevent severe pain that will interfere with ADLs.
      (3) Initiate bowel regimen and medications with opioid use.
      (4) Use pain rating scales to identify serious pain levels.
   e. Assess availability of appropriate pain medication.
   f. Review use of nonpharmacologic cognitive behavioral measures (e.g., relaxation, imagery, distraction, and peer support).

2. Secondary prevention occurs when pain is present. Reduction and control of pain and control of pain are appropriate goals (chronic pain).
   a. Reassess pain experienced over period of time.
   b. Assess use of additional medication for breakthrough pain, which presents between analgesic doses.
   c. Discuss concept of tolerance to opioids with patient and family.
   d. Explain the importance of around-the-clock administration of pain medication.
   e. Discuss use of alternative coping measures.
      (1) Humor, music, reading, mild exercise as distractions.
      (2) Complementary therapies such as relaxation, hypnosis, guided imagery.
      (3) Use of noninvasive cutaneous stimulation (e.g., massage).

3. Tertiary prevention (severe, chronic, and terminal pain): once pain has reached constant and/or unrelenting proportions, reassessment and further medical evaluation and intervention are required.
   a. Assess pain objectively using a pain scale.

    b. Set a "comfort goal" the patient identifies as tolerable (e.g., a score of < 4 on a scale of 0 to 10).

    c. Determine, if possible, the cause of pain and increased intensity.

    d. Discuss new treatment plan with patient.

    e. Reassess frequently, pre- and postintervention, with necessary pain treatment plan modifications.

        (1) At regular intervals after starting treatment plan.

        (2) With each report of new pain.

        (3) At appropriate intervals after each pain control intervention (e.g., 15 to 30 minutes after parenteral drug administration and 1 hour after oral administration). (Jacox, et al., 1994, p. 28)

C. Clinical procedures to relieve pain.

  1. Plans for management of pain associated with painful procedures should address the following:

    a. Why is the procedure being performed?

    b. What is the expected intensity and duration of pain?

    c. What is the expected intensity and duration of anxiety?

    d. What are the planned interventions to decrease pain and anxiety?

    e. How often will the procedure be repeated?

    f. What reaction can the patient expect for the procedure?

    g. What is the meaning of the procedure to the patient/family (Jacox, et al., 1994).

  2. General principles for procedure related pain.

    a. Provide adequate preparation for patient and family.

    b. Adhere to the planned procedure schedule to reduce patient anxiety.

    c. Manage preexisting pain before starting the procedure.

    d. Treat procedure pain prophylactically.

    e. Be attentive to the environment and the need for privacy.

    f. Tailor treatment options to patient/family needs and preferences.

    g. Integrate pharmacologic and nonpharmacologic pain management options.

    h. If possible administer pharmacologic agents by a painless route (Jacox, et al., 1994).

    i. Provide adequate monitoring and resuscitative equipment if conscious sedation is used for the procedure.

    j. Encourage parents to be present during a child's procedure if parents' wish.

    k. The presence of a support person for the patient may be helpful.

    l. Review the experience with patient/family, after the procedure.

    m. After the procedure, assess the effectiveness of pain management.

  3. Noninvasive methods.

    a. Cutaneous stimulation.

        (1) Application of dry or moist heat.

        (2) Application of cold.

        (3) Heating/cooling methods.

        (4) Massage/vibration.

     b. Sites for cutaneous stimulation.
       (1) Directly over or around pain.
       (2) Proximal to pain site.
       (3) Distal to pain site.
       (4) Contralateral to pain.
     c. Nursing responsibility for superficial heating and cooling.
       (1) Protect skin from extremes of temperature.
       (2) Test water temperature with wet or moist application.
       (3) Use layers of cloth between skin and hot pack.
       (4) Wrap ice pack with waterproof material.
       (5) Instruct patient/family to inspect area frequently.
       (6) Monitor area for patient with decreased skin sensation.

4. Invasive methods.
     a. Subcutaneous continuous infusion of opioids for patient unable to tolerate oral medication without IV access.
     b. Intravenous routes provide immediate relief for acute, severe, or escalating pain.
       (1) Bolus.
       (2) Continuous infusion.
       (3) Patient-controlled analgesia (PCA).
       (4) Continuous infusion with the addition of PCA.
     c. Intraspinal routes to deliver medication to spaces or potential spaces surrounding the spinal cord.
       (1) Intrathecal catheter for short-term acute pain management.
       (2) Epidural catheter is tunneled subcutaneously for intermittent or continuous infusion for severe intractable chronic pain.
       (3) Surgical implantation of intraspinal catheters with implanted port for long-term use.
     d. Nursing responsibilities during intraspinal catheter placement.
       (1) Assess patient/family ability to care for system at home.
       (2) Educate patient/family before catheter insertion.
         (a) Signs and symptoms of catheter displacement/migration.
         (b) Prevention of intraspinal neurotoxicity.
         (c) Prevention of intraspinal infection.
         (d) Signs and symptoms of intraspinal infection.
       (3) Explain the steps of the procedure to the patient.
       (4) Position patient in sitting or side lying position.
       (5) Support patient.
       (6) Assist anesthesiologist.
       (7) Observe site for bleeding postinsertion.
       (8) Monitor vital signs.
       (9) Monitor neurologic status for changes.

5. Neuroablation.
     a. Dorsal rhizotomy: selective ablation of the dorsal nerve root, for localized pain in the trunk or abdomen.

    b. Anterolateral cordotomy: ablative procedure of pain conducting tracts involving sensory and thermal fibers.

    c. Commissural myelotomy: disruption of pain-conducting fibers and polysynaptic pain pathway running through the center of the spinal cord.

D. Collaboration/resource identification and referral.

  1. Numerous pain facilities exist for treatment of chronic pain and cancer pain.

    a. Acute pain services are available in hospitals and can be accessed for patients in the ambulatory setting.

    b. The pain services can offer pain management for acute, chronic, and terminal cancer pain.

  2. Professional organizations and state cancer pain initiatives.

    a. American Academy of Pain Management, http://www.aapainmanage.org/index.html

    b. American Pain Society, http://www.ampainsoc.org

    c. American Alliance of Cancer Pain Initiatives, aacti@aacti.org

    d. Hospice Foundation of America, http://www.hospicefoundation.org

    e. American Academy of Hospice and Palliative Care, http://www.aahpc.org

    f. Agency for Health Care Policy and Research (AHCPR), www.ahcpr.gov

    g. Joint Commission on Accreditation of Health Care Organizations, www.jcaho.org

  3. Patient organizations.

    a. American Cancer Society, http://www.cancer.org

    b. American Chronic Pain Association (ACPA), http://coolware/health/medicalreporter/pain.html

    c. Cancer Information Service, www.nci.nih.gov

    d. Hospice Helpline, www.nhpco.org

E. Care management.

  1. Analgesic ladder (Figure 17-2). The World Health Organization (WHO) analgesic ladder identifies pain intensities. Patients do not necessarily progress up the ladder in an orderly manner.

    a. Step 1: Nonopioid analgesics.

      (1) Mild pain relieved by nonopioid analgesics with or without an adjuvant analgesic. Adjuvant analgesics and adjuvant drugs have primary indication other than pain control. Adjuvant drugs are used to enhance the analgesic effect of opioids, provide independent analgesia for specific types of pain, or diminish side effects of pain medications.

      (2) Examples of adjuvant analgesics are: acetaminophen, nonsteroidal antiinflammatory agents, and aspirin.

    b. Step 2: opioid analgesic with/without nonopioid or adjuvant.

      (1) Moderate pain or increasing persistent pain.

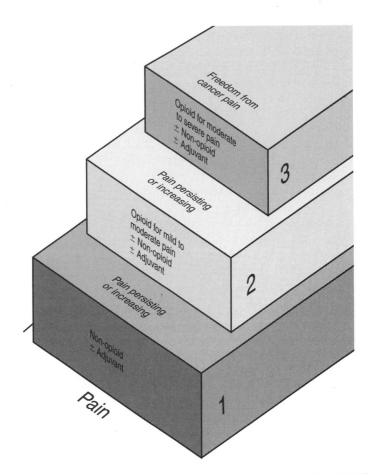

FIGURE 17-2 ■ WHO analgesic ladder. (From World Health Organization [1996]: *Cancer pain relief.* [2nd ed.]. Geneva: WHO.)

> (2) Oral analgesics in a fixed combination are often given (e.g., Tylenol No. 3, Percocet, Vicodin).
>
> (3) Caution should be used to avoid exceeding recommended maximum acetaminophen dose of 4 to 6 g/24 hours.
>
> (4) Agonist-antagonist may reverse analgesia and are not appropriate for cancer pain.
>
> **c.** Step 3: strong opioid.
>
> > (1) The opioid should be available in oral and other routes to avoid change of opioid if route of administration needs to be changed.
> >
> > (2) The opioids should have a short half-life so they can be titrated upward rapidly for severe, escalating pain.
> >
> > (3) Controlled-release opioids should be used for chronic pain so dosing intervals can be lengthened after the appropriate dose is determined with immediate-release formulations (McCaffery and Portenoy, 1999).

■ TABLE 17-1
■ ■ Adjuvant Analgesics

Drug Classification	Indication
Antidepressants	Neuropathic pain
	Postherpetic pain
	Depression secondary to pain experience
Anticonvulsants	Neuropathic pain
	Postherpetic pain
Antihistamines	Pain complicated by anxiety or nausea
Antispasmodics	GI, bladder spasm
Corticosteroids	Pain from nerve compression, lymphedema, bone pain
Muscle relaxants	Musculoskeletal pain
Nonsteroidal antiinflammatory agents (NSAIDs)	Bone metastases, soft tissue infiltration
Biphosphates	Bone pain
Strontium-89	Bone pain

Adapted from Jacox A, Carr D, Payne R, et al. (1994): *Management of cancer pain. Clinical practice guideline, Number 9*, AHCPR Publication No. 94-0592. Rockville, MD: US Department of Health and Human Services, Agency for Health Care Policy and Research; Otto S (1997): *Oncology nursing*, ed 3. St. Louis: Mosby.

    (4) Examples of Step 3 opioids are morphine, oxycodone, hydromorphone, and fentanyl.

    (5) Avoid meperidine for cancer pain management as the metabolite normeperidine may accumulate and cause central nervous system toxicity.

  2. Adjuvant analgesic describes a drug that has a primary indication other than pain but is analgesic in some painful conditions. The potential benefit is usually suggested by the characteristics of the pain (Coyle, Cherny, and Portenoy, 1995). Adjuvant analgesics may also be used to relieve side effects of opioid analgesics. Examples of adjuvant analgesics are (Table 17-1):

    a. Antidepressants.

    b. Anticonvulsants.

    c. Anxiolytics.

    d. Corticosteroids.

    e. Bisphosphonates.

  3. Nonsteroidal antiinflammatory drugs (NSAIDS) or COX2-inhibitors (Celebrex, Vioxx) are effectively used as initial therapy in mild pain. They can be used in combination with opioids and adjuvant analgesics if pain intensity increases. NSAIDs have a ceiling effect, so specified doses should be followed. Most NSAIDs interfere with platelet aggregation and should be used cautiously with patients undergoing surgery, chemotherapy, or a history of bleeding diatheses.

  4. Route of administration.

      a. The oral route is the preferred route because it is the most convenient and cost-effective.

      b. When the oral route is not possible, rectal or transdermal route should be attempted.

          (1) Rectal route.

              (a) Safe, inexpensive route.

              (b) Good route when nausea and vomiting are present.

              (c) Inappropriate with diarrhea, anal/rectal lesions.

              (d) Do not use if the patient is neutropenic or thrombocytopenic.

          (2) Transdermal route.

              (a) Good route for stable pain.

              (b) Not suitable for rapid pain relief or dose titration.

              (c) Drug concentration increases over 12 to 24 hours, then levels off.

              (d) Skin irritation may be a problem.

          (3) Intravenous or subcutaneous routes should be used when rapid incremental doses of analgesia are required.

              (a) Continuous analgesia will provide the most consistent level of analgesia.

              (b) An IV bolus provides the most rapid onset of analgesia, but a shorter duration of relief.

          (4) Intraspinal route: when other routes do not provide relief or side effects limit dose escalation.

F. Patient education.

  1. Give patient permission to report pain.

  2. Explain the importance of good pain management.

  3. Pain self-assessment questions.

    a. Where is the pain? List all sites of pain.

    b. What does the pain feel like? Ache, throb, burn, tingle?

    c. How bad does the pain feel? Give an objective scale rating.

    d. What makes the pain better or worse? What is the patient successfully doing to relieve pain?

    e. How well does the present pain treatment work?

    f. Has the pain changed? Is it better, worse, changed over time?

  4. Analgesia education.

    a. Establish with patient an acceptable pain rating level (i.e., 2 on a scale of 10).

    b. Identify which medications are used for each pain source (e.g., headache versus arthritis).

    c. Provide written instructions for patient and family.

      (1) Name of medication, both brand and generic names.

      (2) Dosage of medication.

      (3) Time to take the medication.

      (4) Side effects of the medication.

    d. Explain rationale for around-the-clock dosing to maintain control of the pain. Assist patient to identify the best time for him/her to take the medication.

    e. Review all medications and medication schedules along with analgesics.

    f. Provide full information when adding a new analgesic to the pain regimen.

    g. Provide written information of phone numbers, appropriate contact persons, and when to call to receive information regarding questions or problems.

G. Advocacy: the nurse must be aware of and recognize barriers to pain management.

    1. Appropriate education, intervention, and advocacy will promote adequate pain intervention and management.

    2. Barriers to effective pain management.

        a. Problems related to health care professionals.

            (1) Inadequate knowledge of pain management. Inadequate curricula in pain management in nursing and medical schools.

            (2) Poor pain assessment skills.

            (3) Concern about controlled substance regulation.

            (4) Concern about patient addiction.

            (5) Inadequate knowledge concerning opioid side effects.

        b. Problems related to patients.

            (1) Reluctance to report pain.

                (a) Fear pain means the disease is worse.

                (b) Concern about taking up physician's time and desire to be a "good" patient.

            (2) Reluctance to take pain medications.

                (a) Fear of addiction or being thought of as an addict.

                (b) Worried about side effects.

            (3) Problems related to the health care system.

                (a) Cancer pain management is given low priority.

                (b) Reimbursement for adequate pain control may not be available.

                (c) Restrictive regulation of controlled substances.

                (d) Problems of opioid availability and access (Jacox, et al., 1994).

H. Telephone practice.

    1. Provision of easy telephone access 24 hours a day.

    2. Nurses educated in pain management to answer the phone.

    3. Clear documentation of telephone advice, treatment, and recommendations in the medical record.

    4. Clear guidelines/protocols to direct nurse in pain management decisions.

        a. Appropriate nursing decisions.

        b. Indicators for referral to physician.

      c. Ongoing quality monitoring of telephone nursing.
  5. Pain diary should be provided to patient and family with instruction on its use.
      a. Pain diary facilitates pain assessment, evaluation of pain control interventions, and further educational needs.
      b. Pain diary will identify success and roadblocks to pain control.
  6. Essential information for telephone intervention.
      a. Patient name and demographics.
      b. Patient telephone number and alternate telephone number.
      c. Pharmacy name and telephone number.
      d. Patient's medication and allergy history.
      e. Assess pain.
         (1) Severity of pain using a number scale.
         (2) Location of pain.
         (3) Description of pain: shooting, throbbing, aching, etc.
         (4) When did pain intensity increase?
         (5) Aggravating and relieving factors.
         (6) Pain diary notations if possible.

I. Communication/documentation.
  1. Multidisciplinary health professionals share areas of expertise to manage pain.
      a. Consistent use of common language.
         (1) Common assessment tools.
         (2) Pain scale ratings.
         (3) Standards for monitoring.
      b. Consistent documentation of pain assessment/reassessment and management.
         (1) Consistent use of documentation tool across the continuum of care.
         (2) Consensus on format of documentation.
         (3) Identify where pain will be documented.
         (4) Identify who will assess/document pain.
         (5) Establish how often pain will be assessed.
         (6) Established communication channels with nurses in other care settings.

J. Outcome management.
  1. Patient outcomes (Johnson and Maas, 1997).
      a. Recognizes symptom/pain onset.
      b. Reports pain.
      c. Recognizes causal factors.
      d. Uses preventive measures.
      e. Uses relief measures.
      f. Uses warning signs to seek health care.
      g. Uses pain diary.
  2. Professional outcomes.
      a. Professionals will assess/reassess pain at each patient encounter.

    b. Pain management is a priority.

    c. Pain protocols are a standard of nursing care.

    d. Pain protocols are a standard for telephone nursing.

    e. Consistent pain management education.

    f. The staff demonstrates proficiency in pain assessment and management.

K. Protocol development/usage.

  1. JCAHO has identified pain management standards as part of total patient care. Mandated standards are to take effect in the year 2000 (JCAHO, 2000; Kowal, 1999). Available through JCAHO website: www.jcaho.org

  2. The Agency for Health Care Policy and Research (AHCPR) Guideline identifying the clinician as responsible for the management and treatment of pain (Kowal, 1999).

  3. Interdisciplinary team approach instituted for the management of pain.

    a. Identify and break down institutional barriers to pain management.

    b. Identify and break down clinician's attitudes concerning pain management.

    c. Select common language for pain control communication.

    d. Staff education on pain, pain medications, and side effect management.

    e. Utilize continuous quality improvement process.

  4. Continuous quality improvement.

    a. Identify the structure.

      (1) Ambulatory setting.

      (2) Hospital outpatient setting.

      (3) Doctor's office.

    b. Identify process.

      (1) Policies and procedures.

      (2) Guidelines.

      (3) Clinical pathways.

      (4) Competency training.

    c. Identify outcomes.

      (1) Patient uses analgesic appropriately.

      (2) Patient reports pain controlled.

      (3) Side effects managed.

      (4) Pain control documented.

    d. Use a continuous quality improvement process.

      (1) Plan.

        (a) Study and collect data on present pain management.

        (b) Identify ways to improve pain management.

        (c) Draft an action plan.

      (2) Do.

        (a) Implement your action plan.

        (b) Monitor process of pain management action plan.

      (3) Check.

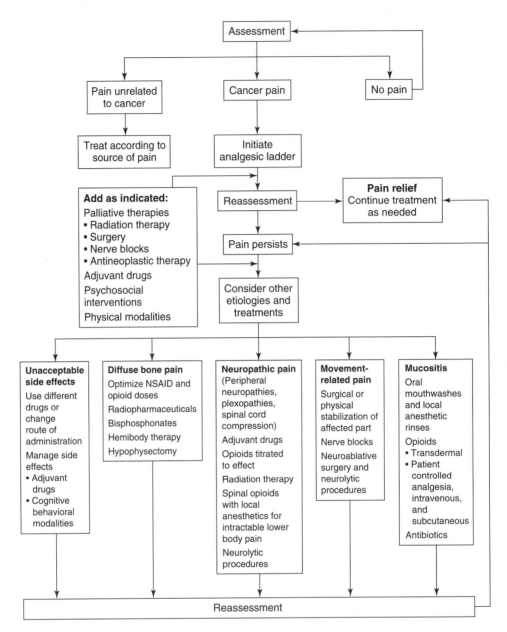

FIGURE 17-3 ■ Flowchart—Continuing Pain Management in Patients with Cancer. (From Jacox A, Carr D, Payne R, et al. [1994]: *Management of cancer pain*. Clinical practice guidelines, No. 9 AHCPR Publication No. 94-0592. Rockville, Md: US Department of Health and Human Services: Agency for Health Care Policy and Research.)

          (a) Compare results of pilot action plan with objectives.

          (b) Repeat *plan* and *do* until expected results are achieved.

      (4) Act.

          (a) Educate staff on results and pain management improvement.

          (b) Continue data collection.

          (c) Continue to monitor for new pain problems.

          (d) Develop a protocol for continuous quality pain care improvement (Figure 17-3).

REFERENCES

Compton P (1999): Substance abuse. In McCaffery M, Pasero C, editors: *Pain, clinical manual.* St. Louis: Mosby, pp. 428-466.

Coyle N, Cherny N, Portenoy R (1995): Pharmacologic management of cancer pain. In McGuire D, Yarbro C, Ferrel B, editors: *Cancer pain management.* Boston: Jones & Bartlett, pp. 89-130.

Goldstein M (1999): Cancer-related pain. In McCaffery M, Pasero C: *Pain, clinical manual.* St. Louis: Mosby, pp. 531-545.

Jacox A, Carr D, Payne R, et al. (1994*): Management of cancer pain.* Clinical practice guideline, No. 9, AHCPR Publication No. 94-0592. Rockville, MD: US Department of Health and Human Services, Agency for Health Care Policy and Research.

Johnson M, Maas M (1997): *Nursing outcomes classification (NOC).* St. Louis: Mosby.

Joint Commission on Accreditation of Healthcare Organizations (JCAHO) (2000): *Pain assessment and management: an organizational approach.* Oakbrook, IL: Author.

Kowal N (1999): Report card for pain management: documentation standards along the continuum of pain care. *Analgesia* 10(11):3-7.

McCaffery M, Portenoy R (1999): Overview of three groups of analgesics. In McCaffery M, Pasero C, editors: *Pain clinical manual,* ed. 2. St. Louis: Mosby, pp. 103-128.

McGuire D, Yarbro C, Ferrell B (1995): *Cancer pain management,* ed. 2. Boston: Jones & Bartlett.

Merskey H (1986): Classification of chronic pain: description of chronic pain syndromes and definitions of pain terms. *Pain,* suppl 3:217.

Otto S (1997): *Oncology nursing,* ed. 3. St Louis: Mosby.

World Health Organization (1990): *Cancer pain relief and palliative care.* Report of a WHO expert committee (World Health Organization Technical Report Series, 804). Geneva, Switzerland: Author.

Other Recommended Readings

American Pain Society (1993): *Principles of analgesic use in the treatment of acute pain and cancer pain,* ed. 3. Skokie, IL: Author.

Brant J (1998): Comfort. In Itano J, Taoka K, editors: *Core curriculum for oncology nursing,* ed. 3. Philadelphia: WB Saunders, pp. 3-13.

Kemp C (1995): Pain: techniques of management. In Kemp C, editor: *Terminal illness.* Philadelphia: JB Lippincott, pp. 123-141.

McGuire D, Sheidler V (!997): Pain. In Groenwald SL, Frogge M, Goodman M, Yarbro C, editors: *Cancer nursing principles and practice,* ed. 4. Boston: Jones & Bartlett, pp. 527-585.

Ruzicka D, Gates R, Fink R (1997): Pain management. In Gates R, Fink R, editors: *Oncology nursing secrets.* Philadelphia: Hanley & Belfus, pp. 284-303.

Spross J, McGuire D, Schmitt R (1990): Oncology nursing society position paper on cancer pain, Part I. *Oncol Nurs Forum* 17(4):595-613.

Spross J, McGuire D, Schmitt R (1990): Oncology nursing society position paper on cancer pain, Part II. *Oncol Nurs Forum* 17(5):751-760.

Spross J, McGuire D, Schmitt R (1990). Oncology nursing society position paper on cancer pain, Part III. *Oncology Nursing Forum* 17(6), 943-955.

Swenson C (1997): Pain management In Otto S: *Oncology nursing,* ed 3. St. Louis: Mosby, pp. 746-791.

18 Neurology

CAROLYN A. BENSON MS, RNC, NP

PATIENT PROTOTYPES

Headache ■ Stroke ■ Back Pain

OBJECTIVES

Study of the information presented in this chapter will enable the learner to:

1. Provide appropriate telephone triage for patients with neurologic complaints.
2. Develop and implement patient education plans.
3. Administer and monitor effect of headache medications per protocol.
4. Function as patient advocate and care coordinator both within and outside the department.
5. Assist department staff in developing their understanding of the patient with headache, stroke, and back pain.

■■■ The patients in the adult ambulatory neurology practice can range in age from 18 to the very elderly. The complaints in this group range from low to very high in complexity. Outpatient neurology is usually a consultative practice, yet will provide long-term management of some patients with neurologic disorders.

For the patient with headache, stroke or back pain the neurology clinic usually becomes a frequent outpatient stop and the main source of treatment and education for the condition. A condition may be acute in its initial presentation and then become a chronic problem. The patient, therefore, must cope with each phase of the neurologic disorder and thus requires the care and education to do so.

HEADACHE

The headache patient is any patient with a new onset or a new type of headache, or has a headache pattern that is persistent in spite of treatment.

    A. Assess/screen/triage.

        1. Assess the patient's headache in all of the following areas:

            a. Location, onset, quality, and intensity of pain.

            b. Associated symptoms including nausea, vomiting, sensory or visual changes.

            c. Previous medications used.

            d. Other therapies used such as antiemetics, icepacks.

    e. Head trauma within the previous 48 hours.

2. Determine the type of headache the patient describes (Diamond, 1998).

    a. Vascular: vascular dilation evokes the headache.

        (1) Triggers include menses, fever, stress, weather, altitude, foods containing vasoactive and vasodilatory substances such as nitrates.

        (2) Main types.

            (a) Migraine with or without aura: two to eight headaches per month, unilateral or bilateral, throbbing with moderate to severe pain. Nausea, vomiting associated symptoms, stress, menses, alcohol, food triggers. Three times more common in females.

            (b) Cluster: one to three attacks per day in cycle, unilateral retroorbital pain severe, excruciating, knife-like. One-sided symptoms. Alcohol, excess sleep can trigger attack. Ten times more common in men.

            (c) Tension-type: characterized by muscle contraction and is episodic or chronic. Can occur daily with constant dull aching pain like a vice around the head. No usual associated symptoms.

            (d) Traction and inflammatory: headaches caused by organic disease such as mass lesions, arteritis, and phlebitis. Neurologic and general examination usually indicates a problem.

3. Determine if the headache meets any of the red flag criteria (Rapport and Sheftell, 1996).

    a. Abrupt onset of a new type of severe headache and any one of the following unresolved symptoms:

        (1) Confusion.

        (2) Difficulty walking.

        (3) Memory problems.

        (4) Weakness or loss of sensation of an extremity or of the face, on one side of the body.

        (5) Visual problems.

        (6) Slurred speech.

        (7) Change in level of consciousness.

    b. Worst headache ever.

    c. Progressive worsening of headache over days or unresponsive to treatment.

    d. Headache triggered by exertion.

    e. Headache accompanied by illness or stiff neck.

4. Communicate information with patient's provider including relief efforts thus far, adequacy and ability of patient to self-manage and triage.

    a. As directed by neurology provider, refer to a routine or urgent clinic appointment or to an emergency department.

    b. If provider not available, to emergency department if any red flag criteria met.

B. Primary, secondary, tertiary prevention.

    1. Assist patient in assessment of headache triggers and strategies to avoid or better live with them. Common headache triggers are:

        a. Menses.

        b. Stress.

        c. Relaxation after stress.

        d. Fatigue.

        e. Sleep changes.

        f. Meal skipping.

        g. Weather changes or extremes.

        h. Glare or flickering lights.

        i. Loud noises.

        j. Perfumes or chemical odors.

        k. Postural changes.

        l. Physical activity.

        m. Coughing.

        n. Food triggers: chocolate, cheeses, alcoholic beverages (especially red wine), citrus fruits, and foods/food-products containing monosodium glutamate, nitrates, and aspartame.

    2. Educate patient in pharmacologic and nonpharmacologic methods of headache control (Silberstein, Lipton, and Goadsby, 1998).

        a. Pharmacologic.

            (1) Prophylactic: medications prescribed to prevent a headache.

                (a) Beta-blockers: propranolol, nadolol, atenolol.

                (b) Antiserotonin: cyproheptadine (Periactin), methysergide (Sansert).

                (c) Calcium channel blockers: verapamil.

                (d) Antidepressants: tricyclics, SSRIs (selective serotonin reuptake inhibitors), lithium.

                (e) Anticonvulsants: divalproex/valproate, gabapentin.

                (f) Nonsteroidal antiinflamatory drugs (NSAIDs): naproxen.

                (g) Monoamine oxidase inhibitors (MAOIs): phenelzine.

            (2) Abortive.

                (a) Selective serotonin agonists: sumatriptan, naratriptan, zolmitriptan, rizatriptan.

                (b) Ergotamine.

                (c) Dihydroergotamine: DHE45 sc and nasal spray.

            (3) Symptomatic.

                (a) Acetaminophen.

                (b) Aspirin.

                (c) Butalbital (caffeine and analgesics).

                (d) Isometheptene.

                (e) Narcotics.

                (f) Nonsteroidal antiinflammatory drugs.

        b. Nonpharmacologic methods.

            (1) Biofeedback.

            (2) Stress reduction training.

(3) Massage.

3. Encourage patient to recognize early symptoms of migraine so abortive treatment can be used early at its most effective time. Common prodromal symptoms and aura are:
    a. Mental state: depressed, fatigued, hyperactive, irritable, euphoric.
    b. Neurologic symptoms: yawning, photophobia, phonophobia, poor concentration.
    c. General: stiff neck, fluid retention, food cravings, anorexia, diarrhea/constipation.
    d. Visual aura: scotoma, C-shaped, objects have motion, colorful or white, bright, fuzzy looking, migrating in visual field.

C. Clinical procedures.
    1. Workup includes vital signs, neurologic examination.
    2. Administer acute headache medication ordered for the patient.
    3. Educate the patient about the medication, effect, and potential adverse effects. Document and communicate effect.

D. Collaboration/resource identification and referral.
    1. Assist patient in obtaining referrals as needed: for clinic visits, testing ordered, and stress reduction, for example.
    2. Reinforce plan of care to help minimize emergency department and urgent care visits.
    3. Referral to support groups: National Headache Foundation 1-800-843-2256, www.headaches.org

E. Patient education.
    1. Educate patient about the different types of headache.
    2. Instruct patient on the headache diary.
    3. Help the patient recognize headache triggers.
    4. Review all medication rationale, potential adverse effects, and appropriate way to take.
    5. List out headache triggers for patient.
    6. Provide headache diet (Diamond, 1998).
    7. Promote lifestyle changes: regular sleeping schedules, regular meal schedules, healthy diet, coping strategies, and stress reduction strategies.

F. Advocacy (also see Patient Education section E above).
    1. May require contact with insurance company for authorization of test and treatments.

G. Telephone practice (Parker and Kelley, 1998).
    1. Triage: assess for headache red flags. Refer to A, 3, a on p. 320.
    2. Patient education: review.
        a. Use of prophylactic medications. Refer to B, 2, a, (1) on p. 321.
        b. Use of abortive medication. Refer to B, 2, a, (2) on p. 321.
        c. Alternative therapies for headache. Refer to B, 2, b on p. 321.
        d. Encourage additional measures such as antiemetics and ice application.
        e. Issues with analgesic rebound: headaches caused by the frequent use of any analgesic (Rapport and Sheftell, 1996).
        f. Issues with narcotic use: tolerance, dependence, abuse.

      g. Avoidance of headache triggers. Refer to B, 1, a-n on p. 321.

      h. Headache diet. Refer to E, 6 on p. 322.

  3. Emotional support.

      a. Reassure patient that medication should help decrease the pain and associated symptoms.

      b. Offer the patient a clear plan to follow if abortive therapy does not work.

      c. Develop plan with patient.

  4. Facilitation.

      a. Facilitate additional acute treatment with primary care and neurology provider.

  5. Coordination.

      a. Coordinate acute visit with primary care provider, neurology provider, and clinic.

  6. Communication/documentation.

      a. Document all telephone encounters.

      b. Communicate via established mechanism with primary care provider and neurology provider.

H. Communication/documentation.

  1. Formally document all patient encounters in clinic including:

      a. Number of times patient had same complaint.

      b. Medications administered and response.

      c. Patient's appearance and behaviors.

      d. Level of discomfort and relief using established scales. For headache, a numeric scale is often used: 0 is no pain, 1 is mild headache, 2 is moderate headache, and 3 is severe headache.

      e. Patient ability to use drug delivery method such as intranasal or self-injection.

  2. Communicate all information via established mechanism to all providers.

I. Outcome management.

  1. Patient identifies and implements methods to prevent acute headaches.

  2. Number of chronic headaches is reduced or eliminated.

  3. Number of rebound headaches is reduced or eliminated.

  4. Care is coordinated across all providers and treatment is consistent with the standard of care.

J. Protocol development/usage.

  1. Headache red flags and triage guidelines. For example, patient with fever and headache is referred to emergency department if provider not available.

  2. Acute headache medication administration.

Terminally Ill Patient with Headache

The terminally ill patient with headache is experiencing a secondary headache disorder caused by a space-occupying lesion of the brain. The patient requires treatment that is palliative in nature and beyond the scope of this outline. Please refer to the vast body of oncology nursing literature that addresses this topic.

STROKE

Acute Stroke

The acute stroke patient is considered a neurologic emergency.
   A. Assessment/screen/triage.
      1. Recognize symptoms of stroke (National Stroke Association, 1999).
         a. Numbness or weakness of arm or leg, especially unilateral.
         b. Confusion or trouble speaking or understanding.
         c. Trouble seeing out of one or both eyes.
         d. Trouble walking, dizziness, difficulty with balance or coordination.
         e. Severe headache, unknown cause.
      2. Call 911 for the patient.
      3. Triage to ED for emergent care.

Subacute Stroke

The subacute stroke patient is neurologically stable and discharged from the acute care hospital and rehabilitation hospital.
   A. Assessment/screen/triage.
      1. Assess for symptoms of new acute stroke and triage to ED. Refer to Acute Stroke section A, 1 above.
      2. Assess for deficits and document.
      3. Assess and document any new problems.
   B. Primary, secondary, tertiary prevention.
      1. Risk factor modification.
         a. Smoking cessation.
         b. Weight reduction.
         c. Heart-healthy diet.
         d. Exercise.
         e. Stress management.
         f. Hypertensive management.
      2. Adherence to antiplatelet therapy. Nonadherence can lead to further stroke.
      3. Recognition of signs and symptoms of further stroke. Refer to Acute Stroke A, 1 above.
      4. Adherence to anticoagulation therapy and prevention of complications of therapy, for example, hemorrhage after a fall.
   C. Clinical procedures.
      1. Not applicable.
   D. Collaboration/resource identification and referral.
      1. Liaison with patient and multiple disciplines to ensure appropriate referrals are made such as:
         a. Rehabilitation: PT, OT, speech/swallowing.

      b. Home skilled and nonskilled care.

E. Patient education.

    1. Risk factor modification. Refer to B, 1 above.

    2. Adherence to antiplatelet and anticoagulant therapy.

    3. Recognition of signs and symptoms of further stroke. Refer to Acute Stroke A, 1 above.

    4. Adherence to anticoagulation therapy and prevention of complications of its use.

F. Advocacy.

    1. May require contact with insurance company for authorization of tests and treatment.

    2. May need intervention for timely referrals and treatment schedules.

    3. May need assistance with community agencies for services such as transportation.

G. Telephone practice.

    1. Triage: assess for symptoms of stroke, triages to ED.

    2. Patient education.

      a. Review signs and symptoms of acute stroke and what to do.

      b. Reinforce importance of minimizing risk factors.

      c. Review importance of medications and adverse effects.

    3. Emotional support.

      a. Reassure patient that medication should help decrease the risk of further stroke.

      b. Refer to stroke support groups, National Stroke Association (NSA) 1-800-Strokes.

    4. Facilitation.

      a. Facilitate rehabilitation, primary care, and other appointments and testing.

      b. Refer to local stroke support groups and NSA 1-800-Strokes.

    5. Coordination.

      a. Coordinate visit with primary care provider, neurology provider, and clinic.

    6. Communication/documentation.

      a. Document all telephone encounters.

      b. Communicate via established mechanism with primary care provider and neurology provider.

H. Communication/documentation.

    1. Formally documents all patient encounters in clinic including:

      a. Medications administered and response.

      b. Note patient's appearance, behavior, and abilities.

      c. Note areas of difficulties.

    2. Communicate all information via established mechanism to all providers.

I. Outcome management.

    1. Progressive improvement in activities of daily living.

    2. Successful use of adaptive techniques and devices to minimize disability.

3. Prevention of complications.

Terminal Stroke

The terminal stroke patient has significant cognitive and physical impairments as a result of stroke.

A. Assessment/screen/triage.
1. Assess for symptoms of new acute stroke and triage to emergency department.
2. Assess for deficits and document.
3. Assess and document any new problems.
B. Primary, secondary, tertiary prevention.
1. Prevent complications of immobility.
a. Pneumonia.
b. Skin breakdown.
c. Contractures.
2. Prevent complications of dysphasia.
a. Malnutrition.
b. Aspiration pneumonia.
3. Recognize signs and symptoms of further stroke.
4. Assess adherence to anticoagulation, antiplatelet therapy and prevention of complications of therapy.
C. Clinical procedures.
1. Provide appropriate support for enteral/parenteral feedings.
D. Collaboration/resource identification and referral.
1. Liaison with patient to ensure appropriate services ordered.
a. Home skilled and nonskilled care.
b. Hospice care.
c. Social work.
d. Placement.
E. Patient education.
1. Family education: work with VNA to identify issues and educate family.
a. Reassure patient and family.
b. Refer to stroke support groups.

BACK PAIN

Acute Back Pain

This common problem is experienced by almost everyone sometime during his or her adult life. It is a common reason for physician office visits and costly in terms of medical treatment, time lost at work and nonmonetary costs such as diminished ability to perform or enjoy usual activities. The panel that developed clinical practice guidelines for acute back problems (AHCPR, 1994, p.1) defined acute back problem as, "activity intolerance due to back-related symptoms and acute as limitations of less than 3 months duration. Back symptoms include pain, primarily in the back, as well as back-related leg pain (sciatica)."

A. Assess/screen/triage.

    1. Assess pain.

        a. Location.

        b. Onset.

        c. Quality.

        d. Severity and impact on activity.

        e. Alleviating factors.

        f. Aggravating factors.

        g. Duration.

    2. Screen "red flags" that suggest underlying spinal conditions such as fracture, tumor, infection, or cauda equina syndrome.

        a. Pain of acute herniated disc.

            (1) Abrupt in onset.

            (2) Brought on by exertion.

            (3) Worse standing.

            (4) Better lying down.

            (5) May radiate into one buttock or down one leg. (Adams, Victor, Ropper, 1998).

        b. Neurologic symptoms.

            (1) Numbness.

            (2) Tingling.

            (3) Weakness.

            (4) Bladder and/or bowel control problems.

        c. Medical history of:

            (1) Use of steroids/cortisone.

            (2) Osteoporosis.

            (3) Cancer.

            (4) Fever.

            (5) Weight loss.

            (6) Injuries.

        d. Nonspinal conditions (vascular, abdominal, urinary, or pelvic pathology) causing referred low back pain.

    3. Attention to psychologic and socioeconomic problems in individual's life because such nonphysical factors can complicate both the assessment and treatment (AHCPR, 1994).

    4. Triage.

        a. Per protocol or consultation.

        b. Emergent visit to clinic or emergency department or urgent visit needed with acute limb paralysis or bowel bladder involvement or sexual dysfunction (Adams, Victor, and Ropper, 1998).

B. Primary, secondary, tertiary prevention based on the outcome of the patient's disease process.

    1. Proper body mechanics instruction.

    2. Back strengthening exercises.

    3. Weight loss.

    4. Employment redesign.

   a. Restricted lifting.

   b. Job retraining.

  5. Back strengthening exercises.

  6. NSAIDs, aspirin, muscle relaxants for comfort.

  7. Call if symptoms worsen.

  8. Follow-up frequently.

  9. Encourage appropriate activities.

 C. Clinical procedures.

  1. Administer acetaminophen or nonsteroidal antiinflammatory drugs (NSAIDs) as directed.

  2. Symptom control methods initially focus on providing comfort to keep patients as active as possible while awaiting spontaneous recovery.

  3. Latter management focuses on activities needed to overcome specific activity intolerance.

 D. Collaboration/resource identification and referral.

  1. Liaison with patient to ensure appropriate care ordered.

   a. Physical therapy.

   b. Follow-up appointments.

 E. Patient education (AHCPR, 1994).

  1. Expectation for both rapid recovery and recurrence of symptoms based on natural history of the disease.

  2. Symptom management.

   a. Review of medications and side effects of: NSAIDs, nonnarcotic and narcotic analgesics.

   b. Appropriate exercises. Safe and reasonable activity modification.

  3. The lack of need for special testing unless red flags are present.

  4. Effectiveness and risk of commonly available diagnostic tests and further treatment measures to be considered should symptoms persist.

 F. Advocacy.

  1. May require discussion with employer regarding ability to work.

  2. Activity modification must be time limited, clear to both patient and employer, and reviewed by clinician on a regular basis.

  3. Help patient establish activity goals in consultation with employer when applicable.

 G. Telephone practice.

  1. Triage.

   a. Assess for signs and symptoms of an acute disc. Refer to red flags, Section A, 2 on p. 327.

   b. Assess for bowel, bladder involvement, sexual dysfunction, or acute weakness.

   c. Refer to ED for urgent visit.

  2. Patient education.

   a. Review use of pain medication, muscle relaxants.

   b. Review use of NSAIDs.

   c. Review importance of appropriate exercise and comfortable positioning.

3. Emotional support.
   a. Reassure patient that medication should help decrease the pain and associated symptoms.
   b. Reassure patient that most back pain usually resolves on its own in 4 to 6 weeks.
4. Facilitation.
   a. Facilitate additional acute treatment with primary care and neurology provider.
5. Coordination.
   a. Coordinate acute visit with primary care provider, neurology provider, and clinic and/or orthopedics.
6. Communication/documentation.
   a. Document all telephone encounters.
   b. Communicate via established mechanism with primary care provider and neurology provider.
H. Communication/documentation.
   1. Formally document all patient encounters in clinic including:
      a. Medication administered and response.
      b. Patient's appearance and behaviors.
      c. Level of discomfort and relief using established scales. General pain scales are numeric with 0 representing no pain and 10 representing extreme pain.
      d. Communicate all information via established mechanism to all providers.
I. Outcome management.
   1. Acute symptoms resolve.
   2. Patient returns to prior level of activity, including activities of daily living and return to work.
   3. Associated symptoms resolve.
J. Protocol development/usage.
   1. Protocols can be facilitated by referral to AHCPR's *Clinical practice guidelines on acute back problems in adults* (1994) and updated research findings.
   2. Areas for development include:
      a. Acute back pain triage to ED or urgent visit.
      b. Acute back pain medication treatment, for example, trying different NSAIDs.

Chronic Back Pain Patient

The chronic back pain patient experiences recurring back pain and related limitations on an ongoing basis, lasting longer than 3 months. Chronic back pain requires a multidisciplinary treatment approach including exercise and behavioral therapy (also see Acute Back Pain section, which starts on p. 326).

A. Patient education.
   1. Proper body mechanics instruction.

      2. Back strengthening exercises.

      3. Weight reduction.

      4. Employment redesign.

        a. Restricted lifting.

        b. Job retraining.

      5. Appropriate use of medications.

      6. Physical therapy.

      7. Use of transcutaneous electrical nerve stimulation (TENS) unit.

B. Telephone practice.

      1. Outreach: refer to chronic pain support groups and for alternative pain management therapies such as acupuncture.

      2. Some organizations and web sites include:

        a. National Arthritis and Musculoskeletal and Skin Disease Information Clearinghouse: serves public, patients, and health professionals by providing information. Available at: http://www/nih.gov/niams/healthinfo/

        b. American Chronic Pain Association: this organization is made up of individuals suffering from chronic pain and health professionals who work in this field. Provides help in coping with chronic pain, and teaches different methods of pain management.

C. Outcome management.

      1. Patient reports satisfaction with symptom management.

      2. Patient takes personal action to control pain.

      3. Disruptive effects of pain are minimized.

REFERENCES

Adams RD, Victor M, Ropper AH (1998): Pain in back, neck and extremities. In Adams RD, Victor M, Ropper A, editors: *Principles of neurology,* ed 6. New York: McGraw-Hill, pp. 194-223.

Agency for Health Care Policy and Research (1994): *Acute low back problems in adults.* Clinical practice guidelines No. 4. Rockville, Maryland: US Department of Health and Human Services Agency for Health Care Policy and Research.

Diamond S (1998): *Diagnosing and managing headaches,* ed 2. Chicago: Professional Communications, pp. 11-121.

National Stroke Association (1999): *Network NSA index of resources and information for those at risk for stroke.* Palo Alto: Syntex Laboratories, pp. 1-32.

Parker C, Kelley SK (1998): Telephone triage in managed care: dispelling the myth of the gatekeeper. *Trends in Nursing* 2(3).

Rapport AM, Sheftell FD (1996): *Headache disorders: a management guide for practitioners.* Philadelphia: WB Saunders, p. 22.

Silberstein SD, Lipton RD, Goadsby P (1998): *Headache in clinical practice.* Oxford: Isis Medical Media, pp. 11-125.

19 Ambulatory Surgery

DEBRA L. JANIKOWSKI MSN, RN, CNA

PATIENT PROTOTYPES

Breast Surgery ■ Child Surgery (ENT) ■ Orthopedic Surgery ■ Moderate Sedation (Conscious Sedation)

OBJECTIVES

Study of the information presented in this chapter will enable the learner to:

1. Describe care coordination for the adult and child ambulatory surgical patient.
2. Identify knowledge and skill sets required for care of the ambulatory surgical patient.
3. Discuss patient and family education for the ambulatory surgery patient.
4. Identify critical factors in the provision of ambulatory conscious sedation.

■■ The concept and practice of ambulatory surgery has evolved rapidly in the past two decades. Consumers have witnessed the surgical experience change from lengthy and often uncomfortable inpatient stays to same-day admission, surgery, recovery, and discharge all within a matter of hours. New anesthetic agents and technologic advances such as conscious sedation and minimally invasive procedures have become the hallmark of ambulatory surgery (Janikowski and Rockefeller, 1998). Nurses practicing in the ambulatory surgical environment provide skilled nursing care for patients across the life span with acuity levels ranging from well to acute, chronic, or terminal and medical histories ranging from simple to complex. According to Brockway (1997), the interactive aspects of ambulatory perioperative nursing flow along a surgical continuum that begins with preoperative assessment and admission, intraoperative surgical skills, sterilization and central processing, postoperative acute phase, and ends with discharge, home planning, and follow-up care. Ambulatory surgery provides the same standard of care but costs an estimated 60% to 70% less than surgery performed in inpatient facilities. The advent of managed care has forced ambulatory surgical programs to focus on consumer needs, convenience, improving outcomes, and decreasing cost without compromising quality of care (Anderson, 1994). The ultimate goal is to provide the patient with a safe, caring environment that is conducive to a positive surgical outcome (Brockway, 1997).

BREAST SURGERY

PATIENT POPULATION: Well and Acute

Definitions

Benign (noncancerous) breast lumps—any noticeable change, thickening, or localized swelling in breast that was not there before.

Fibrocystic breasts—fibrous tissue reacting to abnormal hormone levels with formation of multiple pockets of fluid and increase of fibrous tissue; are the most common cause of lumps in women aged 35 to 50. Responsible for 80% of all breast operations performed. Tenderness and lump size increase during week before menstruation and decrease a week after. Usually disappears after menopause.

Simple cysts—single or multiple fluid-filled sacs. No significant increase in fibrous tissue. Tenderness and lump size fluctuate with menstrual cycle.

Fibroadenoma—single solid tumor consisting of fibrous and glandular tissue, usually movable when palpated, not usually tender. Occurs in women ages 18 to 35. Nearly all breast tumors in women under age 25 are fibroadenomas.

Papillomas—small, wartlike growths in lining of mammary duct near nipple. Can produce clear or bloody discharge from nipple.

Malignant (cancerous) lumps—single, hard, painless. Develop in mammary duct or glands. Commonly found in upper, outer quadrant of breast, may occur anywhere in breast. Grow in an uncontrolled manner, with time will spread beyond the breast.

Early breast cancer—small tumor less than an inch in size, located in breast only. Early diagnosis and treatment increases chance of survival.

Advanced breast cancer—spread to axillary lymph nodes, reduced chance of cure.

Disseminated breast cancer—spread to lymph nodes and other areas such as bones, lungs, and liver. Cure rate is low.

    A. Assess/screen/triage.

        1. Breast and lung cancers are leading causes of death from cancer in American women.

            a. Majority of all breast lumps are benign (noncancerous).

            b. Approximately one woman in eight (12% of all women) will develop breast cancer at some time in her life.

            c. Less than 1% of all breast cancers occur in males.

            d. Breast cancer risk increases with:

                (1) Family history of disease.

                (2) Previous biopsy indicating precancerous condition, or having a prior history of breast cancer.

                (3) Age (greater after 50).

                (4) Giving birth first time after age 30 or never having given birth.

                (5) Beginning periods before age 12 or reaching menopause after age 50.

                (6) Obesity (weight 40% more than ideal weight). More than 30% of daily calories come from fat.

                (7) Drinking alcohol.

                (8) Using or having used hormone replacement therapy (Redman, 1997).

   2. Breast changes requiring attention.
      a. Distinct single lumps (either hard or soft).
      b. Changes in skin texture or color (redness, pebbly skin, thickening, roughness, or puckering).
      c. Changes in breast shape (dimpling, depression, bulges, or flattening).
      d. Changes in nipple location or shape.
      e. Bloody or cloudy nipple discharge.
      f. Breast sores that do not heal (Redman, 1997).
B. Primary/secondary/tertiary prevention.
   1. Primary prevention.
      a. Breast cancer is not preventable but can be detected early.
      b. Risk for breast cancer increases with age (75% of all breast cancers occur in women over the age of 50) and with positive family history (although 80% of women who get breast cancer have no family history).
      c. Monthly breast self-examination (BSE).
         (1) Perform BSE in front of mirror, in the shower, and lying down.
         (2) More than 90% of all breast lumps are discovered by women themselves.
      d. Annual clinical breast examination (CBE) by health care professional.
      e. Lower risk of breast cancer by living a healthy lifestyle.
         (1) Eat a low-fat, low-salt, high-fiber diet.
         (2) Avoid or limit caffeine and alcohol.
         (3) Exercise at least 30 minutes 3 days a week.
         (4) Do not smoke.
         (5) Do regular BSE and have CBE and mammograms as recommended for age.
   2. Secondary prevention.
      a. Ultrasound. Produces images of breast tissue to distinguish between solid and fluid-filled lumps.
      b. Mammography. Low-radiation x-ray that can detect lumps before lumps are felt. Recommend first mammogram age 35 to 40 (or younger if at risk), every 1 to 2 years for ages 40 to 49, annually age 50 and over (Redman, 1997).
         (1) Costs are often covered by private insurance, HMOs, or Medicaid.
         (2) Some programs provide free mammograms.
         (3) Medicare will pay up to 80% of the Medicare-approved amount for screening mammograms.
      c. Tips to obtain a good mammogram.
         (1) Ask if the facility is certified by the FDA.
         (2) Use a facility that specializes in mammograms or does several a day.
         (3) If changing facilities or doctors, request old mammograms.
         (4) Schedule mammogram for time of month when breasts will be least tender.
         (5) Do not wear deodorant, talcum powder, or lotion under arms.

(6) Bring information concerning previous mammograms, biopsies, or other breast treatments.

(7) Ask when results will be available and call facility or doctor if you do not receive them (National Cancer Institute, 1996).

3. Tertiary prevention.
   a. Clinical procedures.
      (1) Needle biopsy/aspiration. Fine needle or core needle used to extract cells from lump. Stereotactic (x-ray guided) biopsy may be used.
         (a) Fluid-filled lump: fluid aspirated, no further treatment may be needed.
         (b) Solid lump: cells and solid tissue removed and evaluated for pathology.
      (2) Open biopsy.
         (a) Excisional biopsy: mass and surrounding margin of normal cells removed and evaluated for pathology.
         (b) Incisional biopsy: affected area partially removed and evaluated for pathology. Further, more extensive surgery may be indicated.

C. Clinical procedures/surgery: it is crucial that the ambulatory care nurse be well versed in the operative process along the continuum of care, because the majority of surgical procedures begin in ambulatory setting such as ambulatory procedure units or same-day surgery units. The smooth coordination of preoperative labs, x-ray, anesthesia interview, physical therapy, and patient education will set the stage for successful outcomes.
   1. Surgical procedures.
      a. Modified radical mastectomy: entire breast and portion of axillary lymph nodes removed; chest muscles left in place.
      b. Simple mastectomy: less extensive than modified radical; only breast removed, chest muscles and axillary lymph nodes remain intact.
      c. Lumpectomy: removal of tumor and margin of surrounding healthy tissue; axial dissection often done in conjunction with lumpectomy (Krames Communications, 1995, 1997).
   2. Same-day surgery.
      a. Schedule arrival time to allow sufficient preparation time.
      b. Complete insurance forms.
      c. Complete preop history and examination, including history of symptoms. Note timing of detection of the lump, size, changes, location, nipple discharge, and breast symmetry (Lowdermilk, Perry, and Bobak, 2000).
      d. Complete lab tests (urine, blood samples as necessary) in advance or same day.
      e. Advise to wear comfortable clothes.
      f. Ensure postprocedure transportation is arranged.
      g. Instruct no food or fluids after midnight.

  h. Notify health care provider if patient feels ill or has elevated temperature.

  3. Pre- and postoperative instructions: provide written and verbal instructions and include caregiver in discussion and demonstrations.

    a. Diet.

        (1) Progress from liquids to semisolid to solid food.

        (2) Good nutrition helps body build tissue and wounds heal.

    b. Self-care.

        (1) Coughing and deep breathing.

        (2) Dressing changes, wound care.

    c. Exercise and driving.

        (1) Remind patient that arm on side of surgery may feel tight.

        (2) Demonstrate active range of motion exercises. Driving may be restricted because of initial decreased range of motion.

    d. Medications.

        (1) Antibiotics

        (2) Pain medications.

    e. Bandages and dressings.

        (1) Keep intact and dry.

        (2) Note drainage, reporting unexpected bleeding or drainage.

    f. Bathing and showering.

    g. Pain (what to expect, what to do).

        (1) Avoid drinking alcohol, driving, and operating machinery while taking pain medications.

        (2) Call medical provider when pain continues after taking medications; feel too sleepy, dizzy, or groggy; experience side effects of nausea, vomiting, or allergic skin reactions.

    h. Stitches, staples, and incision care.

        (1) Expectations regarding physical appearance.

        (2) Equipment usage (emptying drains, changing bandages).

    i. Signs of infection.

        (1) Redness.

        (2) Swelling.

        (3) Fever.

        (4) Foul-smelling discharge.

    j. Emotional support: arrange for visit with a representative of Reach for Recovery. (Local numbers may be obtained from physician, nurse or directory assistance.)

    k. Follow-up visit (usually within 5 days).

        (1) Reinforce education and emotional support.

        (2) Encourage continuation of BSE on unaffected breast.

    l. Return to work.

        (1) Individual and job related.

        (2) Days after minor surgery, weeks after major surgery (Krames Communications, 1995, 1996).

D. Collaboration/resource identification and referral.

1. Identify, document, and share potential patient problems with health team members.
2. Complete a comprehensive discharge needs assessment before surgery.
3. Initiate case management, social work, and home health care or visiting nurse consultations as needed before surgery.
4. Provide local Reach for Recovery phone numbers and other resources as appropriate.
   a. Women's national toll-free breast care helpline 1-800-I'M AWARE.
   b. National Cancer Institute Information Service 1-800-4-CANCER.
   c. American Cancer Society 1-800-ACS-2345.
   d. Medicare Office of Beneficiary Relations (1-800-638-6833).

E. Care management.
   1. Assess and evaluate patient medically, surgically, and cognitively during all phases of the surgical course.
      a. Preoperative.
         (1) Blood tests, EKG, urinalysis (chest x-ray is no longer seen as cost effective or medically necessary). Should be individualized based on the purpose of the procedure and underlying medical conditions.
         (2) Preoperative educational needs assessment, teaching/instruction, and evaluation.
      b. Intraoperative.
         (1) IV access.
         (2) Anesthetic medications for comfort.
         (3) Cardiac and oxygenation monitoring.
      c. Postoperative phases I, II, and home.
         (1) Physiologic vital sign monitoring.
         (2) Walking, eating, breathing, and coughing.
         (3) Postoperative evaluation, pain management.
      d. Rehabilitation as necessary.
      e. Use of external prosthesis.
   2. Biopsy patients.
      a. Pain medications for comfort.
      b. Fitted bra for support.
      c. Observe operative site for infection.
      d. Stitches dissolve or removed.
   3. Mastectomy patients.
      a. Pain medication for comfort.
      b. Drains to prevent fluid accumulation.
      c. Dressings over incision site.
      d. Numbness of chest wall and underarm region will decrease.
      e. Arm and hand swelling may occur.
      f. Shoulder motion and strength may be limited. Arm exercises taught to stretch scar tissue, increase strength, and restore normal range of motion (Krames Communications, 1995, 1996, 1997).
   4. Radiation therapy or chemotherapy may be indicated.
   5. Reconstructive surgery may be indicated.

F. Patient education.
  1. Adults learn when the educational content and experience:
    a. Is goal-oriented (helps solve a problem).
    b. Has clear objectives (provides clarity regarding what is going to be taught).
    c. Is interactive (two-way involvement).
    d. Allows a feeling of success while learning.
  2. Assess patient readiness to change.
    a. Prochaska's stages of change (Linnell, 1998).
      (1) Precontemplation: patient cannot see problem but others can; cons of changing out-weigh pros.
      (2) Contemplation: patient acknowledges problem and begins serious thinking to solve it; pros begin to outweigh cons; possibilities surface.
      (3) Preparation: problem is made public; actions are planned.
      (4) Action: obvious activity; strategies implemented; requires time and energy commitment.
      (5) Maintenance: consolidation of earlier gains, strategies implemented to prevent relapse.
      (6) Termination: patient exits change cycle; new behavior is now a habit such as monthly breast self-examination (BSE).
  3. Education helps individuals detect cancer, aids in treatment regimes, pain management and rehabilitation, and cope with changes in body image (anatomy, physiology, and sexual).
    a. Educational needs include:
      (1) Information on type and extent of cancer, underlying reasons for symptoms, what symptoms to expect, physical needs, nutritional needs, medications, psychologic needs, activity needs, and combating fatigue, what to expect in the future, treatment of side effects, community resources.
      (2) Ways to reassure and encourage, deal with decreased energy, unpredictable future, depression, and fears, cope with stress and diagnosis, be patient and tolerant, maintain a normal family life, discuss death.
    b. Types of cancer pain intervention education include:
      (1) Progressive muscle relaxation.
      (2) Meditation.
      (3) Hypnotherapy.
      (4) Systematic desensitization.
      (5) Biofeedback.
      (6) Behavior modification or reinforcement.
      (7) Psychotherapy and counseling.
G. Advocacy.
  1. At every opportunity, encourage women to do breast self-exams (BSE), have clinical breast exams (CBE), and mammography as recommended (Kemper, 1997).
  2. Health belief model.

      a. Tool for understanding patient's perception of disease and their decision-making process in seeking and using health care services.

      b. Predicts consumption of health care services when patients:

         (1) Perceive they have a disease or condition or are likely to contract it.

         (2) Perceive disease or condition is harmful and has serious consequences.

         (3) Believe suggested health intervention is of value.

         (4) Believe effectiveness of treatment is worth the cost and barriers that may be confronted.

  3. Types of resources and nursing actions that assist breast cancer patients in coping.

      a. Physical resources (health and energy): reinforcing importance of good diet to maintain strength.

      b. Psychologic resources (positive beliefs, problem-solving): reinforcing positive attitudes concerning treatment and cure.

      c. Social resources (social skills, social support): referral to support groups like I Can Cope and Reach to Recovery or counseling. Mobilize family and friends.

      d. Material resources (money, goods, and services): referral to social services, discharge planning (Rankin and Stallings, 1996).

H. Telephone practice.

  1. Initiate preoperative interview and instructions.

  2. Postoperative discharge contact should be attempted within 24 hours.

      a. Assess pain control.

      b. Reinforce self-care instructions.

      c. Assess and respond to coping and emotional needs.

      d. Evaluate patient and family satisfaction with the episode of care.

I. Communication/documentation.

  1. Coordination and timely execution of care along the continuum.

      a. Preoperative evaluation and teaching interview.

      b. Verification of surgical consent.

      c. Patient's response to interventions.

J. Outcome management.

  1. Efficacy: effect of a treatment or intervention under ideal, controlled situations.

  2. Effectiveness: results of an intervention when administered under usual practice conditions.

  3. Examine processes and care outcomes to explain variation resulting from differences in implementation of treatments or innovations.

      a. Process: timeliness, accuracy, completeness, appropriateness, efficiency, responsiveness, empathy.

      b. Outcomes: satisfaction, clinical results, patient knowledge and performance, functional status and quality of living, access/utilization, cost/financial (Hastings, 1997).

  4. Develop, institute, and evaluate use of clinical/critical pathways and/or care maps to decrease variability in processes and care outcomes.

K. Protocol development/usage.
 1. Clinical/critical pathways/care maps (Howe, 1997).
  a. Facilitate the progress of patients from admission through discharge.
  b. Increase predictability of outcomes.
  c. Increase compliance with standard plan of care.
  d. Provide documentation of patient and family education.
  e. Decrease length of stay.
 2. Patient care maps.
  a. Increase patient and family participation in postoperative care.
  b. Increase understanding of expected interventions and outcomes.
  c. Decrease anxiety over discharge and home/self-care (Whedon, 1995).

CHILD SURGERY (ENT)

PATIENT POPULATION: Chronic Manifestation of Acute Problem.

Children are individuals in various stages of rapid growth and development.

Definitions

Otitis media—Inflammation of the middle ear caused by bacteria or virus, common in children, can cause severe pain, temporary or permanent hearing loss, and delayed speech development if not treated. May recur as a result of chronically infected sinuses, adenoids, and tonsils. Serous otitis media may be present without infection.

Adenoiditis—Infection of the lymphoid tissues located at the back of the nose above the palate and near the opening of the Eustachian tubes that drain middle-ear secretions into nasal passages. Become enlarged as they fight infection in the upper-respiratory tract or in response to allergies. If adenoids become too large, they can block opening of the Eustachian tube and increase the likelihood of ear infections.

Tonsillitis—Infection of the lymphoid tissues located on both sides of the back of the throat. Become enlarged as they fight infection in the upper-respiratory tract. Largest between ages of 4 and 7 because of large number of upper-respiratory infections in this age group.
 A. Assess/screen/triage.
  1. Assess family's support mechanisms, coping styles, comprehension of surgery and child's developmental stage. If available, encourage parents and patient to tour facility and interact with caregivers before day of surgery.
  2. Identify barriers to communication: cultural and socioeconomic factors, primary language, education, parenting experience.
  3. Complete laboratory screening tests in advance to minimize anxiety and distress on day of surgery (Lancaster, 1997). Be aware of any bleeding tendencies.
  4. Reasons for placing pressure equalizing tubes (myringotomy) (Schmidt, 1999).

        a. Frequent middle ear infections (usually more than four per year) that fail to respond to treatment with continuous antibiotics.

        b. Fluid has been continuously present greater than 4 months, both ears are involved, has caused a documented hearing loss or speech delay.

        c. Eustachian tube dysfunction (Eustachian tubes do not allow proper ventilation of the middle ear to equalize air pressure, creates negative pressure behind the eardrum, causing reduced movement of the eardrum and subsequent pain).

        d. Ear infections with other complication factors such as mastoiditis.

        e. Significantly reduces incidence of recurrent ear infections.

    5. Reasons for removing adenoids (adenoidectomy).

        a. Frequent ear infections. Adenoids may be a bacterial reservoir that leads to bacterial infections in the ear. Enlarged adenoids may obstruct the Eustachian tube orifices.

            (1) If ear infections are caused by allergies, children generally do not profit from an adenoidectomy.

            (2) If adenoidectomy is indicated, there is no need to remove the tonsils during the operation as they serve different functions.

        b. Airway/nasal obstruction interfering with breathing.

        c. Airway/nasal obstruction interfering with intelligibility of speech.

    6. Reasons for removing tonsils (tonsillectomy).

        a. Frequent, severe tonsillitis, recurrent abscesses of the tonsils.

        b. Tonsil enlargement. Tonsils are not too large unless they are touching. Peak size is reached between 8 to 12 years, then usually spontaneously shrink.

        c. Persistent mouth breathing.

        d. Severe snoring, airway or throat obstruction/sleep apnea.

        e. Abnormal speech.

        f. Persistent swallowing difficulties.

        g. Asymmetric tonsils (possible neoplasm of the tonsils).

B. Primary/secondary/tertiary prevention.

    1. Otitis media is most common diagnosis recorded for doctor visits in children.

        a. Approximately one third of all children have more than three ear infections in their first 3 years of life.

        b. Otitis media is most common cause of hearing loss in children.

        c. Early detection and treatment, which may include surgical intervention, can prevent unnecessary hearing loss (American Academy of Otolaryngology—Head and Neck Surgery, 1999).

    2. Encourage routine health maintenance visits, timely acute care attention, and consistent chronic care follow-up.

C. Clinical procedures.

    1. Otoscopic examination: pneumatic otoscopy, acoustic reflectometry.

    2. Audiogram: tones are sounded at various pitches. Measures how much hearing loss has occurred by measuring response to sounds of various pitches at different levels of intensity.

3. Tympanogram: measures air pressure in the middle ear and mobility of the eardrum. Indicates how well Eustachian tube is functioning and if mobility of the eardrum and relative ability to conduct sound has been impaired.
4. Myringotomy: operation involves a small surgical incision into the eardrum to promote drainage of fluid and to relieve pain. A small hollow tube may be placed into the opening in the eardrum to help equalize air pressure and prevent accumulation of fluid in the middle ear (most commonly referred to as PE tubes).
    a. Usually done in operating room under general anesthesia as same-day surgery.
    b. Surgery lasts 5 to 15 minutes (plus time required for general anesthesia).
    c. Under a microscope, a small incision is made in each eardrum and a tube is inserted in this incision.
    d. Patients usually go home shortly after surgery. Following general anesthesia, patients must be awake and comfortable before discharge. Not all institutions require voiding and taking liquids by mouth before discharge as it may induce vomiting. Urinary retention is rare in pediatric surgical population.
    e. Tubes can be placed even if a patient has an ear infection. A respiratory infection or other severe illness may require delaying surgery.
    f. One disadvantage: patient must avoid getting water in the ear while the tubes are in place.
5. Adenoidectomy and/or tonsillectomy.
    a. Usually done in operating room under general anesthesia as same-day surgery. Some surgeons admit overnight for children under 3 years of age with significant obstructive sleep apnea or craniofacial problems.
    b. Surgery lasts 15 to 30 minutes (plus time required for general anesthesia).
    c. Performed through mouth (no external incisions).
    d. Discharge a few hours after surgery. Following general anesthesia, patients must be awake and comfortable without signs of bleeding or protracted nausea and vomiting. Not all institutions require voiding and taking liquids by mouth before discharge as it may induce vomiting. Urinary retention is rare in pediatric surgical population.
D. Collaboration/resource identification and referral.
    1. Ensure age-appropriate equipment is available.
        a. Accurate height and weight measures are essential. Medications are calculated on kilogram weight. Kilogram scales avoid conversion and medication errors.
        b. Correctly sized blood pressure cuffs and pulse oximeter sensors are needed for accurate baseline readings.

      c. Neonatal and pediatric sized bells for stethoscopes are necessary for proper heart and lung auscultation.

      d. Most important age-appropriate equipment: airways. Source of difficulties is usually respiratory in children. Pediatric sized ambu bags, masks, endotracheal tubes, and infant to child size nasal and oral airways must be readily accessible for emergencies (Lancaster, 1997).

      e. Pediatric size defibrillator paddles on crash cart.

  E. Care management.

    1. Day of surgery.

      a. Evaluate child and family's preparation and readiness for surgery.

      b. Keep operative delays to a minimum.

      c. Talk directly to the child to elicit cooperation and a sense of trust.

      d. Be honest about the sensations and pain child will experience.

      e. Give child as many choices as possible to foster independence.

      f. Reward child for cooperation.

      g. Complete physical assessment.

      h. If sedation is administered, child must be continuously monitored.

    2. Post surgery recovery.

      a. Assess/evaluate vital signs, operative site.

      b. When stable and awake, allow parent at recovery bedside.

      c. Nausea and vomiting are the most frequent problems after general anesthesia.

        (1) Most common reason for delay in discharge from PACUs.

        (2) Most common reason for unanticipated admission to hospital after same-day surgery.

      d. Children are prone to disorientation, hallucinations, and at times, uncontrollable physical activity upon emergence from general anesthesia.

        (1) Most effects wear off quickly, but irritability and hyperactivity may linger for up to 24 hours.

        (2) Close observation by an informed adult may be warranted.

      e. Assess and treat pain.

    3. Discharge and home care.

      a. Preparation for discharge begins with preadmission visit.

      b. Review verbal and written instructions. Address questions and concerns. Ensure parental confidence with:

        (1) Care of surgical site and dressings.

        (2) Residual nausea and vomiting.

        (3) Pain management.

      c. Provide phone numbers for routine questions and urgent situations.

        (1) Fever is most common problem within 24 hours of surgery and general anesthesia. Fever that occurs 5 to 10 days after surgery is more likely to indicate a wound infection or an unrelated problem.

      d. Telephone parent within 24 hours after surgery.

(1) Review postoperative care instructions.

(2) Assess for: bleeding, nausea and vomiting, intake and output, activity level, pain level, effectiveness of medications, parent and child coping skills.

(3) Evaluate satisfaction with process (Lancaster, 1997).

   e. Pressure equalizing tubes home instructions.

(1) Postop pain: usually mild, may be treated briefly with acetaminophen (e.g., Tylenol) or ibuprofen (e.g., Motrin).

(2) Postop bleeding from ear: uncommon and would be a very small amount.

(3) Postop drainage from ear: occasionally occurs, may prescribe antibiotics.

(4) Return visit in 4 to 6 weeks.

(5) Audiogram and tympanogram repeated.

(6) 10% of children who have PE tubes placed continue to have ear infections.

   f. Adenoidectomy and tonsillectomy home instructions.

(1) Tonsil area becomes coated with a white material for 10 to 14 days.

(2) Pain: Very sore throat for 7 to 10 days (more so with tonsillectomy than adenoidectomy). Ear pain often occurs as a result of throat pain being referred to ears. Acetaminophen (e.g., Tylenol) is recommended pre- and postop. Caution for children under 18 years: aspirin, ibuprofen (e.g., Motrin, Advil) may increase risk of bleeding. Narcotics may be prescribed for more severe pain.

(3) Bleeding: Small amount of bleeding (less than 1 teaspoon of bright red blood) may occur day of surgery and about 1 week later. Do gentle cold-water gargling. Health care provider should be notified of any bleeding over 1 teaspoon.

(4) Fever: Low-grade fever (101°) is common after surgery.

(5) Voice: Some patients note a nasal voice, particularly after adenoidectomy (throat is adjusting to pain and removal of the tonsils/adenoids). May notice liquid in nose when drinking and swallowing (usually improves in several weeks).

(6) Phlegm: Mucus and phlegm build up after a T&A. Gargling, coughing, and clearing throat can cause pain and bleeding (may swish warm water in mouth).

(7) Nausea: Common day of and night after surgery (may be caused by anesthesia medications or swallowed blood in stomach).

(8) Diet: Soft nonacidic foods and adequate hydration.

F. Patient education.

   1. Schedule assessment visit and surgical suite tour.

   a. Prepare child for impending surgery, treatments, and anesthesia prior to surgery.

b. Prepare child for postoperative sensations and treatments.

2. Pressure equalizing tubes.

a. Diet: normal, no restrictions.

b. Activity: as tolerated, keep ears dry for 2 weeks after surgery (no swimming, may recommend ear plugs while bathing).

c. Tubes usually stay in eardrums about 1 year, times vary. Tubes usually fall out on their own.

d. May be necessary to remove tubes if intact after about 2 years. May cause scarring or perforation.

e. Ear infections are still possible after tube placement, check for drainage from the ear. Reduction in number of occurrences is possible.

f. Some bleeding may occur when tube falls out of eardrum.

g. Teach parents/child care providers signs of hearing loss.

(1) Newborn (birth to 6 months).

(a) Does not startle, blink, move, cry, or react to unexpected loud noises.

(b) Does not awaken to loud noises.

(c) Does not freely imitate sound.

(d) Responds to loud noises as opposed to the voice.

(e) Cannot be soothed by voice alone.

(f) Does not turn head in direction of voices.

(g) General indifference to sound.

(2) Young infant (6 to 12 months).

(a) Does not point to familiar persons or objects when asked.

(b) Does not babble or babbling has stopped.

(c) By 12 months is not understanding simple phrases such as "wave by-bye" and "clap hands" by listening alone.

(3) Infant (13 months through 2 years).

(a) Does not accurately turn in direction of a soft voice on the first call.

(b) Is not alert to environmental sounds.

(c) Does not respond appropriately on first call.

(d) Does not respond to sound or locate where sound is coming from.

(e) Responds more to facial expressions and gestures than verbalizations.

(f) Uses gestures rather than verbalization to express desire, especially after age 15 months.

(g) Does not begin to imitate and use simple words for familiar people and things around home.

(h) Yelling or screeching to express needs.

(i) Does not sound like or use speech like other children of similar age.

(j) Does not listen to TV at a normal volume.

(k) Does not show consistent growth in understanding and the use of words to communicate (American Academy of Otolaryngology—Head and Neck Surgery, 1994).

3. Post-tonsillectomy and adenoidectomy patient education.
   a. Activity: rest for several days, increase activity as tolerated, avoid exercise or heavy exertion for at least 2 weeks.
   b. Pain control: take pain medications every 4 to 6 hours for first day or two; acetaminophen (e.g., Tylenol) is recommended because aspirin, ibuprofen (e.g., Motrin, Advil) may increase risk of bleeding.
   c. Brush teeth, rinse mouth with warm water or warm salt water (1/2 tsp. in 8 oz. of water); avoid use of gargles or vigorous toothbrushing.
   d. Diet: eating and drinking generally hurt after T&A; begin with liquids and advance to soft diet.
      (1) Avoid dry, hard foods that might irritate and cause bleeding.
      (2) Avoid red beverages and chocolate; may be confused with blood if vomiting occurs.
      (3) Do not drink through straws; can cause negative pressure and cause bleeding.
      (4) Avoid milk and dairy products because they coat the throat causing the patient to clear the throat more often and may initiate bleeding.
      (5) Encourage cool liquids, sports drinks of electrolyte solution, and soft tepid foods such as pasta and mashed potatoes.
G. Informed consent.
   1. Pressure equalizing tubes.
      a. Risks.
         (1) Possible injury to tympanic membrane and nearby structures such as hearing-balance organs, nerves, blood vessels.
         (2) Perforation in eardrum even after tubes fall out.
         (3) Drainage from ears or continued infections.
         (4) Possible need for other treatments such as continued antibiotics or placing another set of tubes in the future.
         (5) Reactions to anesthesia and other medications.
   2. Adenoidectomy and tonsillectomy.
      a. Risks.
         (1) Bleeding (3% to 5% of patients have some bleeding after surgery that requires treatment).
         (2) Nasal voice/velopharyngeal incompetence. (After surgery throat re-learns to close off nose from mouth for swallowing and speaking. On rare occasions, may cause permanent voice or swallowing problems requiring treatment).
         (3) Nasopharyngeal stenosis (scarring and tightening of throat).
         (4) Injury to mouth; throat area and teeth, or other structures in area.
         (5) Dehydration.

        (6) Infections.

        (7) Injury to Eustachian tubes which connect ears to throat.

        (8) Reactions to anesthesia and other medications.

        (9) Avoid aspirin, ibuprofen (e.g., Motrin, Advil) because they may increase risk of bleeding (acetaminophen [e.g., Tylenol] is recommended pre- and postop).

H. Telephone practice.

  1. Initiate preoperative reminder call to parents/caregiver day before surgery.

    a. Review oral restrictions (NPO restrictions have become much less rigid in recent years to decrease anxiety and irritability).

    b. Ask caregiver about:

      (1) Presence of rashes, bites, sore, or abrasions in surgical area.

      (2) Symptoms of cold, fever, runny nose, or cough.

      (3) Exposure to chickenpox: calculate incubation dates, if within 8 to 21 days of contagion, may postpone elective surgeries to decrease risk of exposure to others (Lancaster, 1997).

  2. Postoperative discharge contact should be attempted within 24 hours of surgery.

    a. Assess pain control, bleeding, nausea and vomiting, and oral intake.

    b. Reinforce self-care instructions.

    c. Evaluate patient and family satisfaction with the episode of care.

I. Communication/documentation.

  1. Coordination and timely execution of care along the continuum.

    a. Preoperative evaluation and teaching interview.

    b. Verification of surgical consent.

    c. Patient's response to interventions.

J. Outcome management.

  1. Desired outcome: child and parent are prepared for each part of surgical experience.

  2. Evaluate requirement for preanesthetic medications.

    a. Infants and young children induced with flavored anesthetics inhaled via face mask.

    b. Older children and adolescents induced with IV sedative/muscle relaxant prior to general anesthesia.

  3. Potential for pulmonary aspiration of gastric contents.

    a. Stop milk, food, solids, and formula 8 hours before arrival.

    b. Stop breast milk 2 to 3 hours before arrival.

    c. Stop clear fluids 2 to 3 hours before arrival (Briggs, 1997, Lancaster, 1997).

K. Protocol development/usage.

  1. Preadmission visit and assessment.

  2. Day of surgery assessment and preparation.

  3. Postoperative recovery care.

  4. Discharge instructions.

  5. Urgent and routine follow-up care.

ORTHOPEDIC SURGERY

PROTOTYPE PATIENT: Arthroscopy Surgery
PATIENT POPULATION: Acute, Chronic

Definition

Arthroscopy is a surgical procedure used to visualize, diagnose, and treat problems inside a joint. A small incision is made in the skin and a pencil-sized instrument containing a small lens and lighting system is inserted to magnify and illuminate the structures inside the joint. Light is transmitted through fiberoptics to the end of the arthroscope that is inserted into the joint. By attaching the arthroscope to a mini television camera, the surgeon is able to see the interior of the joint. The television camera displays the image of the joint on a television screen allowing the surgeon to look at the cartilage, ligaments, and under the kneecap. The surgeon can then determine the amount or type of injury and what type of repair is necessary (American Academy of Orthopedic Surgeons, 1995).

  A. Assess/screen/triage.
    1. Common conditions found during arthroscopic examination of joints.
      a. Inflammation.
      b. Injury (acute or chronic).
      c. Loose bodies of bone and/or cartilage.
    2. Most frequently examined joints.
      a. Knee.
      b. Shoulder.
      c. Elbow.
      d. Ankle.
      e. Hip.
      f. Wrist.
    3. Disorders treated with a combination of arthroscopic and standard surgery.
      a. Rotator cuff procedure.
      b. Repair or resection of torn cartilage (meniscus) from knee or shoulder.
      c. Reconstruction of anterior cruciate ligament in knee.
      d. Removal of inflamed lining (synovium) in knee, shoulder, elbow, wrist, ankle.
      e. Release of carpal tunnel.
      f. Repair of torn ligaments.
      g. Removal of loose bone or cartilage in knee, shoulder, elbow, ankle, or wrist.
    4. Physical assessment.
      a. Presenting complaint.
      b. General medical history.
      c. Physical examination.
      d. Laboratory and imaging procedures.
  B. Primary/secondary/tertiary prevention.
    1. Primary prevention.

        a. Weight lifting safety.

        b. Jogging/running safety.

        c. Appropriate protective gear (shoes, helmets, padding).

        d. Change in lifestyle to increase physical activity.

    2. Secondary prevention.

        a. Sports medicine.

        b. Physical therapy.

    3. Tertiary prevention.

        a. Change in lifestyle may be required to decrease activities causing repetitive injuries.

        b. Joint replacement may be indicated.

C. Clinical procedures.

    1. Preoperative preparation.

        a. Rest.

        b. Quadriceps strengthening exercises.

        c. Crutch walking instructions initiated.

        d. Analgesics, no aspirin or anticoagulants for 3 to 5 days preoperatively.

        e. Anesthesiology evaluation with American Society of Anesthesiologist (ASA) classification for safe provision of conscious sedation.

    2. Day of surgery.

        a. Patient identifies knee to be operated on.

        b. Tourniquet positioned high on thigh.

        c. Leg scrubbed per protocol.

        d. General anesthetic administered, documented, and monitored.

        e. Procedure completed.

        f. Postoperative care.

            (1) Operative site monitored for bleeding.

            (2) Management of complications.

            (3) Vital signs monitored per protocol.

        g. Discharge.

            (1) Patient alert, pain controlled.

            (2) Crutch walking instructions reinforced.

            (3) Patient accompanied by responsible adult.

            (4) Written instructions given for pain control, activity level, ice to operative site, pressure dressings, leg-raising exercises, return visit.

D. Collaboration/resource identification, and referral.

    1. Physical therapy.

    2. Pain management.

E. Care management.

    1. Role of the perioperative nurse.

        a. Preadmission.

            (1) Screen for red flags (physical, emotional, environmental).

            (2) Identify potential problems and plan interventions.

        (3) Emphasize restrictions, medications, surgical preparations, need for transportation and responsible adult in attendance postoperatively.

    b. Day before surgery.

        (1) Preoperative reminder call.

        (2) Confirm time of surgery.

        (3) Reinforce oral and medication restrictions.

    c. Day of surgery.

        (1) Establish rapport with patient and family.

        (2) Provide reassurance and keep patient informed of any anticipated delays.

        (3) Provide need-to-know information, explain all procedures and how day will progress.

        (4) Model appropriate behaviors: calm, positive demeanor.

        (5) Provide written instructions and emergency phone numbers.

        (6) Demonstrate use of equipment.

    d. Postoperative phone call.

        (1) Follow up on physical condition and emotional state.

        (2) Be receptive to perceptions and concerns (identified trends offer opportunities for improvement) (Lancaster, 1997).

F. Patient education.

  1. Perioperative teaching considerations.

    a. Anxiety and stress.

        (1) Personality types influence amount of anxiety and stress experienced, which affects patient's ability to retain information.

        (2) Knowing the patient's state of mind is important: some stress heightens awareness, whereas a lot of stress interferes with retention of information.

        (3) Nurse must provide the right amount of caring, concern, and information.

    b. Learning needs and styles.

        (1) Learning is more effective when it is in response to a need.

        (2) Active involvement is essential for learning to occur.

        (3) Material/information presented must be meaningful and geared to the educational level of the patient.

        (4) Learning must be reinforced.

        (5) A combination of methods is more effective (written, verbal, videos).

        (6) Provide an opportunity for the patient and family to ask questions (Lancaster, 1997).

G. Advocacy and informed consent.

  1. Determine if patient is an appropriate candidate for ambulatory procedure.

    a. Assess emotional status.

    b. Cognitive assessment.

   c. Social assessment.

   d. Cultural assessment.

   e. Special assessments.

    (1) Geriatrics.

    (2) Pediatrics.

    (3) Mental retardation.

   f. Patient Self-Determination Act.

    (1) Bill of Rights.

    (2) Consents.

    (3) Refusal of blood products (Williams, 1997).

 H. Telephone practice.

  1. Postoperative telephone follow-up:

   a. Assists in evaluating postoperative conditions/outcomes.

   b. Reinforces postoperative teaching.

   c. Can be used to elicit patient and family satisfaction with the process.

   d. May be used to obtain performance feedback (Kleinpell, 1997).

 I. Communication/documentation.

  1. Clinical pathway for ambulatory surgery.

   a. Outcome-based timelines that offers consistent standards of care for ambulatory surgery patients.

   b. Reduce documentation needs, decrease length of stay, and provides autonomy for nursing staff.

   c. Standardize nursing assessment, interventions, patient and family education, preanesthesia assessment, discharge criteria, home-care instructions.

 J. Outcome management.

  1. Improving outcomes.

   a. Preventing unanticipated hospital admission.

   b. Assessing recovery time after anesthesia.

   c. Postoperative physician or emergency room visit.

   d. Evaluating mortality, major morbidity occurrences.

  2. Ambulatory surgery physical outcomes.

   a. Postoperative nausea and vomiting.

   b. Pain/surgical site discomfort.

   c. Drowsiness.

   d. Dizziness.

   e. Sore throat.

  3. Analyzing patient outcomes after ambulatory surgery provide opportunities to:

   a. Describe the impact of care on return to usual activity level.

   b. Assess patient satisfaction.

   c. Establish a more accurate and reliable basis for clinical decision-making.

   d. Evaluate the effectiveness of care and efficacy of clinical pathways.

   e. Identify opportunities for improvement (Kleinpell, 1997).

MODERATE SEDATION (CONSCIOUS SEDATION)

PATIENT POPULATION: Well, Acute, Chronic (Child, Adult, Elderly)

Definition

Conscious sedation is the use of medication resulting in amnesia and/or analgesia to sufficiently blunt but not remove a patient's protective reflexes in order to allow the performance of a procedure or test. The patient should exhibit a state of reduced consciousness that allows the patient to tolerate unpleasant procedures while retaining the ability to independently and continuously maintain cardiorespiratory function and appropriately respond to physical stimulation and/or verbal commands (ASA, 1996).

  A. Assess/screen/triage.

    1. The assessment, screening, and triage of ambulatory surgical patients receiving conscious sedation is essential for a safe and uneventful experience.

      a. The ASA classification system is a widely used screening tool (Table 19-1).

      b. Accurate patient classification identifies patients with disease processes that may require hospitalization and management by anesthesiology. Typically, ASA class III and IV patients are not candidates for ambulatory RN management.

    2. The age range and developmental level of patient populations receiving conscious sedation must be considered.

      a. Adult and pediatric patients differ in:

        (1) Physical and psychologic needs.

        (2) Type of medications and dosages.

        (3) Emergency resuscitation measures and equipment sizes.

■ TABLE 19-1
■ ■ **American Society of Anesthesiology (ASA) Classification System**

Classification	Description
ASA-1	Normal healthy patient
ASA-2	Patient with mild systemic disease (mild diabetes, controlled hypertension, anemia, chronic bronchitis)
ASA-3	Patient with severe systemic disease that limits activity but is not incapacitating (angina, obstructive pulmonary disease, prior myocardial infarction)
ASA-4	Patient with severe systemic disease that is a constant threat to life (heart failure, renal failure, acute myocardial infarction)
ASA-5	Moribund patient not expected to survive (ruptured aneurysm, head trauma with increasing ICP, shock caused by myocardial ischemia)
E	Emergency

Source: Somerson SJ, Husted CW, Sicilia MR (1995): Insights into conscious sedation. *Am J Nurs* 95(6):28.

(4) Staff training requirements.

    b. Disabled and psychologically immature patients may require deep sedation or general anesthesia for safety and compliance.

  3. Thorough medical record review and patient interview are essential and should include:

    a. Patient diagnosis.

    b. Medical illness history, including use of alcohol and tobacco and drug allergies. Last oral intake and a focused physical exam including cardiac, respiratory, and airway.

    c. Prior surgical procedures: previous uncomplicated procedures cannot be taken as a guarantee of a problem-free course.

    d. Specialty consultations to ascertain that other medical conditions are optimally treated.

    e. Use of over the counter (OTC) medications or dietary supplements.

    f. History of prior anesthesia or conscious sedation.

      (1) Medications and dosages used.

      (2) Airway management used.

      (3) Drug reactions including latex products and anesthetic complications.

    g. Determination of availability of postprocedure transportation.

B. Primary/secondary/tertiary prevention.

  1. Primary prevention.

    a. Early detection of potential complications can decrease the likelihood of adverse outcomes (ASA, 1996).

    b. Continuous monitoring of the patient's physiologic and psychologic status is required.

    c. Documentation of intraoperative monitoring at 5-minute intervals (may increase to 15-minute intervals as the patient progresses through the recovery process).

    d. The most important monitor is the person designated to do the monitoring. The person assigned to monitor the patient should not be hands-on involved in the procedure.

  2. Secondary prevention.

    a. Appropriate training and competencies in operation of emergency equipment.

    b. Knowledge of and immediate access to emergency resuscitative drugs.

  3. Tertiary prevention.

    a. Immediate access to a higher level of care should patient's condition warrant.

C. Clinical procedures.

  1. Desired goals of conscious sedation include:

    a. Maintenance of consciousness.

    b. Alteration in mood.

    c. Relaxation.

    d. Cooperation.

  e. Elevation of pain threshold.

  f. Minimal variation of vital signs.

  g. Some degree of amnesia.

  h. Decreased verbal communication.

  i. Initiation of slurred speech.

  j. Arousable sleep.

  k. Rapid safe return to baseline awareness and vital signs (AORN, 1996, p. 206; Ringler, 1995, p. 638).

 2. Undesirable effects of conscious sedation include:

  a. Loss of consciousness.

  b. Respiratory depression.

  c. Hypotension.

  d. Apnea.

  e. Unarousable sleep.

  f. Severely slurred speech.

  g. Agitation.

  h. Combativeness (AORN, 1996, p. 206 ; Ringler, 1995, p. 638).

 3. Essential monitoring equipment for ambulatory surgery patients should include:

  a. Functional source of oxygen (and a back-up source).

  b. Positive-pressure ventilation (bag valve mask).

  c. Suction equipment and appropriate-sized suction catheters.

  d. Sufficient electrical outlets and clearly labeled emergency power supply.

  e. Adequate illumination with backup battery-powered equipment.

  f. Emergency cart with equipment appropriate for patient's age and size (defibrillator, emergency drugs, airway equipment, and IV solutions and supplies).

  g. Equipment to monitor cardiac rate and rhythm, blood pressure, pulse rate, respiratory rate, oxygen saturation (pulse oximetry).

  h. Reliable means of two-way communication to summon help (Janikowski and Rockefeller, 1998).

D. Collaboration/resource identification and referral.

 1. Statements and standards for the provision of conscious sedation in the ambulatory setting.

  a. American Nurses' Association (ANA).

  b. Association of Operating Room Nurses (AORN).

  c. Association of PeriAnesthesia Nurses (ASPAN).

  d. Emergency Nurses Association (ENA) (Odom, 1997).

  e. Local standards per medical policy and procedure committees.

  f. American Society of Anesthesiology Guidelines on Sedation and Analgesia by Non-Anesthesiologists.

E. Care management.

 1. If any reversal agents are used, patient must be observed for up to 2 hours postprocedure to ensure that respiratory depression does not occur.

2. Patients receiving conscious sedation should not drive or take public transportation within 24 hours after surgery or discharge from the facility (JCAHO, 1998).
3. Patient evaluation is ongoing until recovery and independence are achieved or chronic care is required.
4. End goal.
   a. Facilitate safe and monitored recovery.
   b. Reduce patient and family anxiety.
   c. Control health care costs.
   d. Facilitate return to preoperative state of functioning or better (Redmond, 1995).

F. Patient education.
   1. Verbal and written preprocedure instructions.
      a. Dietary restrictions, NPO status, preps.
      b. Skin care for operative site.
      c. Exercises required postoperatively.
      d. Medication instructions.
   2. Verbal and written discharge instructions.
      a. Provide to patient and responsible adult caregiver/escort.
      b. Document in medical record.
   3. Discharge instructions.
      a. Self-care of operative site(s).
      b. Activity level and limitations.
      c. Symptoms to expect following procedure.
      d. Symptoms that need to be brought to the health care professional's attention.
      e. Signs and symptoms of infection or bleeding.
      f. Dietary restrictions.
      g. Medication instructions.
      h. Avoidance of operation of motor vehicles, electric equipment, or heavy equipment as advised by health care provider.
      i. Avoidance of alcohol consumption, tobacco, and making important decisions for 24 hours post-procedure.
      j. Follow-up care (time, place, and date).
      k. Phone number(s) for assistance in the event of post-procedure problems (Odom, 1997; Janikowski and Rockefeller, 1998).

G. Advocacy.
   1. JCAHO Standards for Conscious Sedation (1998).
      a. Patients receiving conscious sedation and subsequent monitoring in an ambulatory setting receive the same quality of care as patients in the traditional operating room.
      b. Provider administering conscious sedation must be qualified, have training, skills, and experience to rapidly recognize adverse events and initiate appropriate and timely response when patient's changing condition requires medical intervention (Constentino, 1996).
      c. A person not involved in performing the procedure must monitor the patient.

H. Telephone practice.

    1. Preoperative phone calls.

        a. Patient convenience.

        b. Provide and reinforce instructions.

        c. Decrease failed appointments.

        d. Obtain medical information.

    2. Postoperative phone calls.

        a. Evaluate progress and obtain medical information.

        b. Comfort level.

        c. General satisfaction.

        d. Provide reassurance and positive reinforcement.

I. Communication/documentation.

    1. Documentation of patient data should be predetermined and standardized.

    2. Terminology to describe the spectrum of consciousness.

        a. Alert and awake.

        b. Sedated and cooperative.

        c. Asleep and easily arousable.

        d. Asleep but slow to arouse to name.

        e. Arousable only to pain.

        f. Unarousable (AORN, 1996; JCAHO, 1998).

    3. Documentation of monitoring data on a time-based record.

        a. Cardiac rate and rhythm (continuous for patients with underlying cardiovascular disease because of increased risk for dysrhythmias).

        b. Blood pressure, pulse rate, respiratory rate (taken every 1 to 2 minutes during onset of sedation and every 5 to 10 minutes during the procedure).

        c. Oxygen delivery route (nasal cannula, face mask) and flow rate, oxygen saturation.

        d. Level of consciousness.

        e. Verbal response.

        f. Medication administered, dosage, time, route, patient response, name of ordering physician or anesthesia provider.

        g. Type and amounts of IV fluids and blood components administered.

        h. Pre- and postprocedural temperatures on patients less than 16 years of age.

        i. Any interventions and the patient's response.

        j. Any significant events or untoward reactions and their resolution (AORN, 1996).

    4. Practical objective criteria, note time frames, ensure uniform, safe recovery and discharge (Chung, 1995).

        a. The postanesthetic recovery (PAR) score is an effective, reliable, and safe assessment and documentation tool but only addresses the early phases of recovery.

        b. The modified postanesthetic recovery (PAR) score additionally determines street fitness and home readiness. Nine items are assessed:

            (1) Activity: ability/inability to move extremities.

    (2) Respiration: ability/inability to breathe and cough.

    (3) Circulation: blood pressure readings within preanesthetic level.

    (4) Consciousness: awake or arousable.

    (5) O_2 saturation: on room air or with oxygen supplement.

    (6) Pain: none, mild, or severe.

    (7) Ambulation: dizziness/vertigo, able to walk.

    (8) Feeding: nauseated/vomiting, able to drink.

    (9) Urine output: voiding/unable to void (Janikowski and Rockefeller, 1998).

c. The postanesthesia discharge scoring system (PADSS) measures the discharge readiness of ambulatory surgical patients. Five items are assessed:

    (1) Vital signs.

    (2) Activity and mental status.

    (3) Pain.

    (4) Nausea and/or vomiting.

    (5) Surgical bleeding.

    (6) Intake and output (Table 19-2).

d. The modified postanesthesia discharge scoring system (MPADSS) does not require voiding and drinking for discharge (Odom, 1997).

■ **TABLE 19-2**
■ ■ **Postanesthesia Discharge Scoring System**

---

1. Vital Signs
   2 = within 20% of preoperative value
   1 = 20%-40% of preoperative value
   0 = 40% of preoperative value
2. Ambulation and mental status
   2 = oriented x 3 and has a steady gait
   1 = oriented x 3 or has a steady gait
   0 = neither
3. Pain, or nausea/vomiting
   2 = minimal
   1 = moderate
   0 = severe
4. Surgical bleeding
   2 = minimal
   1 = moderate
   0 = severe
5. Intake and output
   2 = has had PO fluids and voided
   1 = has had PO fluids or voided
   0 = neither

The total score is 10. Patients scoring ≥9 are considered fit for discharge.
Source: Chung F (1995): Discharge process. In Twersky R, editor: *The ambulatory anesthesia handbook*. St. Louis: Mosby, p. 438.

   e. The modified circulation Alderete score may be used for children 12 years or less. A minimum Alderete score of eight is generally required for discharge.
J. Outcome management.
   1. Outcomes are what happens to patients after an interaction with the health care system. Includes patient's perception of the success/failure of the surgery.
   2. Measurable outcomes.
      a. Disease-specific.
         (1) Physiologic signs and symptoms (i.e., headaches, asthma attacks).
      b. General health.
         (1) Functional or general well being (i.e., mobility, return to work/activities, productivity, self-image).
      c. Patient performance.
         (1) Understanding and compliance with medical treatment plan (i.e., take medications correctly, wound self-care).
      d. Patient satisfaction.
         (1) Based on perceptions (i.e., amenities, caring, results).
         (2) Dissatisfiers: waiting times, inadequate pain relief, lack of preoperative and postoperative information, respect for patient's preferences (Benson, 1992).
K. Protocol development/usage.
   1. Conscious sedation training programs should be standardized, competency-based, have established baseline educational requirements, and ensure comparable training throughout an institution. Key components of a conscious sedation education program include:
      a. Current basic cardiac life support certification (BCLS) and advanced cardiac life support certification (ACLS).
      b. Review of anatomy and physiology.
      c. Preprocedural sedation assessment, ASA physical status classifications, and patient selection criteria.
      d. Conscious sedation vs. deep sedation, general anesthesia, and local anesthesia.
      e. Medications, dosages, administration rates, onset/duration, adverse effects, contraindications, and reversal agents.
      f. Management and monitoring of patients before, during, and after conscious sedation.
      g. Management of emergency cases.
      h. Competency in operating and troubleshooting essential equipment.
      i. Patient education.
      j. Discharge criteria.
      k. Documentation and medicolegal issues.
      l. Pre- and posttesting, preceptorship to practice newly acquired skills, and regularly scheduled recertification (Janikowski and Rockefeller, 1998).

2. Protocol for management of patients susceptible to malignant hyperthermia.
   a. Malignant hyperthermia is a syndrome with a distinctive set of signs and symptoms that may occur in susceptible individuals when given certain drugs for general anesthesia or muscle relaxation (approximately one in every 20,000 patients).
   b. Episode may begin immediately or later in PACU.
   c. Succinylcholine is one of the most common triggers of MH, especially when used in conjunction with an inhaled anesthetic agent. Other anesthetic agents to avoid using in MH susceptible patients: halothane (most frequent), enflurane, ether, desflurane, methoxyflurane, cyclopropane, sevoflurane, and isoflurane.
      (1) Medical history.
      (2) Family history of malignant hyperthermia, unexpected deaths, or complications from anesthesia.
      (3) History of muscle disorders (muscle weakness).
      (4) Dark or cola-colored urine after anesthesia.
      (5) Unexplained high fever after surgery (Williams, 1997).
3. Protocol for management of patients with latex sensitivity.
   a. Obtain thorough medical history: food allergies, childhood or adult eczema, and asthma. Gender: 75% of latex sensitive individuals are women.
      (1) Surgical history: multiple surgeries, intraoperative events consistent with anaphylaxis, hypotension, reactions during dental or radiologic procedures.
      (2) Occupational history: history of exposure, work-related symptoms, upper and lower respiratory symptoms.
      (3) Other symptoms: itchy hands, localized angioedema, urticaria after touching poinsettia plants.
      (4) Pharmacy to prepare latex-free injectable medications when applicable.
   b. Provide latex-free environment (no direct patient contact with latex products).
      (1) List of safe alternative products.
      (2) Set up a latex-free cart.
      (3) Provide patient warning signs and alert bracelets (Williams, 1997).

REFERENCES

Anderson LC (1994): Outpatient surgery center accreditation. *AORN J* 60: 959-967.

American Academy of Otolaryngology—Head and Neck Surgery (1999): *Doctor, why does my child's ear ache?* Alexandria, VA: Author.

American Academy of Otolaryngology—Head and Neck Surgery (1994): *Is my baby's hearing normal?* Alexandria, VA: Author.

American Society of Anesthesiologists (1996): Practice guidelines for sedation and analgesia by non-anesthesiologists: a report by the American Society of Anesthesiologists task force on sedation and analgesia by non-anesthesiologists. *Anesthesiology* 84(2):459-471.

Association of Operating Room Nurses (1996): *Recommended practices for monitoring the patient receiving intravenous conscious sedation. 1996 standards and recommended practices.* Denver: Author.

Association of Operating Room Nurses (1991): Issues surrounding intravenous conscious sedation. *AORN J*54(1):105-107.

Benson DS (1992): *Measuring outcomes in ambulatory care.* Chicago: American Hospital Publishing.

Briggs MB (1997): Nurse practitioners manage pre-admission testing. *AAACN Viewpoint* 19(6):4-5.

Brockway PM (1997): The ambulatory surgical nurse: evolution, competency, and vision. *Nurs Clin North Am* 32(2):387-394.

Chung F (May 1995): Recovery patterns and home-readiness after ambulatory surgery. *Anesthesia and Analgesia* 80(5): 896-902.

Constentino A (1996): Tucson Medical Center develops uniform conscious sedation policy. *Inside Ambulatory Care* 3(1):1, 4-5.

Hastings C (1997): Outcomes measurement: the challenge for ambulatory care nursing. *AAACN Viewpoint* 19(4):6-7.

Howe RS, editor (1997): Case management of ambulatory surgery patients: one size fits all. *Clinical pathways for ambulatory care case management.* Gaithersburg, MD: Aspen, pp. 1-13:1.

Janikowski D, Rockefeller C (1998): Awake and talking: ambulatory surgery and conscious sedation. *Nurs Econ* 16(1):37-43.

Joint Commission on Accreditation of Healthcare Organizations (1998): *1998 Comprehensive Accreditation Manual for Hospitals.* Oakbrook Terrace, IL: Author.

Kemper DW (1997): *Healthwise handbook,* ed 13. Boise, ID: Healthwise, pp. 229-233.

Kleinpell RM (1997): Improving telephone follow-up after ambulatory surgery. *J PeriAnesthesia Nurs* 12(5):336-340.

Krames Communications (1995): *Breast surgery from biopsy to reconstruction.* San Bruno, CA: Author.

Krames Communications (1996): *The post-op book. A guide for surgical patients.* San Bruno, CA: Author.

Krames Communications (1997): *Breast lumps. A guide to understanding breast problems and breast surgery.* San Bruno, CA: Author.

Krames Communications (1997): *Common breast conditions. Understanding benign breast problems.* San Bruno, CA: Author.

Lancaster KA (1997): Care of the pediatric patient in ambulatory surgery. *Nurs Clin North Am* 32(2):441-454.

Lancaster KA (1997): Patient teaching in ambulatory surgery. *Nurs Clin North Am* 32(2):417-427.

Linnell KE (1998): Patient health education in the changing ambulatory care environment. *AAACN Viewpoint* 20(1):1, 6-8.

Lowdermilk D, Perry S, Bobak I (2000): *Maternity & women's health care,* ed 7. St. Louis: Mosby.

National Cancer Institute (1996): *Chances are you need a mammogram.* National Institutes of Health Pub. No. 96-3836, Bethesda, Md: Author.

Odom J (1997): Conscious sedation in the ambulatory setting. *Crit Care Nurs Clin North Am* 9(3):361-370.

Rankin SH, Stallings KD (1996): *Patient education issues, principles, practices,* ed 3. Philadelphia: Lippincott-Raven, pp. 105-110.

Redman BK (1997): *The practice of patient education,* ed 8. St. Louis: Mosby, pp.106-118.

Redmond MC (1995): Using home health agencies to meet patient needs in phase III recovery. *J Post Anesthesia Nurs* 10(1):21-26.

Ringler JD (1995): The use of diazepam and ketamine for IV conscious sedation in outpatient surgery settings. *AORN J* 62(4):638-546.

Schmitt B (1999): *Instructions for pediatric patients,* ed 2. Philadelphia: WB Saunders.

Somerson SJ, Husted CW, Sicilia MR (1995): Insights into conscious sedation. *Am J Nurs* 95(6):26-33.

Whedon MA (1995): Practice corner. *Oncol Nurs Forum* 22(1):147-150.

Williams GD (1997): Preoperative assessment and health history interview. *Nurs Clin North Am* 32(2):395-416.

Whaley LF, Wong DL (1997): *Essentials of pediatric nursing,* ed 5. St. Louis: Mosby.

Nurse-Managed Clinics

Compiled by JOAN ROBINSON, MS, RN, CNAA

PATIENT PROTOTYPES

Wound Care ■ Anticoagulation ■ Incontinence

OBJECTIVES
Study of the information presented in this chapter will enable the learner to:

1. Identify the principle roles of the ambulatory care nurse in a nurse-managed clinic for wound care, anticoagulation management, and continence.

2. Identify one primary, one secondary, and one tertiary preventive intervention.

3. Identify criteria that, when present, would indicate the patient needs immediate care.

4. Identify areas of patient teaching for patients in wound care, anticoagulation, and continence clinics.

5. Relate nurse competencies to services offered by nurse-managed clinics.

6. Identify issues and barriers to practice encountered by nurse-managed clinics.

7. Identify factors that place a patient at risk for developing a wound and/or wound complications.

8. Identify therapy for over- and under-coagulation.

■■
■■■ Nurse-managed clinics are not a new concept. They are as old as Sanger and Breckenridge, who in 1895 developed the first prospective payment system at the Frontier Nursing Service (Frenn, Lundeen, Martin, Riesch, and Wilson, 1996). Nurse-managed clinics (nurse-run or nurse-led clinics) also are considered a contemporary role for nurses. Nurse-managed clinics refers to a variety of practices: from independent entities, where patients have direct access to the nurse and the practice is controlled by the nurse, to clinics where patients are referred to a nurse and the clinic exists within a larger health care organization under the direction of the parent organization. As the health care system has continued to undergo dramatic change, social and economic factors have created a constant state of evaluation of care delivery. Nurses and others, within and outside formal organizations, have responded by creating innovative approaches to increase access to care for patients. In the nurse-run clinic, the patient sees a nurse for care. The role

of the nurse may be independent or a collaborative relationship with a physician where care is guided by protocol, depending upon the education and experience of the nurse, the state's nurse practice act and other laws, and practices of the state and/or institution. Practices may be interdisciplinary involving many members of the health care team. The three authors of this chapter discuss the role dimensions of the nurse in a specialty practice nurse-managed clinic.

WOUND CARE

David R. Crumbley, MSN, BS, RN, CWCN

The recent development of outpatient wound care clinics is in response to the proliferation of wound care knowledge and technology over the past 10 years, the high cost of managing chronic wounds, and recent insistence by third party payers to provide an increasing amount of care in the outpatient setting (Crumbley, Ice, and Cassidy, 1999). Outpatient wound care clinics specialize in the management of the patient with disorders of the integument. Disorders of the integument include acute and chronic wounds, which may incorporate surgical wounds healing by primary, secondary, or tertiary intention, vascular ulcers (venous and arterial), inflammatory ulcers/tissue-collagen ulcers, pressure ulcers, diabetic ulcers, and burns. Many of these disorders/wounds are preventable or can be limited in severity if managed appropriately using a multidisciplinary collaborative effort (Frykberg, 1998; Reiber, Boyko, and Smith, 1995). The multidisciplinary wound care team generally includes, but is not limited to the following specialties: general, vascular, and plastic surgery; family practice; internal medicine; orthopedics; dermatology; wound care; podiatry; orthotics; physical therapy; dietary; and home health. However, patient care requires coordination in this multidisciplinary setting to prevent fragmentation, and to allow effective outcomes to be recognized (Steed, Edington, Moosa, and Webster, 1993; Jaramillo, Elizondo, Jones, Corfero, and Wang, 1997; Crumbley, 1997; Crumbley, et al., 1999). Therefore the role of the ambulatory care nurse in this setting requires not only the clinical expertise of a health care provider, but also depends on the nurse's ability to function as a care manager/case manager for the patient with a wound.

    A. Assessment/screen/triage.
        1. Risk factors for disorders of the integument (Wysocki and Bryant, 1992; Bonham, 1999). (The terms disorder of the integument and wound will be used interchangeably throughout this section.)
           a. Diabetes.
           b. Peripheral neuropathy.
           c. Autoimmune disease.
           d. Chronic illness/disease.
           e. Obesity.
           f. Poor nutritional status.
           g. Sedentary lifestyle.
           h. Immobility.
           i. Decreased mentation.

    j. Incontinence.

    k. Increasing age.

    l. History of coronary artery disease and or arterial insufficiency, or venous insufficiency.

    m. History of long-term steroid therapy.

    n. Infectious agent.

    o. Recent surgery.

    p. Recent trauma.

2. A thorough patient history should include medical, surgical, pharmacologic, lifestyle, and wound (current and past wounds including treatment) histories. This data provides the nurse with the necessary information to formulate an effective treatment plan.

3. Physical exam/assessment (Bonham, 1999).

    a. Height should be assessed initially but weight is requisite for each visit.

    b. Assess the patient's hygiene status to determine if this is an area where amplified efforts toward patient/family education will need to be focused.

    c. Assess for steadiness, mobility, and the need for assistive devices. Observe footwear for signs of excessive wear or inadequate fit.

    d. Mentation and sensory assessment should include evaluation for peripheral neuropathy.

    e. Assess skin turgor, mobility, and overall appearance of the skin.

        (1) Is the skin warm to touch with good capillary refill to the extremities?

        (2) Assess potential problem areas such as bony prominences (i.e., ischial spine, femoral head, coccyx) of the immobile or sensory-impaired patient.

        (3) It may be necessary to assess the entire integument if the patient is sensory-impaired.

    f. Assess the patient for cardiovascular or respiratory insufficiency (blood pressure, pulse oximetry).

        (1) Does the patient have adequate blood pressure, capillary refill, pulses, skin changes or hair loss to extremities that would indicate peripheral vascular disease?

        (2) Assess for central and peripheral edema.

        (3) If the wound is to the foot, what is the ankle brachial index (ABI)? (ABI is a measurement comparing the systolic pressure in the brachial artery to the systolic pressure in the ankle. A 1 to 1 ratio, or an ABI of 1.0 is ideal. Lesser values could indicate arterial disease. However in the patient with diabetes, an abnormally high ABI could indicate calcification of arteries. Consultation/collaboration with a vascular specialist may be necessary.)

    g. Lab work (potential) (Konstantinides, 1992; Doughty, 1992).

        (1) Wound culture.

(2) CBC with differential.

(3) Total lymphocyte count.

(4) Serum albumin, transferrin, or prealbumin.

(5) Hemoglobin A_{1c}, and/or blood glucose.

h. Assessment of wound characteristics (Sussman, 1998; Cooper, 1992).

(1) Location of the wound.

(2) Dimensions of the wound can be determined by measuring the open area of the wound in centimeters along the vertical and horizontal axis. This is accomplished by measuring the wound length at its greatest distance and the wound width at its greatest distance (Figure 20-1). Clarity is enhanced through simple drawings that indicate wound shape and the location of wound measurements. More sophisticated measuring techniques are available; however, the previously mentioned technique is possibly the simplest and requires limited resources.

(3) Appearance of the wound.

(a) Assess the color of the wound bed. Red is healthy; Yellow, unhealthy; Black, unhealthy and ischemic; Pale, unhealthy and poorly perfused.

(b) Assess for the following signs of infection: redness, erythema, or warmth to surrounding tissue, pain, purulent drainage, and/or inflammation.

(4) Assess the wound drainage for appearance, amount, and odor.

(5) Assess the surrounding tissue (periwound) and the wound

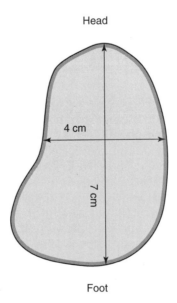

Head

4 cm

7 cm

Foot

FIGURE 20-1 ■ Measurement of the Wound (Developed by David R. Crumbley.)

edges for inflammation, maceration, etc. If calloused tissue is present in surrounding tissue, suspect the wound may be in response to repeated pressure.

(6) Assess the quantity and quality of pain experienced by the patient. Use pain scale appropriate for client (pediatric, non-English speaking, etc.).

B. Primary, secondary, tertiary prevention (Clemen-Stone, McGuire, and Eigsti, 1998).

  1. Primary prevention.

  a. Institute an awareness campaign that focuses on healthy lifestyle behaviors and disease prevention.

  b. Incorporate health promotion activities that reinforce healthy behaviors and disease prevention.

  2. Secondary prevention.

  a. Perform risk assessments using validated tools for screening to determine those individuals at risk for acquiring a wound (refer to risk factors under section A, 1 on pp. 362-363).

  b. Provide preventive and informative educational programs tailored to each risk factor group. For example, an educational program for the diabetic patient with peripheral neuropathy should focus on daily foot care and shoe selection.

  c. Educate fellow health care providers regarding the early signs of a potential or worsening wound in order to enhance rapid detection and early treatment.

  d. Provide prompt, appropriate care based on accurate diagnosis.

  e. Perform routine evaluation of progress and make adjustments/recommendations as necessary.

  3. Tertiary prevention.

  a. Schedule routine follow-up visits to monitor wound progression or recurrence.

  b. Ensure referrals for appropriate aftercare personnel or supplies are instituted. For example, compression stockings for the venous leg ulcer patient following wound resolution, or orthotics for the patient with diabetes who has a resolved foot ulcer.

C. Clinical procedures.

  1. Topical therapy* (Doughty, 1992) pertains to the coverings or dressings used to manage a wound. Numerous topical therapies/dressings are available for use in wound management, each having unique properties. See Table 20-1 for examples of topical therapies and Box 20-1 for goals of topical therapy.

  a. Determine the etiology of the wound.

  b. Determine the appropriate topical therapy and cleansing solution for

---

*Topical therapy is an vast subject area, which is too extensive to be covered in this endeavor. It is *highly* recommended that the nurse managing an outpatient wound clinic seek further information and education in regard to topical wound care.

TABLE 20-1
■ Examples of Topical Therapies

Dressing	Application	Properties	Absorptive Capabilities	Contraindications
Transparent film dressing	Covering	Protects, insulates, maintains moist environment, and assists in autolytic debridement of wound	None	Moderate/large amount of drainage, sensitivity or infection
Polyurethane foam dressing	Covering	Protects, insulates, absorbs, maintains moist environment, and assists in autolytic debridement	Moderate	Large amount of drainage, sensitivity, or infection
Gauze	Covering, or to fill space in a wound	Protects, insulates, absorbs, assists in mechanical debridement	Minimal to moderate	Dry wound
Calcium alginate	Placed under a cover dressing or gauze; used to fill space in wound	Protects, insulates, maintains moist environment and assists in autolytic debridement of wound	Moderate to large	Dry wound
Hydrogel (amorphous)	Placed in wound to promote moist environment	Maintains moist environment and assists with autolytic debridement of wound	None to minimal	Heavily draining wound, or sensitivity
Hydrogel (sheets)	Covering	Protects, insulates, maintains moist environment and assists in autolytic debridement of wound	Minimal to moderate	Heavily draining wound, sensitivity, or infection
Hydrocolloids	Covering	Protects, insulates, maintains moist environment and assists in autolytic debridement of wound	Minimal to moderate	Heavily draining, sensitivity, or infection

Adapted from Sussman C, Bates-Jensen B, editors (1998): *Wound care: a collaborative practice manual for physical therapists and nurses.* Gaithersburg, MD: Aspen. Doughty D (1992): Principles of wound healing and wound management. In Bryant R, editor: *Acute and chronic wounds: nursing management.* St. Louis: Mosby, pp. 31-68.

■ BOX 20-1
■ **GOALS OF TOPICAL THERAPY**

1. Remove necrotic tissue
2. Eliminate infection
3. Eliminate dead space
4. Absorb excess exudate
5. Insulate wound bed
6. Protect wound from trauma or secondary contamination
7. Maintain moist environment

Adapted from Bonham P (1999): *Wound care specialty course.* Unpublished manuscript, Medical University of South Carolina.

wound care based on the wound etiology and the following wound characteristics:

(1) Amount of wound drainage.
(2) Location of the wound.
(3) Presence of infection.
(4) Client and family receptiveness (user friendliness).
(5) Cost.

c. Make adjustments to topical therapy as wound characteristics change.

2. Pharmacologic management.
   a. Antibiotics (infection).
   b. Topical steroids (inflammation).
   c. Glucocorticoid (severe inflammation).
   d. Diuretics (edema).
   e. Hemorrheologic agent (assists in management of peripheral vascular disease by reducing blood viscosity and improving red blood cell flexibility).
   f. Nonsteroidal antiinflammatory drugs (NSAIDs) or narcotics (pain relief).

3. Lifestyle management.
   a. Nutritional/dietary support to include increased amounts of protein from meats, milk products, or nutritional drinks; vitamin A from green and yellow vegetables; vitamin C from citrus fruits; and zinc from seafood.
   b. Evaluate diabetic patients for increased blood sugar, which can impede the wound-healing process.
   c. Discuss the need to increase or decrease activity, dependent on wound etiology and location. For example, the patient with a diabetic ulcer on the plantar surface of the foot should limit excessive walking. However, the patient with venous insufficiency and a venous leg ulcer should be encouraged to walk, consequently promoting venous return through the pumping properties of the calf muscle.
   d. Modify sleeping or seating habits. For example, in venous insuffi-

ciency raise foot of bed (unless contraindicated, e.g., congestive heart failure) and elevate extremity when seated; in the paraplegic with ulcer on ischial spine, practice pressure relief while seated and obtain special seating devices.

    e. Modify bathing practices to coincide with dressing changes.

    f. Evaluate whether treatment plan is conducive to patient's lifestyle. For example, it is improbable that a single mother with two small children will comply with bed rest for 2 weeks. Avoid use of the term noncompliant as a substitute for inadequate treatment planning!

D. Collaboration/resource identification and referral.

    1. Provide concise and timely feedback concerning patient care and progress to members of multidisciplinary treatment team either through verbal, written, or electronic medium.

    2. Identify and facilitate activation of ancillary resources required for effective treatment and aftercare.

    3. Initiate/facilitate referrals as needed.

    4. Collaborate with the patient and family in treatment planning (refer to lifestyle management in section C, 3 on p. 367 and above).

E. Care management. (Also refer to collaboration/resource identification and referral in section D above as well as primary, secondary, and tertiary prevention in section B, 1-3 on p. 365.)

    1. Coordinate care, ensuring multidisciplinary care does not become fragmented care.

    2. Use clinical/critical pathways to plan care of patient.

    3. Maintain a database of all patients, which includes name and contact information.

    4. Schedule periodic follow-up visits to ensure that aftercare is accomplished and no new problems develop.

    5. Participate actively in multidisciplinary care management team meetings.

    6. Assign each patient a backup provider who is familiar with the case in an effort to promote continuity of care.

F. Patient education (education should always include significant others and caregivers).

    1. Topical therapy.

        a. Discuss the topical therapy to be used. Include the following characteristics of the therapy:

            (1) Dressing change and wound cleansing technique.

            (2) Rationale for the therapy.

            (3) Benefits of the therapy.

            (4) Adverse effects to observe for during therapy.

            (5) Explain to the patient and/or caregiver what they should expect to see, feel, and/or smell before, during, and after a dressing change. For example, calcium alginates may have a fishy odor.

            (6) Discuss the projected rate of healing.

        b. Discuss alternative therapies in the event that wound characteristics change or the therapy causes adverse effects.

    2. Pharmacologic therapy.
      a. Discuss rationale for therapy.
      b. Discuss benefits as well as adverse reactions.
      c. Discuss dosage and regimen for administration.
    3. Lifestyle therapy.
      a. Discuss rationale for nutritional intake, activity modifications, and other lifestyle modifications.
      b. Discuss benefits and adverse reactions associated with specific lifestyle modifications.
      c. Identify risk factors that can be controlled and develop a collaborative plan to modify these factors.
    4. Wound healing characteristics.
      a. Discuss expectations of treatment in regard to healing rate, pain, and wound appearance.
        (1) Decrease in size of wound.
        (2) Decrease in necrotic tissue.
        (3) Decreased pain.
        (4) Free of signs and symptoms of infection.
    5. Healthcare access.
      a. Discuss signs and symptoms that necessitate *emergent* care.
        (1) Fever, chills, increased warmth to wound or surrounding tissue, or purulent drainage.
        (2) Increased bleeding or pain.
        (3) Decreased sensation to an extremity with a wound.
        (4) Paresthesia, pallor, or coolness to an extremity with a wound.
        (5) Dehiscence of a wound that had previously been closed.
      b. For aftercare, discuss *early* signs and symptoms that indicate the need for professional health care intervention to prevent recurrence of wounds.
G. Advocacy. (Also refer to the collaboration/resource identification section D on p. 368 and the referral as well as care management section E on p. 368.)
    1. Assist patient in accessing the health care system as necessary.
    2. Assist patient in resolving barriers to care as necessary. Barriers include:
      a. Access to healthcare (assistance may take the form of education or facilitation).
      b. Adequate financial resources. Numerous modern topical therapies are expensive and treatment for a chronic wound may encompass several months; consequently treatment can become costly. Advocacy may take the form of assisting the patient to procure financial resources to ensure care. For example, contacting vendors who might provide samples or supplies at a discounted rate.
      c. Access to supplies. Before prescribing a topical dressing ensure that it is available through local vendors.
H. Telephone practice.
    1. Ensure that patients are aware of the symptoms or signs that necessitate contacting a health care provider (refer to healthcare access section F, 5 above).

2. Establish and implement protocols for triaging patients via the telephone.

3. Ensure that *all* clinic personnel are aware of telephone triage protocol and emergent symptoms that require urgent intervention.

I. Communication/documentation.

1. Develop a documentation method for patient assessment, treatment, and progress, that facilitates communication among all members of the treatment team and provides a complete narrative of care.

   a. Document all encounters (i.e., office and telephone).

   b. Include wound images as a part of documentation if possible. Images are beneficial for wound healing documentation, outcome tracking, education, and for protection from liability.

2. Communicate and coordinate treatment plans with patient and significant others, as well as other team members.

3. Protect patient confidentiality.

J. Outcome management.

1. Determine which outcomes will be measured in an outcome management plan. Those outcomes being monitored should be considered important to your organization, your patients, and yourself. Outcomes must be measurable and meaningful (e.g., healing rates [time and percent healed], decreased amputations in the diabetic population, decreased amount of skin grafting, and/or patient satisfaction).

2. Include individual and aggregate outcomes.

3. Monitor outcomes daily. Your job and the future of your clinic depend on it!

4. Evaluate outcomes at least quarterly.

K. Protocol development/usage (Wound Ostomy and Continence Nurses Society, 1992, 1993; AHCPR, 1992; Crumbley, et al., 1999).

1. Use current practice standards, research, and practice findings to develop clinical/critical pathways for each wound category seen in your clinic.

2. Ensure patient has a pathway in his or her treatment record that pertains to his or her particular type of wound. For example, each venous leg ulcer patient should have the same critical pathway. Pathways can and should be individualized; however, treatment should be consistent among groups.

3. Evaluate patient progress according to his or her clinical/critical pathway. If progress is not sufficient, adjustments should be incorporated.

ANTICOAGULATION

Assanatu I. Savage, BSN, RNC, MA
Bobbie McCarthy, RN

Long-term anticoagulation therapy has continued to increase as a successful adjunct to care for persons with clotting disorders and as standard management for persons with cardiovascular disease. Increased use has led to the development of systematic and coordinated approaches in outpatient management of these persons.

The registered nurse in physician-supervised anticoagulation clinics must have the ability to assess, teach the patient, communicate with the health care team, and provide optimal coordination and management of therapy. The information and support provided must enable patients to integrate anticoagulation therapy into their lifestyle. The establishment of an anticoagulation clinic requires a transdisciplinary approach. Team players may include, but are not limited to, the medical staff, nurse, pharmacy, laboratory, medical records, and administration.

Warfarin (Coumadin) is the most widely used anticoagulant in the United States. It has been found to provide a more stable anticoagulation effect than other oral anticoagulants in the outpatient setting (Spandorfer and Merli, 1996). Warfarin for injection is now available for intravenous administration for patients who are unable to receive oral drugs (Dupont Pharmaceutical, 1999). Aspirin, clopidogrel (Plavix), and ticlodipine (Ticlid) are powerful oral platelet aggregation inhibitors, commonly used for prevention and recurrence of myocardial infarction and stroke (*Physician's Desk Reference* [PDR], 1999). Other anticoagulants in use are heparin, enoxaparin (Lovenox), and dalteparin (Fragmin), the latter two derivatives of heparin given subcutaneously (Raimer, Thomas, and Lake, 1995). This section will focus mainly on the use of warfarin; however, a brief discussion on aspirin, heparin, and enoxaparin (Lovenox) will be provided.

A. Assessment/screen/triage (for the most common cases seen in a nurse-managed anticoagulation clinic).
   1. Risk factors/indications for anticoagulation therapy.
      a. Patients with bleeding disorders (Duke Coagulation Consult Service, 1999).
         (1) History of abnormal bleeding.
         (2) Prolonged bleeding or clotting times.
         (3) Factor deficiencies.
         (4) Thrombocytopenia.
         (5) Complex coagulopathies.
      b. Patients with recurrent thrombosis (Duke Coagulation Consult Service, 1999).
         (1) Recurrent venous thrombosis.
         (2) Recurrent arterial thrombosis.
         (3) Early onset of deep vein thrombosis (DVT) or pulmonary embolus (PE) without a predisposing factor.
         (4) Lupus anticoagulants and anticardiolipin antibodies.
         (5) Deficiencies of natural anticoagulants (protein C, protein S, antithrombin III).
      c. Patients with cardiac disorders/diseases (Spandorfer and Merli, 1996).
         (1) Atrial fibrillation/atherosclerotic heart disease.
         (2) Cardiac valve replacement/disorder.
         (3) Prosthetic valve replacement.
         (4) Myocardial infarction.

    2. A thorough screening process is necessary for individualized and effective management of therapy. It will include:
      a. A review of the history and physical exam.
      b. A review of past medical and surgical histories.
      c. Assessment of medication usage: prescribed, over-the-counter, herbs, and history of allergies.
      d. Assessment of nutrition and lifestyle.
      e. Assessment and evaluation of body mass (weight).
      f. Presence of other diseases/illnesses.
      g. Assessment of psychosocial support (especially for the elderly).
    3. Management is based on the results of individualized international ratio (INR) and prothrombin (PT) for warfarin and activated partial thromboplastin time (APTT) for heparin. Triage will depend on the following baseline data and periodic assessment of lab values.
      a. INR and PT/APTT lab results.
      b. Hemoglobin and hematocrit.
      c. Urinalysis.
      d. Occult blood.
      e. Platelet count.
B. Primary, secondary, tertiary prevention.
    1. Primary prevention.
      a. Provide training and resources that promote a healthy lifestyle and encourage disease prevention.
    2. Secondary prevention.
      a. Screening susceptible population for risk factors.
      b. Constant monitoring and provision of early intervention and thorough follow-up to avoid further complications.
      c. Awareness of special considerations for the elderly (Marine and Goldhaber, 1998) and provision of necessary interventions.
        (1) Auditory and visual deficits.
        (2) Fine and gross motor deficits.
        (3) Cognition and memory deficits.
        (4) Risk for fall/injury.
        (5) Dietary inconsistencies: vitamin K.
        (6) Polypharmacy: increased risk of drug interactions.
        (7) History of noncompliance with medications.
      d. Interact with other disciplines/community outreach programs to provide support and assist in optimal care.
    3. Tertiary prevention.
      a. Maintenance of a thorough follow-up program, for example, use of flow sheet for documentation of medication dosage, lab values, and missed doses.
      b. Achievement of therapeutic goal, for example, acceptable INR range, in most cases 2-3 and PT level 18-21.
      c. Individualized maintenance therapy.
      d. Prevention and management of bleeding.

      e. Patient education.

      f. Interventions for over- and under-coagulation.

C. Clinical procedures.

  1. Ensure that nurse clinic privileges are within boundaries of the state nurse practice act. Usually patients will transition from an intravenous anticoagulant (heparin) or subcutaneous anticoagulant (enoxaparin) to an oral anticoagulant (warfarin). The first visit should develop rapport and involves the following activities:

      a. History taking and obtaining baseline labs.

      b. Patient/significant other(s) education.

         (1) Review reason(s) for therapy.

         (2) Explain drug pharmacology.

         (3) Review current medications and use of herbs.

         (4) Educate to generic and brand names of medications.

         (5) Provide printed materials suitable to patient's reading level and visual acuity.

         (6) Consider use of pictures for functionally illiterate patients.

         (7) Instruct in maintenance of drug record and need for accessibility.

         (8) Instruct on drug-drug and food-drug interactions.

         (9) Provide information and need for Medic Alert bracelet.

         (10) Instruct on overall lifestyle and management therapy.

         (11) Side effects.

         (12) Definition of INR/PT and patient's target INR.

         (13) Importance of compliance to medication.

      c. Set goals and expectations for therapeutic range for labs.

      d. Set dates for reevaluation and end of therapy.

      e. Assess psychosocial barriers.

         (1) Transportation issues.

         (2) Meals.

         (3) Work.

         (4) Finances.

         (5) Literacy.

  2. Subsequent visit.

      a. Assess for bleeding or clotting problems.

      b. Review drug dosage (may have patient, especially the elderly, to bring all of their medications).

      c. Note any change in other drug therapies.

      d. Review lab results.

      e. Document patient's progress on a flow sheet.

      f. Update provider on patient's progress and implement dosage adjustment as necessary.

      g. Schedule next visit.

D. Collaboration/resource identification and referral.

  1. Involve patient and significant other(s) in the plan of care.

  2. Collaborate with the health care team through verbal, written, or electronic communication.

3. Gain support of ancillary services to facilitate safe and effective care.
4. Initiate psychosocial support, especially for the elderly, as needed, for example, Meals on Wheels, transportation, visiting nurse, and daily telephone checks.
5. Make other referrals as necessary (e.g., nutritionist).
6. Provide constant updating, adjustment, and goal setting with the patient, significant other(s), and the health care team members.

E. Care management. (Also refer to the primary, secondary, and tertiary prevention section B on pp. 372-373, the clinical procedures section C on p. 373, and the collaboration/resource identification and referral section D on p. 373 and above). Anticoagulation therapy, in most cases, is managed using heparin, enoxaparin, aspirin, or warfarin. Clinical status determines follow-up care requirements (Raimer, et al., 1995).

1. Pharmacologic agent, monitoring, and management.
   a. Heparin: given subcutaneous for patients unable to tolerate oral anticoagulant, pregnant and nursing women (Spandorfer and Merli, 1999).
      (1) Establish baseline and monitor activated partial thromboplastin (APTT)/prothrombin (PT) time.
      (2) Assess for soft tissue bleeding.
      (3) Monitor for heparin-induced thrombocytopenia and thrombosis (HITT), also known as *white clot syndrome.*
      (4) Stop heparin and give protamine sulfate for over-anticoagulation (heparin reversal) (Raimer, et al., 1995).
   b. Enoxaparin: a heparin derivative causing same adverse conditions but with decreased incidence of HITT relative to heparin.
      (1) Monitor as for heparin.
      (2) Enoxaparin does not alter APTT or PT, and routine labs not required.
      (3) May perform periodic hemoglobin, hematocrit, and platelet count.
      (4) Treat over-anticoagulation with slow intravenous protamine sulfate (Raimer, et al., 1995).
   c. Aspirin: oral antiplatelet used mainly for prevention of recurrent myocardial infarction and decreased incidence of stroke (PDR, 1999).
      (1) Assess for bleeding (e.g., petechiae, ecchymosis, bleeding gums).
      (2) Assess for drug-drug interaction to avoid overdosing.
      (3) Monitor periodic platelets, hematocrit, PT, blood urine salicylate, hepatic and renal function test.
      (4) Treat toxicity by inducing emesis, or gastric lavage. In some cases, hemodialysis may be indicated for adults, peritoneal dialysis for children, and exchange transfusion for infants.
   d. Warfarin: most commonly used oral anticoagulant; acts by preventing the manufacture of vitamin K-dependent clotting factors; these

include factors II, VII, IX, X, and anticoagulant proteins C and S (PDR, 1999).

(1) Obtain baseline labs.

(2) Monitor PT and INR.

(3) Assess for bleeding: blood in urine, bruising, blood in stool, bleeding gums, low platelet, hemoglobin, and hematocrit counts (Raimer, et al., 1995).

(4) Identify patient at risk for bleeding.

   (a) Elderly.

   (b) Patient with history of hemorrhagic stroke, gastrointestinal (GI) bleeding, possibly liver or peptic ulcer disease, alcoholism, use of nonsteroidal antiinflammatory drugs (NSAIDs), aspirin use, diabetes, anemia, renal insufficiency hypertension (Spandorfer and Merli, 1996).

   (c) Postpartum females, teenagers, and young adults who need warfarin education specific to their needs and lifestyle, for example, sports, menses, teratogenicity, and adolescent adjustment behaviors.

(5) Assess and monitor for dermatologic conditions such as warfarin-induced skin necrosis, purple toes syndrome, alopecia, dermatitis, and maculopapular erythematous rash. These conditions resolve once warfarin is discontinued (Spandorfer and Merli, 1996).

(6) Over-anticoagulation caused by warfarin is treated with vitamin K (Raimer, et al., 1995).

e. Unlike heparin and enoxaparin, the effect of warfarin is influenced by many drugs, foods, and presence of other illnesses (PDR, 1999; Brosnan, 1996).

(1) Some factors that may increase the effect of warfarin include various medications (e.g., antibiotics, cholesterol, and seizure medications), alcohol, decreased intake and absorption of vitamin K, liver dysfunction, diarrhea, infectious disease, and hyperthyroidism.

(2) Some factors that may decrease the effect of warfarin include certain medications (barbiturates, corticosteroids, rifampin, estrogen-containing products, etc.), increased vitamin K intake (e.g., spinach, kale, herbal teas), edema, hyperlipemia, and hypothyroidism.

(3) Contraindications for warfarin include: pregnancy, hemorrhagic tendencies, or blood dyscrasia, threatened abortion, eclampsia, and preeclampsia.

(4) Consult a nursing drug handbook or *Physician's Desk Reference* for more information and contraindications for warfarin therapy.

F. Patient education. (Also refer to the clinical procedures, section C on p. 373 and the care management section E on p. 374 and above.)

1. Include patient, significant other(s), and/or care provider in plan of care.
2. Explain basic physiology and reason for therapy.
3. Explain clotting mechanism.
4. Discuss factors that affect therapy: diet, medications, illnesses, lifestyle, age, body size.
5. Offer video viewing and written instructions appropriate to patient.
6. Explain and discuss signs and symptoms of over- and under-anticoagulation.
7. Discuss health care and emergency access during and after working hours.

G. Advocacy. (Also see the collaboration/resource identification, and referral section D on pp. 373-374 as well as care management, section E on pp. 374-375.)
   1. Develop rapport and assist patient in accessing this service.
   2. Provide ongoing education, monitoring, and support.
   3. Collaborate and give feedback to the rest of the health care team.
   4. Assist (especially the elderly) in maintaining compliance. This may involve consulting with social work to arrange for a visiting nurse or developing a calendar and/or a seven-day pill box.

H. Telephone practice
   1. Be knowledgeable about the different colors and dosages of warfarin (some patients know their drugs only by the color).
   2. Establish standing orders for medication.
   3. Call patients with their lab results and inform them of any need for dosage adjustment and next lab work.
   4. Remind patients of next visit.
   5. Contact patient for missed appointments.
   6. Develop a telephone triage protocol, for example, abnormal lab values and adverse reactions.
   7. Train staff in telephone triage and how to identify and handle emergencies.
   8. Develop quality monitoring process for telephone triage.

I. Communication/documentation.
   1. Communicate, coordinate, and document plan of care as agreed upon by all team members.
   2. Develop or adapt an assessment tool for initiation, evaluation, and monitoring of therapy.
   3. Document all encounters.
   4. Document and communicate missed doses, appointments, lab results compliance, and/or psychosocial issues with the rest of the health care team.
   5. Call patients for missed appointments or contact via letter to reschedule.
   6. Make other arrangements for patients without telephone for continuity of care.

J. Outcome management: outcomes must be measurable and significant to the plan of care and clinic's mission.
   1. Timely recognition and management of over/under-anticoagulation.

2. Maintenance of lab values within stated parameters.
3. No evidence of drug interactions.

K. Protocol development/usage.
  1. Adhere to current practice and licensure standards.
  2. Individualized therapy based on clinical status.
     a. Usual initial loading dose is 5 mg (patients sensitive to warfarin may be started on a lower dose).
     b. Warfarin is taken in the evening.
     c. Dosage is adjusted by the nurse, based on PT/INR values and patient assessment, according to protocols or with direct consultation of the physician.

INCONTINENCE

Patricia A. Rutowski, MSN, RN, CS

Urinary incontinence (UI) is a "condition in which involuntary loss of urine is a social or hygienic problem and is objectively demonstrable" (Bates et al.,1979). The prevalence of UI in the United States in 1994 was 13 million people (AHCPR Guidelines, 1996). According to Wagner and Hu (1998) the societal cost of incontinence for individuals aged 65 and older was $26.3 billion, or $3565 per incontinent individual. This condition is a significant financial burden for individuals and for society.

Key to the management of UI is recognition that UI is a condition whose cause must be diagnosed before treatment. The most common types of UI are stress incontinence (SUI), urge incontinence, and a combination of SUI and urge incontinence symptoms known as mixed incontinence. The incidence of UI is more prevalent in females than males. More specifically, UI is more experienced by and diagnosed in females who have given birth more than four times, in hysterectomized women, the elderly, and men who have had a prostatectomy. The condition of UI can be treated. Symptoms can be eliminated or improved with behavioral treatment, including fluid management, habit training, timed voiding, pelvic muscle strengthening (Kegel exercises) and/or support devices (pessaries), medication, and surgery. A significant barrier to UI evaluation and treatment is the social stigma of UI. Patients are reluctant to discuss this problem with providers and UI is often overlooked in routine review of systems. Moreover, many providers are unaware of how to do primary care evaluation and initial behavioral treatment. Most often medication, rather than behavioral treatment, is the first treatment of choice in the primary and specialty settings. The lack of treatment for UI can lead to social isolation, financial burden for absorbent pads, other health care problems, and increased national cost of health care.

The U.S. Department of Health and Human Services through its Agency for Health Care Policy and Research (AHCPR) recognized the importance and the growth potential of the health problem of UI by publishing management guidelines in 1992 and 1996 (Fantl, Newman, and Collins, 1996). These guidelines were among the first group of researched, nationally published, health care guidelines for providers. The ANA hosted a task force of leading nurse experts in the field of incontinence. Subsequently, curriculum guidelines for all levels of nursing education and competencies were developed (Jirovec, Wyman, and Wells, 1998) (Box 20-2).

In the United States, nurses have run continence clinics since the 1980s. In Great Britain, the existence of the continence nurse specialist is even older. Continence nurses have a range of educational preparation. Many of these nurses are certified by nursing organizations that have a special interest in continence care. Sites for nurse-run continence clinics and services include ambulatory care, acute care hospitals, extended care facilities, nursing homes, and home care settings. Continence nurses also provide consultations to institutions, patients, and families. They

■ BOX 20-2
■ **EDUCATIONAL COMPETENCIES FOR CONTINENCE CARE: BASIC PREPARATION FOR BEGINNING PROFESSIONAL PRACTICE**

A professional nurse will be able to independently:
1. Obtain a focused health history to include:
   a. the presence of risk factors for urinary incontinence (UI) and medical conditions that may be contributing to UI and identifying patients at risk for the development of UI
   b. confirming the presence and effect of UI subjectively
   c. a detailed exploration of the symptoms of UI and associated factors including symptoms of leakage, frequency, urgency, and nocturia (failure to store); and retention and overflow (failure to empty)
   d. medication review including prescription and nonprescription drugs to identify those patients whose medications may negatively affect urine control
   e. bowel pattern to include frequency, consistency, and usage of any assistive products (e.g., dietary measures, prescription and nonprescription medications including suppositories and enemas)
   f. functional, environmental, social, and cognitive factors that may contribute to or result in UI
2. Obtain an intake and output record that includes:
   a. voiding records from patients that include time and onset of incontinent episodes, voiding pattern, 24-hour recording with diurnal and nocturnal frequency, amount voided, amount leaked, activity when leakage occurred, and presence of inadequate or excessive output
   b. intake record with 24-hour pattern of fluid intake that includes amount, frequency, and type of oral intake
3. Obtain diagnostic measures to detect evidence of urinary tract infection and other disorders contributing to incontinence that may include:
   a. urinalysis or the use of a chemically treated dipstick to detect hematuria, pyuria, bacteriuria, glycosuria, or proteinuria
   b. obtaining clean catch or catheterized urine specimen for culture and sensitivity
   c. obtaining catheterized urine specimen to detect amount of urine in bladder or post void residual (PVR) urine volume
4. Conduct a physical examination that includes:
   a. focused abdominal exam to estimate suprapubic fullness; to rule out palpable hard stool, and to evaluate bowel sounds

From Jirovec MM, Wyman JF, Wells TJ (1998): Addressing urinary incontinence with educational continence care. *Image J Nurs Sch* 30(4):375-378.

also participate in program development for communities and organizations (Jacobs, Wyman, Rowell, and Smith, 1998). Most often, but not always, nurse-run continence clinics provide behavioral treatment and medication evaluation services after a diagnosis of the cause and type of UI is made by a primary or specialty health care provider (Jacobs, et al., 1998).

Barriers to nursing continence care in all settings include a lack of understanding by physicians, administrators, payers, legislators, regulators, and consumers about treatment for incontinence, the competencies of professional nurses, and about nurse-run clinics. Medicare approved reimbursement to nurse practitioners and

---

■ BOX 20-2
■ **EDUCATIONAL COMPETENCIES FOR CONTINENCE CARE: BASIC PREPARATION FOR BEGINNING PROFESSIONAL PRACTICE—cont'd**

   b. examination of the genitals including skin integrity of perineum, appearance of urethral meatus, and presence of prolapse
   c. rectal exam including evaluation of sphincter tone, perineal sensation, and presence or absence of fecal impaction
   d. confirming the presence of UI objectively and evaluation of the force and character of urine stream during voiding with observation of actual toileting of client
   e. a functional assessment including mobility, self-care ability, cognitive ability (mental status exam), and communication patterns
5. Assess environment
6. Initiate nursing interventions that include:
   a. strategies that promote bladder health (fluid hydration, caffeine reduction, bowel programs, dietary strategies, weight reduction, smoking and alcohol reduction)
   b. educating and counseling patients and families (e.g., anatomy and physiology of genitourinary system, factors affecting continence, etiologic factors related to UI, treatment options available to patients who may benefit from scheduled voiding regimens without further testing)
   c. identifying patients who require further evaluation before therapeutic intervention; collaborating with physicians or advanced practice nurses regarding diagnosis, intervention plan, expected outcomes, and ongoing evaluation
   d. implementing scheduled toileting programs for functional incontinence and evaluating its effectiveness
   e. supervising nursing staff in the implementation of prompted voiding and scheduled toileting programs and evaluation of its effectiveness
   f. evaluating patients with indwelling catheter for voiding trial and initiation of bladder training
   g. teaching pelvic muscle exercises to patients at risk for developing stress incontinence
   h. implementing bladder training programs for early symptoms of stress or urgency
   i. implementing of scheduled toileting programs for patients at risk for developing functional incontinence before UI develops
   j. identifying patients who would benefit from assistive devices to maintain continence
   k. recommending appropriate containment devices and topical therapy for prevention and management of perineal skin breakdown

clinical nurse specialists in 1999 (Jacobs, et al., 1998). However, payment for behavioral procedures such as biofeedback remains an issue for all providers. The challenge is to educate the public about incontinence, its impact on the individual, society, and health care costs. Moreover, marketing nurses as primary, first line clinicians for UI treatment is an ongoing priority.

A. Assess/screen/triage.

   1. History (in addition to a routine review of systems) assessment should be made for:

     a. Risk factors.

       (1) Chronic disease, lung disease, strokes, neurologic disease such as multiple sclerosis, disseminated lupus erythematosus, Parkinson's disease, and spinal cord injury. Trauma to head, spinal column, or pelvis.

       (2) Kidney, bladder, vaginal, and vulvar disease/infections.

       (3) Constipation, diarrhea, and irritable bowel syndrome.

       (4) Fluid intake, type, amount and time of day, number and amount of voids, and if applicable, bowel movements (a voiding diary or record that is completed by the patient is used to collect this data).

     b. Current medications.

     c. Allergies: medications and/or environmental.

     d. Surgical history with special emphasis on reproductive and abdominal, neurologic, and prostatectomy surgery.

     e. Reproductive history with note of large babies and difficult deliveries.

     f. History of abuse: verbal, physical, and/or sexual (both male and female).

     g. Patient description of urine and/or fecal loss problem.

       (1) Onset: acute or chronic.

       (2) Duration.

       (3) Frequency.

       (4) Nocturia.

     h. Coping mechanisms that affect function: physical, social, and psychologic.

       (1) Wearing absorbent products/adaptation of clothing.

       (2) Frequent toileting.

       (3) Social withdrawal/decreased social networking.

       (4) Beliefs, knowledge, and need for UI education about incontinence, anger or acceptance because of age or indifferent attitude about improving symptoms.

         (a) Should be considered in the assessment and the plan of care.

         (b) Behavioral treatment requires patient and/or family or caregiver action, cooperation/motivation.

     i. Mobility and manual dexterity.

     j. Environment: bathroom facilities and accessibility, privacy.

    2. Physical assessment.

      a. Abdomen, including bowel sounds, suprapubic tenderness, and observable and/or palpable masses and organomegly.

      b. Skin integrity of the perineum, lower extremities, and abdomen and genitalia.

      c. Neurologic: sensory (speech, hearing, and eyesight), orientation and cognition, reflexes, gait, sensitivity to sharp and dull, and muscle strength.

      d. Pelvic: lymph nodes, external genitalia, vaginal and rectal tone and strength.

        (1) Observation of organ prolapse cystocele, uterine prolapse, rectocele, urethrocele, or enterocele.

        (2) Do a wet mount on women with suspected vaginitis. Observe for atrophic tissue in women.

        (3) Perform cough test.

          (a) Cough test done in the lithotomy or standing position.

          (b) Patient is asked to cough with a full bladder; this is intended to reproduce UI symptoms under stress.

      e. Rectal: sphincter tone, presence of stool, rectal mass, prostate.

      f. Skin.

        (1) Men: abnormalities of the foreskin and glans penis.

   3. Triage the following to primary care facility, urology medical specialty, or emergency room.

      a. Acute onset of dysuria, urinary frequency, hematuria, fever, and suprapubic pain (unless assessment and treatment is in the scope of practice of the nurse or management is included in the clinic protocols).

      b. Inability to urinate.

      c. Persistent hematuria.

      d. Failure to respond to first-line treatments.

B. Primary, secondary, tertiary prevention.

   1. Primary prevention.

      a. Assessment for pelvic muscle strength and patient awareness of the use and purpose of pelvic floor muscles (levator ani group).

        (1) This should be done digitally with routine pelvic exams.

        (2) Pelvic muscle strength should be documented and reviewed with the patient.

        (3) Women with weaker pelvic musculature, who are identified early and are taught strengthening exercise (Kegel's), may avoid UI later in life (Sampselle and Brink, 1990).

      b. Patient and public education regarding UI incidence, impact, assessment, and treatment.

   2. Secondary prevention.

      a. Pelvic muscle assessment and strengthening (Kegel's) before and after surgery for prostatectomy and bladder cancer.

      b. Prenatal and postpartum incontinence assessment, including the measurement of pelvic strength; anticipatory guidance about incontinence.

    3. Tertiary prevention.

      a. Behavioral treatment after UI type is diagnosed postpartum, post-prostatectomy, after spinal cord injury, stroke, or symptom development with chronic disease.

      b. Women who have had corrective surgery for symptomatic organ prolapse or hysterectomy may develop or have UI symptoms recur.

C. Clinical procedures.

    1. Urinalysis and culture and sensitivity (if indicated by abnormal UA).

    2. Bladder record or voiding diary.*

    3. Postvoid residual (PVR). This is done with catheterization or an ultrasound scanner. Depending on the limits of the protocol, refer patients with a PVR of 70-100 ml to urology.

    4. Urodynamic testing to assess bladder emptying, capacity, bladder wall compliance, and bladder sensation.

      a. Currently routine urodynamic testing is controversial.

      b. The AHCPR Guidelines (Fantl, Newman, and Collins, 1996) and research (Burgio, et al., 1998) support behavioral treatment of reversible UI as a safe and effective conservative intervention and as a first-line treatment for UI.

    5. Cytology for evaluation of malignancy with symptoms of persistent hematuria and bladder pain.

D. Collaboration/resource identification/referral.

    1. Most UI clinics have a collaborative agreement or relationship with a physician and other health professionals. This provides an opportunity to work as a member of a multidisciplinary team. Multidisciplinary teams are made up of:

      a. Primary care providers: physicians, nurse practitioners, nurse midwives.

      b. Nurse specialists: rehabilitation, women's health, men's health, enterostomal therapists, geriatrics.

      c. Urologists, urogynecologists, physical therapists.

    2. Referral: AHCPR Guidelines (Fantl et al.,1996) identify criteria for further evaluation.

      a. Uncertain diagnosis based on a lack of correlation between symptoms and clinical evaluation.

      b. Treatment failure, including a lack of patient satisfaction.

      c. Evaluation for surgical intervention.

      d. Persistent hematuria, persistent symptomatic urinary tract infection and pain.

---

*A prototype of a voiding diary can be found on page 147, Attachment B, of the AHCPR 1996 UI Guidelines.

    e. Other conditions, including suspicion of prostate cancer, pelvic prolapse, persistent difficult bladder emptying.

E. Care management.

  1. Behavioral management of incontinence, both urinary and fecal, is within the scope of practice for registered nurses.

  2. Managing medications for UI is within the scope of nursing practice.

    a. The scope of practice of the nurses managing behavioral UI treatment including medications depends on their education, the nursing practice act in the state in which they practice and

    b. The collaborative practice agreement developed with the supervising physician.

  3. The AHCPR UI guidelines call for behavioral therapy for incontinence before medication or surgery, except when critical health outcomes require surgery (Fantl, et al., 1996).

  4. Stress urinary incontinence (SUI).

    a. Definition: "urine loss coincident with an increase in intra-abdominal pressure, in the absence of a detrusor contraction or an over distended bladder" (Fantl et al., 1996, p. 16).

    b. Symptoms: leakage of urine with cough, laugh, exercise, lifting.

    c. Treatments.

      (1) Behavioral* (Bump, Hurt, Fantl, and Wyman, 1991).

        (a) Pelvic muscle strengthening exercises (Kegel's).

        (b) Surface EMG biofeedback.

        (c) Vaginal or anal biofeedback.

        (d) Electrical stimulation biofeedback.

        (e) Vaginal cones.

        (f) Fluid intake evaluation and management.

          (i) Done with the use/evaluation of the patient data from a completed voiding diary.

          (ii) Common findings on a bladder diary are high intake of caffeinated beverages, above or below average fluid intake, and use of alcohol and caffeine-containing beverages after 5 PM.

          (iii) Intake of these bladder irritants can cause urinary urgency and nocturia.

        (g) Bowel management.

          (i) Impaction relief.

          (ii) Management of irritable bowel syndrome.

          (iii) Management of constipation.

         (h) Bladder training.

      (2) Pessaries are devices placed in the vagina for women who have prolapse of the bladder, uterus, rectum, and/or vagina.

---

*Items a to d are directed toward increasing the strength and control of the pelvic floor muscles.

(3) Medications.
  (a) Estrogen, intravaginal
  (b) Alpha-adrenergic agonists increase tone of urethral sphincter. Common drugs: pseudoephedrine (e.g., Sudafed) and phenylpropanolamine. Side effects include elevated blood pressure and trouble sleeping.
  (c) Imipramine.
(4) Collagen implants.
(5) Surgery.
5. Urge UI and mixed UI.
  a. Definitions: *Urge UI* is involuntary loss of urine associated with a strong desire to void (AHCPR, 1996). *Mixed UI* is a combination of stress UI and urge UI.
  b. Symptoms: urgent desire to void, urinary frequency, nocturia.
  c. Treatments.
    (1) Behavioral.
      (a) Pelvic muscle strengthening (Burgio, et al., 1998). Often biofeedback in the form of electrical stimulation is successful.
      (b) Bladder training.
      (c) Visualization.
      (d) Relaxation.
    (2) Drug therapy.
      (a) Anticholinergic agents (e.g., oxybutynin [Ditropan]).
      (b) Drugs affecting the sympathetic and parasympathetic nervous system (e.g., imipramine).
      (c) Muscarinic antagonists (e.g., tolterodine [Detrol]).
      (d) Estrogenation of the vagina.
6. Overflow UI.
  a. Definition: "involuntary loss of urine associated with overdistention of the bladder" (Fantl, et al., 1996, p. 16).
  b. Symptoms.
    (1) Frequency.
    (2) Nocturia.
    (3) Passive dribbling.
    (4) Feeling of bladder pressure or fullness.
    (5) May have symptoms of urge and/or stress UI.
  c. Treatments.
    (1) Self-catheterization education (ISC).
    (2) Medication for men with benign prostate hypertrophy (BPH): alpha-blocker for urethral sphincter relaxation; phenoxybenzamine, finasteride (Proscar), doxazosin (Cardura), terazosin (Hytrin), tamsulosin (Flomax).
7. Functional/environmental UI: a diagnosis of exclusion, after evaluation has ruled out all other causes of UI.
  a. Definition: inability to reach toilet or remove clothes in time to void

in the toilet. This may be the result of impairment of physical or cognitive functioning, or both.
  b. Treatment.
    (1) Bedside commodes.
    (2) Male and female urinals.
    (3) Timed voiding, assisted.
F. Patient education.
  1. Anatomy, physiology, and pathophysiology of the genitourinary system.
  2. Factors affecting or contributing to incontinence, such as constipation; bladder irritants such as caffeine, alcohol, tobacco; and chronic disease, such as diabetes.
  3. Pelvic muscle exercises (PME).
    a. These exercises should be taught digitally (Bump, et al., 1991).
    b. Graduated program of exercise should be initiated based on the patient's current level of muscle strength and ability to identify the pelvic muscles.
    c. Written instructions should be given that include the number of PMEs to be done in a set and the number of sets per day.
    d. Endurance of contractions is also given (hold the contraction for 2 seconds, then rest for 4 seconds).
    e. If the patient is not able to develop pelvic muscle strength with digital training, biofeedback-assisted training can be used.
  4. Relaxation.
  5. Visualization.
G. Advocacy: many organizations exist that give the public and clinicians information and assistance. Several are listed below.
  1. National Association for Continence (NAFC), formerly Help for Incontinent People (HIP). This organization publishes a quarterly newsletter and an annual guide to UI products and resources. These are provided to all members.
(800) BLADDER
website: http://www.nafc.org
  2. The Simon Foundation for Continence
P.O. Box 835
Wilmette, IL 60091
(800) 23-SIMON
website: http://www.simonfoundation.org
  3. Agency for Health Care Policy and Research
(Urinary Incontinence in Adults Guideline Update Panel)
P.O. Box 8547
Silver Spring, MD 20907
(800) 358-9295
website: http://www.ahcpr.gov
H. Telephone practice.
  1. Evaluate progress toward outcomes.
  2. Screen for infection or other acute condition.

3. Screen for the need for referral (see referral section D, 2 on pp. 382-383).
I. Communication/documentation.
   1. Demographic information including age, sex, address.
   2. History and physical.
   3. Impression/diagnosis, including any nursing diagnoses that apply.
   4. Plan of care, including patient goals for the outcome of care.
   5. SOAP notes for each visit after the initial intake.
   6. Letter to referring clinician giving pertinent information, plan of care, and projected timeframe for continence clinic services.
J. Expected outcomes.
   1. Stress UI: decrease or eliminate urinary leakage as evidenced by decreasing use of pads, voiding diary records, or urodynamic studies.
   2. Urge UI and mixed UI: increase bladder capacity, less frequent voids, decrease in the use of pads as evidenced by voiding diary, urodynamic studies.
   3. Functional UI: decrease or eliminate in use of pads, decrease in wetting episodes as evidenced by patient records or reports of caregivers/patient.
   4. Patient satisfaction with care.
K. Protocol development/usage.
   1. Protocols are individually developed between supervising physicians, organizations, institutions, and the providers of UI care.
   2. They can be detailed or broad.
   3. Potential items for inclusion in protocols include:
      a. Medical history.
      b. Physical exam.
      c. Types and number of treatments for the types of incontinence.
      d. Laboratory testing.
      e. Urodynamic testing.
      f. Patient education.
      g. Use of home biofeedback units.
      h. Referral guidelines.
      i. Outcome review.

REFERENCES

Agency for Health Care Policy and Research (1992): *Pressure ulcers in adults: prediction and prevention*. Rockville, Md: US Department of Health and Human Services.

Bates-Jensen B (1998): Management of exudate and infection. In Sussman C, Bates-Jensen B, editors: *Wound care: a collaborative practice manual for physical therapists and nurses*. Gaithersburg, MD: Aspen, pp. 49-82.

Bates P, Bradley W, Glen E, et al. (1979): The standardization of terminology of lower urinary tract function. *J Urology* 121:551-554.

Bonham P (1999): Wound care specialty course. Unpublished manuscript, Medical University of South Carolina.

Brosnan J (1996): A patient-focused pathway for ambulatory anticoagulation care. *J Nurs Care Qual* 11(2):45.

Bump RC, Hurt WG, Fantl A, Wyman JF (1991): Assessment of Kegel pelvic muscle exercise performance after brief verbal instruction. *Am J Obstet Gynecol* 165(2):322-327.

Burgio KL, Locher JL, Goode PS, et al. (1998): Behavioral versus drug treatment for urge urinary incontinence in older women: a randomized controlled trial. *JAMA* 280(23):1995-2000.

Clemen-Stone S, McGuire S, Eigsti DL, editors (1998): *Comprehensive community health nursing: family, aggregate and community practice*, ed 5. St. Louis: Mosby.

Cooper D (1992): Wound assessment and evaluation of healing. In Bryant R, editor: *Acute and chronic wounds: nursing management.* St. Louis: Mosby, pp. 69-90.

Crumbley D (1997): Reflections of a certified wound care nurse. *J Wound Ostomy Continence Nurs* 24:189-190.

Crumbley D, Ice R, Cassidy R (1999): Nurse-managed wound clinic: a case study in success. *Nursing Case Management* 4:168-180.

Doughty D (1992): Principles of wound healing and wound management. In Bryant R, editor: *Acute and chronic wounds: nursing management.* St. Louis: Mosby, pp. 31-68.

Duke Coagulation Consult Service, Division of Hematology, Department of Medicine, Duke University Medical School (http: geryon.mc.duke.edu/coag/dukeccs.html), 29 November 1999.

Dupont Pharmaceuticals (1999): Coumadin tablets, Coumadin for injections (package insert). Wilmington, DE: Dupont Pharmacy.

Fantl JA, Newman DK, Collins J (1996): *Urinary incontinence in adults: acute and chronic mnagement.* Clinical practice guideline no. 2, 1996 Update. AHCPR Publication No. 96-0682. Rockville, MD: U.S. Department of Health and Human Services, Public Health Service, Agency for Health Care Policy and Research.

Frenn M, Lundeen S, Martin K, et al. (1996): Symposium on nursing centers: past, present and future. *J Nurs Educ* 35(2):55-62.

Frykberg R (1998): The team approach in diabetic foot management. *Adv Wound Care* 11:71-77.

Jacobs M, Wyman J, Rowell JP, Smith D (1998): Continence nurses: a survey of who they are and what they do. *Urol Nurs* 18(1):13-20.

Jaramillo O, Elizondo J, Jones P, et al. (1997): Practical guidelines for developing a hospital-based wound and ostomy clinic. *Ostomy/Wound Management* 43:28-39.

Jeter K, Faller N, Norton C (1990): *Nursing for continence.* Philadelphia: WB Saunders.

Jirovec MM, Wyman JF, Wells TJ (1998): Addressing urinary incontinence with educational continence-care. *Image J Nurs Sch* 30(4):375-378.

Konstantinides N (1992): Principles of nutritional support. In Bryant R, editor: *Acute and chronic wounds: nursing management.* St. Louis: Mosby, pp. 288-300.

Marine JE, Goldhaber SZ (1998): Controversies surrounding long-term anticoagulation of very elderly patient in arterial fibrillation. *Am Coll Chest Physician* 113(4):1115-1118.

Physician's Desk Reference, ed 53 (1999): *Coumadin tablets, Coumadin injections.* Montvale, NJ: Medical Economics Co.

Raimer F, Thomas M, Lake C, (1995): Clot stoppers using anticoagulants safely and effectively. *Nursing* 95:36-38.

Reiber G, Boyko E, Smith D (1995): *Diabetes in America,* ed 2. Bethesda, MD: National Institutes of Health.

Sampselle CM, Brink CA (1990): Pelvic muscle relaxation: assessment and management. *J Nurse-Midwifery* 35(3):127-132.

Spandorfer JM, Merli GJ (1996): Outpatient anticoagulation issues for the primary care physician. *Managed Care Office Practice* 80(2):475-487.

Steed D, Edington H, Moosa H, Webster M (1993): Organization and development of a university multidisciplinary wound care clinic. *Surgery* 114:775-779.

Sussman C (1998): Assessment of the skin and wound. In Sussman C, Bates-Jensen B, editors:

Wound care: a collaborative practice manual for physical therapists and nurses. Gaithersburg, MD: Aspen, pp. 49-82.

Sussman G (1998): Management of the wound environment. In Sussman C, Bates-Jensen B, editors: *Wound care: a collaborative practice manual for physical therapists and nurses.* Gaithersburg, MD: Aspen, pp. 49-82.

Wagner TH, Hu TW (1998): Economic costs of urinary incontinence in 1995. *Urology* 51(3):355-361.

Wound Ostomy and Continence Nurses Society (1992): *Standards of care patient with dermal wounds: pressure ulcers.* Costa Mesa, CA: Wound Ostomy and Continence Nurses Society.

Wound Ostomy and Continence Nurses Society (1993): *Standards of care patient with dermal wounds: lower extremity ulcers.* Costa Mesa, CA: Wound Ostomy and Continence Nurses Society.

Wysocki A, Bryant R (1992): Skin. In Bryant R, editor: *Acute and chronic wounds: nursing management.* St. Louis: Mosby, pp. 1-30.

ADDITIONAL RESOURCE

Additional information regarding standards of practice, practice guidelines, and wound care courses and schools are available from the Wound Ostomy and Continence Nurses Society at http://www.wocn.org/

21 Telehealth Nursing Practice

MAUREEN ESPENSEN, BSN, RN

OBJECTIVES

Study of the information presented in this chapter will enable the learner to:

1. Define telehealth nursing practice and understand its origin, purpose, and role as a dimension of ambulatory clinical practice.

2. Identify the framework and parameters for the practice of telehealth nursing.

3. Discuss the use of protocols, guidelines, and algorithms for assessing and triaging patients.

4. Describe the fundamentals of telehealth nursing practice, professional competencies, and professional practice.

5. Discuss the scope of practice for telehealth nursing.

6. Describe unique communication, assessment, and documentation applications.

7. Recognize nursing intervention classifications (NIC) and nursing outcome classifications (NOC) for telehealth nursing.

8. Recognize the need for population assessment prior to implementation of a telehealth nursing program.

9. Identify practice issues affecting the safe practice of telehealth nursing.

■
■■ In this chapter, telehealth nursing in ambulatory practice is described. Information is presented on the telehealth nursing framework and parameters for practice. Significant issues affecting practice are described and information is presented on this growing nursing subspecialty.

    A. Definition of telehealth nursing practice.
        1. The proposed definition of telehealth nursing practice is "nursing practice using the nursing process to provide care for individual patients or defined patient populations over a telecommunication device" (American Academy of Ambulatory Care Nursing [AAACN], 2001a).
    B. Definition of telephone triage.
        1. Telephone triage: identifying the order of patient needs according to urgency and appropriate disposition (AAACN, 1997).
        2. Telephone triage is one of several activities used in telehealth nursing practice.

C. Terminology differences of telephone and telehealth.
1. The use of the word *telephone* limits nursing practice to the traditional telephone.
2. Today's technologies employed by consumers and patients include the telephone, e-mail, Internet, facsimile, telephone device for deaf (TTD/TTY), and telemedicine.
3. The use of the word *telehealth* expands nursing practice to include the telecommunication technologies just mentioned.
D. Defined criteria for telehealth nursing practice includes:
1. Using protocols, algorithms, or guidelines to systematically assess and address patient needs.
2. Prioritizing the urgency of patient needs.
3. Telehealth nursing practice includes assessment, triage, documentation, education, prioritization, collaboration, and evaluation.
4. Developing a collaborative plan of care with patients and their support systems. The plan of care may include:
   a. Wellness promotion.
   b. Prevention education.
   c. Advice and care counseling.
   d. Disease management.
   e. Care coordination.
5. Evaluating outcomes of practice and care (AAACN, 1997).
E. Purpose and benefits of telehealth nursing.
1. Telehealth nursing practice is an extension of the clinical setting with its own set of assessment, communication, documentation, and evaluation techniques. The purpose and benefits include:
   a. Patient advocacy.
   b. Provider support.
   c. Enhancement of care delivery such as decreasing inappropriate emergency department and provider visits.
   d. Increased patient satisfaction by providing another dimension to care access.
   e. Management of scarce resources by enhancing patient flow and provider efficiencies (Matherly and Hodges, 1992).
F. Origins of telephone nursing practice.
1. An often repeated story is that the first telehealth interaction occurred during a telephone call by Alexander Graham Bell. He was calling for Mr. Watson, his assistant, to come and help him with an injury to his hand.
2. In the last half of the 1970s, Kaiser-Permanente health organization began using a system of telephone triage as a means for patients to access care (McKesson-HBOC, 1997).
3. Beginning in the early 1980s ASK-A-NURSE® types of marketing programs were developed and sold to hospitals to attract callers for the purpose of physician referral (McKesson-HBOC, 1997).

4. The rise of health maintenance organizations (HMOs) has increased the use of telecommunication for:
   a. Demand management of patient's access to care including triage, health information, and decision support.
   b. Medical management support for precertification and referral authorization.
   c. Customer services including benefits, eligibility, and provider relations.
   d. Member services including enrollment, health risk appraisals, primary care provider selection (Briggs, 2000).
5. Hospital-based delivery systems have embraced telehealth services to support multiple functions including:
   a. Marketing hospital services and physicians and registering callers for classes/seminars.
   b. Providing traditional physician answering services enhanced by nurse triage.
   c. Supporting activities to manage financial and clinical risk in capitated populations.

G. Telehealth nursing practice today.
   1. Recognized as a nursing subspecialty by AAACN and American Nurses' Association (ANA).
   2. *Telephone Nursing Standards of Practice* developed in 1997 by AAACN. Revised in 2001 to *Telehealth Nursing Standards of Practice*.

H. Practice settings for telehealth nursing.
   1. Primarily associated with ambulatory care settings.
   2. Single provider/practice office and multispecialty clinics.
   3. Hospital emergency departments.
   4. Organized hospital-based call centers.
   5. Health maintenance organization (HMO) settings.
   6. National call centers for health care organizations or consumer service bureaus.
   7. Anywhere there is a telecommunication device through which the patient may communicate with the nurse (Briggs, 2000).

FRAMEWORK AND PARAMETERS FOR TELEHEALTH NURSING PRACTICE

Standards provide the framework and parameters that define the scope of practice for telehealth nursing practice and the functions within the ambulatory care setting. "Nursing standards are a written value statement that defines a level of performance or a set of conditions determined to be acceptable by some authority" (Marker, 1988).

A. Purposes of standards.
   1. Formalizes practice information for easy reference.
   2. Defines acceptable levels of performance, patient care, and system operations.

    3. Provides definition of nursing care and impediments to care.

    4. Delineates professional accountability.

  B. Standards applicable for telehealth nursing.

    1. Legal standards such as state nurse practice act.

      a. Each state nurse practice act defines the function and scope of practice.

      b. The professional nurse is responsible for knowing the state nurse practice act.

    2. Professional standards.

      a. Developed by professional organizations such as the ANA and the AAACN.

      b. Specific standards applicable to telehealth and telephone nursing. AAACN Telephone Nursing Administration and Practice Standards (1997).

      c. General standards applicable to telephone nursing: American Association of Office Nurses (AAON), *Office Nursing Practice Standards for Quality Care of Patients* (1996).

      d. Position statement applicable for telephone nursing: Emergency Nurse Association (ENA), *Position Statement Telephone Advice,* developed in 1991, revised in 1996 (ENA, 1991; 1996).

    3. Regulatory standards.

      a. Developed by local and state health departments.

      b. Developed by national organizations such as:

        (1) Joint Commission for Accreditation of Healthcare Organizations (JCAHO, 1998).

        (2) American Accreditation Healthcare Commission/URAC (2000) have developed "24 Hour Telephone Triage and Health Information Standards" for managed care telephone triage settings.

    4. Organizational standards.

      a. Defines performance expectations for the telehealth practice nurse within the organizational structure.

      b. Organizational standards include:

        (1) Policies.

        (2) Job descriptions.

        (3) Performance standards.

        (4) Standards of care.

        (5) Protocols, guidelines, and algorithms (Marker, 1988).

PROTOCOLS, GUIDELINES, ALGORITHMS

Protocols, guidelines, and algorithms are used for assessing and triaging patients, along with critical thinking and judgment. Throughout this chapter, the global term *guideline* is succinctly used to describe protocols, algorithms, and guidelines.

  A. Definitions of protocols, algorithms, and guidelines.

    1. Protocols: "Often used interchangeably with Algorithm and Guideline.

Defines the ongoing care or management of a broad problem or issue in six areas:

    a. Assessment/data collection/caller interview process.

    b. Classification/determination of acuity.

    c. Nature/type/degree of advice/intervention/direction to callers.

    d. Information/education of callers.

    e. Validation of patient understanding/verbal contracting.

    f. Evaluation/follow-up/effectiveness of advice or intervention.

A protocol directs the advice/triage/education/counseling process, assisting in the organization of large amounts of significant information in priority order. It helps show the interrelationship of data, forcing consideration of all possible or likely decision choices. It directs decision making to be based upon data" (AAACN, 1997, p. 25).

    2. Algorithms: "Written clinical questions using a branch chain logic (flow chart). Algorithms prescribe what steps to take given particular circumstances or characteristics. Some algorithms also include designed points in the decision-making process where physicians and other caregivers need to discuss with patients or families their preferences for particular options. Algorithms rely on nurses' ability to analyze and interpret patient responses to clinical questions" (AAACN, 1997, p. 24).

    3. Guideline: "Guideline is sometimes seen to be a more narrative description of assessment steps that includes education and counseling text to support nurses during calls" (AAACN, 1997, p. 25).

        a. A vehicle that directs the nurse to individualize a plan of care to meet the needs of the customer. Guidelines provide flexibility and allow for modification of nursing practice (McGear and Simms, 1998).

        b. "Guidelines structure the use of the nursing process, are symptom-based, include disposition criteria, home care advice with education and counseling text designed to support nurses" (McKesson-HBOC, 1997).

B. Common ambulatory care situations requiring protocols, guidelines, algorithms.

    1. Telephone triage, counseling, and education.

    2. Case management.

    3. Ambulatory procedures (e.g., ocular examinations, auditory evaluation, glucose tolerance testing).

    4. Anticipatory guidance sessions with parents.

    5. Preoperative preparations.

    6. Posthospitalization follow-up.

C. Contents of protocols, guidelines, and algorithms.

    1. Symptom based. Do not medically diagnose (e.g., a guideline for extremity injury, not sprained ankle).

    2. Description of the guideline and symptoms that are included in this guideline.

3. Symptom discussion that describes symptoms in this guideline.
4. Triage categories or acuity levels that classify the urgency of symptoms (e.g., emergent, urgent, non-urgent, and so forth).
5. Warning signs that describe symptoms to watch for and when to seek care if these symptoms occur.
6. Disposition information that describes the disposition of care, such as:
   a. Emergent: 911 or send to the emergency department immediately.
   b. Urgent: seek medical care within the next few hours.
7. Home care measures that provide detailed information on first aid, home care, or health improvements for symptoms.
8. Reference list for more information or references that were used to develop the guideline.

D. Purpose and benefits of using guidelines for assessment and triaging of patients.
   1. Meets goal of providing safe, effective, appropriate care and disposition of patient.
   2. Provides standardization of care.
   3. Provides structure in nurse performance.
   4. Decreases common practice errors such as omission of assessment steps.
   5. Ensures documentation ease, efficiency, and retrievability.
   6. Increases consistent, quality care and nursing performance.
   7. Increases legal protection.
   8. Meets accreditation standards.
   9. Enhances evaluation of performance.

E. Factors influencing guideline depth and scope.
   1. Community standards for medical care.
   2. Advances in medical technology.
   3. Practice settings: physician's office or large formalized managed care call center.
   4. Changing philosophy of care: depth of assessment and care provided by telephone.
   5. Increasing knowledge of the telehealth practice profession.

F. Perceived disadvantages of using guidelines for assessment and triaging of patients.
   1. For professional registered nurse.
      a. Nursing judgment used must stay within the framework of the guidelines.
      b. Requires in-depth training and experience to become proficient.
      c. Patient interaction is more structured.
      d. Assessment is limited to single sense gathering of information.
   2. For physician or provider.
      a. Less individualized triaging because of using triage indicators.
      b. Perceived loss of control for each patient's plan of care.
      c. Conflict in allowing professional registered nurse empowerment in assessment and triage decisions.
   3. For management.

        a. Concern of guidelines being expensive to develop, maintain, or purchase.

G. Guideline characteristics.

    1. Comprehensive enough to include a vast majority of symptoms for the telehealth population.

    2. Current for practice setting and standards of care.

    3. Reviewed and approved by medical director and physician specialists.

    4. User-friendly, easy to read and understand.

    5. Revisable for specific population needs.

H. Guideline development considerations.

    1. Should follow a standardized developmental framework.

    2. Created in "sets" based on body systems and correlated to population groups.

    3. Generic enough to include a broad range of secondary symptoms.

    4. Developed by nurses with telehealth nursing experience.

        a. Focused on the unique assessment process for telehealth nursing.

        b. Awareness that patients must be triaged to "right place, right time, right care."

    5. Created collaboratively with nurses and physician specialists.

    6. Process to develop guidelines is labor-intensive: usually 8 to 10 hours for a practice group to develop one guideline.

FUNDAMENTALS OF TELEPHONE PRACTICE

A. Systematically assessing and addressing patient needs with protocols, algorithms, or guidelines.

B. Prioritizing the urgency of patient needs (triaging).

C. Educating and communicating with patients using telecommunication devices.

D. Developing a collaborative plan of care with patients, their support systems, and providers of health care.

E. Documenting the telecommunication interaction.

F. Understanding technical issues regarding telecommunication.

G. Demonstrating knowledge of legal issues specific to telehealth nursing.

H. Evaluating outcomes of practice and quality measurements.

I. Maintaining confidentiality (AAACN, 1997).

SCOPE OF PRACTICE FOR TELEPHONE NURSING

The scope of practice for telehealth nursing demonstrates the professionalism of practice and includes a broad variety of nursing functions.

A. Scope of practice.

    1. Triage and disposition: assessment is performed through a telecommunication device instead of physically seeing and touching the patient.

    2. Guidance: direction and supervision of the patient with the patient or significant other acting as the care assessor and care provider.

3. Education: instructing and providing information to the patient on care issues.
4. Counseling: conferring with the patient on these plans and creating plans of care.
5. Coordination: using other health care resources and providing referrals and dispositions to appropriate levels of care.
6. Evaluating patient understanding and ability to participate in plans of care.

B. Includes using the nursing process of assessment, planning, implementation, and evaluation during telehealth interactions.
   1. Assessment.
      a. The reason for the call or patient's chief complaint.
      b. History of symptoms and associated symptoms.
      c. Allergies and medical history.
      d. Comprehensive assessment of the patient.
   2. Analysis.
      a. The clinical guidelines, protocols, or algorithms used and triage category (e.g., emergent, urgent, non-urgent, etc).
   3. Planning.
      a. The disposition of the patient based on acuity of symptoms (e.g., 911, emergency department, walk-in clinic).
      b. Any recommendations for further care, referrals or teaching (e.g., referral made to diabetes educator).
   4. Intervention.
      a. The nurse's intervention (e.g., transferring calls to 911, coordination of provider appointment).
      b. Information and education provided (e.g., providing home care measures for symptoms).
      c. Documentation of nursing process.
   5. Evaluation.
      a. Patient's acceptance and understanding of the plan of care (e.g., agrees to try home care and call back in 1 day if no improvement).
      b. Follow-up actions and plans of the nurse (e.g., prescription telephoned to pharmacy; patient will call back tomorrow to report status).
      c. The plan of the patient (e.g., patient agrees to appointment; will have husband drive her).

PROFESSIONAL COMPETENCIES AND PROFESSIONAL DEVELOPMENT

Telehealth nurses must demonstrate professional nursing competencies as well as ongoing knowledge enhancement and skill development. The competencies should be measurable and include:

A. Performance criteria in:
   1. Clinical knowledge for populations served.

2. Age-specific competencies.
3. Assessment skills for telephone and other telecommunication devices employed in setting.
4. Communication skills including effective listening, assertiveness, negotiation, and counseling.
5. Critical thinking and decision-making.
6. Educational/teaching effectiveness.
7. Demonstration of excellent customer service skills.
8. Knowledge and use of internal and external resources.
9. Effective use of current documented protocols or guidelines.
10. Accurate and expedient documentation.
11. Documented use of the nursing process.
12. Demonstration of effective use of computers, telephones, fax machines, etc. (AAACN, 1997).

B. Registered nurse knowledge experience criteria.
 1. Clinical knowledge required for critical decisions.
 2. Clinical nursing experience.
  a. Minimum of 3 years of applicable clinical nursing experience is the industry average before employment in a telephone nursing position.

C. Professional development.
 1. Ongoing enhancement of own clinical, telehealth, technical, medical-legal knowledge.
  a. Core education is included in the telehealth nursing practice core curriculum of the AAACN (2001b). Release date: 2001.
  b. Requirements to take telephone nursing practice certification examination include 2 years of experience in telephone nursing, which comprises a minimum of 2000 hours (Jerabeck, 2000).
 2. Researching and defining practice as further concepts in medical management are developed including personal health management, disease management, quality management, and outcome management.
 3. Remaining abreast of telehealth changes and recommending improvements for practice.
 4. Designing and shaping telehealth nursing for the future by demonstrating professional clinical knowledge, critical thinking, and judgment.

TELEHEALTH NURSING INTERVENTIONS AND OUTCOMES

Telehealth nursing includes nursing interventions "based upon clinical judgment and knowledge, that a nurse performs to enhance patient/client outcomes" (McCloskey and Bulechek, 2000).

A. Approved nursing intervention classifications (NIC) for telephone nursing (McCloskey and Bulechek, 2000).
 1. Telephone consultation.
  a. Definition: "Eliciting patients' concerns, listening and providing support, information, or teaching in response to patient's stated concerns, over the telephone" (McCloskey and Bulechek, 2000, p. 659).

    b. Activity examples: identify self with name and credentials, inform patient about call process, establish level of caller's knowledge, provide means of overcoming identified barriers to learning.

  2. Triage: telephone.

    a. Definition: "Determining the nature and urgency of a problem(s) and providing directions for the level of care required, over the telephone." (McCloskey and Bulechek, 2000, p. 675).

    b. Activity examples: direct, facilitate and calm caller, prioritize reported symptoms, use standardized symptom-based guidelines, maintain confidentiality, discuss and resolve problems with collegial help.

  3. Telephone follow-up.

    a. Definition: "Providing results of testing or evaluating patients' response and determining potential for problems as a result of previous treatment examination, or testing, over the telephone" (McCloskey and Bulechek, 2000, p. 661).

    b. Activity examples: obtain consent to disclose test results to non-patient, provide information on community resources, document education provided and resultant self-care responsibilities.

  4. Surveillance: remote electronic.

    a. Definition: "Purposeful and ongoing acquisition of patient data via electronic modalities (telephone, video conference, e-mail) from distant locations, as well as interpretation and synthesis of patient data for clinical decision making with individuals or population" (McCloskey and Bulecheck, 2000, p. 663).

    b. Activity examples: determine patient's health risk(s), identify data with problematic or population implications, monitor data for validity and reliability, monitor patient coping strategies.

B. Nursing outcome classifications (NOC) that can be linked for telephone nursing. A detailed description of the NIC/NOC system for telephone nursing is available in the *Nursing Interventions Classification,* 2000.

  1. Telephone consultation, examples of NOCs: acceptance: health status, anxiety control, caregiver outcomes, compliance behavior, information processing.

  2. Triage: telephone, examples of NOCs: decision making, self-care outcomes, suicide self-restraint.

  3. Telephone follow-up, examples of NOCs: coping, participation: health care decisions, well-being.

  4. Telephone surveillance, examples of NOCs: risk control, risk detection (Haas and Androwich, 1999).

TELEHEALTH ASSESSMENT

Registered nurses do not medically diagnose but assess patients and make critical decisions on care. The assessment of patients through telecommunication devices is unique because the locus of assessment changes.

A. The nurse must guide and not "lead the patient on" in assessing symptoms.
    1. There must be clear delineation between the patient being an active participant in assessment and the patient self-diagnosing.
B. The locus of care is not physically with the nurse. The patient/caregiver is the provider of care.
C. The locus of assessment shifts to the patient.
    1. The nurse becomes the listener, interpreter, teacher, and coach for the assessment.
    2. The patient is an active partner in the assessment and is the primary assessor (e.g., the patient must actively determine and point to the pain site and then put into words where the pain is located).
    3. The locus of assessment may not even be with the patient, but with the caller/caregiver who assesses the patient.
        a. The caregiver becomes the eyes and ears for the nurse.
        b. The nurse directs the caregiver to describe what they see and observe.
D. The telecommunication encounter is time-limited.
    1. Must be focused and limited to moving the caller to the next best step or level of intervention.
    2. The nurse cannot meet each and every need of the caller but must focus on the most important needs for this encounter.
    3. Extensive needs of a caller/patient may indicate that an in-person assessment is required (Dahl, personal correspondence).

TELEHEALTH COMMUNICATION

The primary telehealth assessment tool is the interaction with the patient or caregiver. Interactions are brief with communication techniques focusing on obtaining detailed information without the use of tactile or visual senses.
A. The nurse directs the caller to examine self or the patient.
    1. Using techniques provided by nurse.
    2. Interpreting the caller's description of symptoms, location, appearance of notable features is done by the nurse.
B. The nurse must establish trust immediately in order to elicit accurate information.
    1. Identifying self to caller with name and title.
    2. Identifying the patient by name and, if the patient is not the caller, the relationship to the caller.
    3. Identifying the patient's relationship to the provider (established patient or new patient).
C. The nurse demonstrates expert communication skills including:
    1. Asking open-ended questions.
    2. Using active listening techniques.
    3. Understanding the reason for call.
    4. Identifying any hidden agendas for the call (e.g., exploring why the patient is really calling and what does the patient want to achieve/obtain with the interaction).

5. Repeating and clarifying the caller's statements in order to understand their descriptions.
6. Asking the caller to quantify and qualify symptoms by using pain scales, using common sizes (e.g., pea size, quarter size).
7. Avoiding ambiguities, vague terms, and in-depth medical terminology.

D. The nurse is alert for a caller's self-diagnosis and/or bias toward treatment.
1. Hearing the caller describe multiple symptoms.
2. Sorting and prioritizing these symptoms.
3. Identifying primary symptoms and secondary symptoms.

E. The nurse maintains confidentiality of interactions.
1. Patient interactions take place in a private environment away from other patients, visitors, and inappropriate personnel.
2. Disclosure statements are signed by patients before information is provided to family members.
3. Records of calls are safeguarded against breach in confidentiality.

TELEHEALTH DOCUMENTATION

The purpose of documenting the telehealth encounter includes medical, administrative, financial, and legal/regulatory issues. The telehealth practice nurse must recognize the truth of the old adage, "if it wasn't documented, it wasn't done."

A. Documentation purposes.
1. Clinical.
   a. Is the basis for planning and maintaining continuity of care.
   b. A means to communicate vital patient information to health care providers.
   c. Shows the clinical decision-making process.
2. Administrative/financial.
   a. Assist in maximizing reimbursement.
   b. Provides information for monitoring of care and evaluation of quality.
3. Legal/regulatory.
   a. Shows evidence of whether care was rendered.
   b. Shows if a legal standard of care was met.
   c. Demonstrates patient care, patient understanding, and events.

B. Specific documentation policies for telehealth encounters.
1. Assessment and triaging of symptoms.
2. Providing of medical information or education.
3. Requests for prescriptions.
4. Over-the-counter dosages of medications.
5. Providing test results.
6. Care coordination issues.
7. Follow-up interactions and outbound calls.
8. Any other type of conversation or telecommunications with patients should also be documented.

C. Documentation of telecommunication encounters need to include the:
1. Patient and record identifiers.
   a. Date and time of call/contact.

b. Patient name, birthdate, and specific identifier (medical record number).

c. Caller name and relationship to patient.

d. The signature of all personnel handling the contact or initials if a signature page is used.

2. Reason for the call. Use quotations from patient if possible.

3. Complete assessment of symptoms.

    a. Primary and secondary symptoms, characteristics, onset, location, aggravated by (foods, medications, positions), relieved by/improved with, time duration, intensity (pain scale).

    b. Clinical guideline/protocol used for assessment and triage category.

    c. Comfort measures/home care provided.

4. Allergies, current medications, medical history.

5. Information and education provided.

    a. Specific education provided (e.g., the incubation period of chickenpox).

    b. Reference material for education (e.g., reference books with book name and page number. Standing orders).

6. Disposition of patient; referrals provided or offered.

7. Disclaimers given to the patient (e.g., "Call back if symptoms worsen, change, or persist. Call back anytime.")

8. Patient's/caller's understanding of care, plan of action, any refusals from patients and nurse's rebuttal to refusal.

9. Reference source used for care coordination issues. Administrative standards of care, physician standing orders.

10. Interventions completed (e.g., "prescription phoned in to . . . ").

11. Follow-up calls. Additional data to document.

    a. Date and time of every follow-up attempt.

    b. Date and time of completed call.

    c. Summary of follow-up conversation.

    d. Patient's understanding of plan of care.

D. Documentation methods and formats.

1. Documentation methods.

    a. Narrative: story-like, free flowing according to caller's response and interviewer's style.

    b. SOAP (Subjective, Objective, Assessment, Plan of Care).

    c. Documentation by exception/inclusion.

2. Documentation formats.

    a. Standardized forms with boxes or trigger questions to cue the nurse to gather specific information.

    b. Computerized systems with software embedded documentation fields.

OPTIMAL TELEPHONE NURSING SERVICES

Each practice setting has unique services and patient populations. It is important to identify the demand for telephone nursing care in order to provide optimal services.

A. Identify the demands and needs for telehealth care.
   1. What patient populations are contacting the service/provider.
   2. Why patients are calling.
   3. What do the patients want from the service and their expectations for telephone care (e.g., are patients calling for symptom assessment, clarification of instructions, reinforcement of education, prescriptions).
B. Identify the specific population being served.
   1. Special needs (e.g., elderly patients, oncology patients, indigent populations).
   2. Cultural issues (e.g., language barriers).
C. Identify the prioritization of call handling.
   1. Systematically sort calls and develop internal triaging so that:
      a. Symptom calls are prioritized by acuity and handled before non-symptom/general calls.
      b. Non-registered nurses are not assessing or triaging patients.
      c. All personnel recognize emergency calls and notify appropriate personnel to handle the call immediately.
   2. Efficiently and effectively answer and return call with notification systems.
D. Analyze telephone call volumes.
   1. Identify peak call days and times.
   2. Identify the "waiting time" for answering the initial call.
   3. Identify the "holding time" after answering the call.
   4. Develop staffing models to meet the call demand.
   5. Identify reasons for abandoned calls.
   6. Identify inappropriate messaging.
E. Create methods to decrease call volume and call demand.
   1. Develop educational brochures for patients on care of illnesses.
   2. Provide ambulatory patients with written discharge instructions.
   3. Provide descriptors of when to call/how to call/how to request a refill.

TELEHEALTH PRACTICE ISSUES

Telehealth practices may vary according to their setting and purpose of service. However, global issues for both formal and informal setting include:

A. Licensure issues to address.
   1. State-to-state nursing practice acts differ in the level of independence of assessment, triaging, and scope of practice.
   2. Communicating with patients resident outside of the state(s) where the nurse is employed may be a violation of a state's nurse practice act.
      a. Mutual recognition model: National Council of State Boards of Nursing (NCSBN) is recommending a mutual recognition model similar to driver's license.
      b. The mutual recognition model is a compact such that:
         (1) Each state is responsible for licensing its registered nurses and determining their scope of practice.

      (2) Each state that has the mutual recognition compact signed into law recognizes the license of the nurse from another state that has the mutual recognition compact.

      (3) The model covers both traditional nursing care and telehealth nursing care. Described in the literature as "interstate compact" or "mutual recognition model" (Haas, 1999).

B. Professional issues to address.

  1. Job descriptions must include:

    a. Detailed and defined scope of responsibilities and minimum qualifications.

    b. Accountability for actions and outcomes of telecommunications.

    c. Chain of authority.

  2. Formal training and education must include:

    a. Detailed orientation to telehealth nursing. Industry average is 2 to 4 weeks full time.

    b. Ongoing competency measurements.

    c. Quality improvement program on assessment, communication, and documentation skills for each employed nurse.

  3. Administrative issues to address with specific policies.

    a. Patient confidentiality and privacy during telehealth interactions.

    b. Callers not affiliated with the provider (non-patients) seeking symptom assessment, triaging, and health information.

    c. Language barriers and provision of interpretive services.

    d. Caregivers calling for patients.

    e. Chronic callers and repetitive callers.

    f. Calls from minors, elderly, and pregnant women.

    g. Third party callers when the patient is not present with caller.

    h. Dissatisfied callers.

  4. Practice issues to address.

    a. Issue: providing advice instead of information and education.

      (1) Patient may misinterpret that the nurse is telling him/her what to do.

      (2) Misrepresents the nurse as the director of care.

      (3) Solution: if the nurse provides information and education instead of advice the patient perceives herself/himself as holding final responsibility for care decision and action.

    b. Issue: providing personal opinions.

      (1) Legal risks are increased when standards of practice, protocols, and guidelines are not used for assessment and care.

      (2) Decreases professionalism of interaction.

      (3) Solution: nurse should verbalize the use of protocols, algorithms, and guidelines (e.g., "According to my guideline for diarrhea . . . ").

    c. Issue: providing a diagnosis (e.g., "Sounds like you have chickenpox").

      (1) Portrays the practicing of medicine without a license.

(2) Solution: nurse should always give a disclosure (e.g., "I am a registered nurse, in order to be diagnosed ____").

   d. Issue: lack of thorough assessment.

     (1) Prematurely triages the disposition of patient.

     (2) May be the result of personal knowledge about the patient and assuming the symptoms and history.

     (3) Solution: judiciously complete assessment steps and use guidelines.

   e. Issue: improper use of guidelines.

     (1) Relying on memory instead of using or reading guidelines.

     (2) Essential assessment questions cannot be skipped.

     (3) Solution: nurse should be diligent in use of guidelines.

   f. Issue: not documenting each call.

     (1) There is no documented proof that care was rendered.

     (2) Solution: nurse must follow administrative policies on documentation.

   g. Issue: promising interventions and outcomes (e.g., "I promise that the doctor will call you this morning").

     (1) Places patient at risk: patient symptoms may worsen and he/she simply waits for the return call.

     (2) With broken promises, a negative perception occurs.

     (3) Solution: nurse should provide reasonable expectations for patients and validate their understanding of plan.

REFERENCES

American Academy of Ambulatory Care Nursing (AAACN) (1997): *Telephone nursing practice administration and practice standards.* Philadelphia: Author.

AAACN (2001a): *Telehealth nursing practice administration and practice standards.* Manuscript submitted for publication.

AAACN (2001b): *Telephone nursing practice core curriculum.* Manuscript submitted for publication.

American Accreditation Healthcare Commission/URAC (2000): *24-hour telephone triage and health information standards.* Washington, DC, Website: www.urac.org

Briggs J (2000): The call center and its impact on health care. In Rosenthal B, editor: *Directory of medical call centers.* New York: Faulkner & Gray, pp. 33-45.

Emergency Nurses Association (ENA) (1991): Position statement: telephone advice. *J Emerg Nurs* 17(5):52A.

ENA (1996): *Position statement telephone advice.* Parkridge, IL: Bulletin. Available: www.ENA.org

Haas S (2000): Update on multistate licensure. *AAACN Viewpoint* 22(1):3-4.

Haas S, Androwich I (1999): Telephone consultation. In Bulechek G, McCloskey J, editors: *Nursing interventions: effective nursing treatments,* ed 3. Philadelphia: WB Saunders, pp. 670-684.

Jerabeck E (2000): Test sites, dates, set for TNP certification exam. *AAACN Viewpoint* 22(6):20.

Joint Commission on Accreditation of Healthcare Organizations (JCAHO) (1998): *1998 Hospital accreditation standards (HAS), standards, intent.* Oakbrook Terrace, IL: Author.

Jones MA, editor (1996): *Office nursing practice standards for quality care of patients.* Montvale, NJ: American Association of Office Nurses.

Marker CS (1988): *Setting standards for professional nursing: the Marker model.* St. Louis: Mosby.

Matherly SC, Hodges S (1992): From costly nuisance to profitable tool. In Barnett F, Meyer GG, editors: *Ambulatory care management and practice.* Gaithersburg, MD: Aspen, pp. 314-333.

McCloskey G, Bulechek J, editors (2000): *Nursing interventions classification (NIC),* ed 3. St. Louis: Mosby.

McGear R, Simms J (1998): *Telephone triage and management.* Philadelphia: WB Saunders.

McKesson-HBOC (1997): *Nurse training manual.* Broomfield, CO: Access Health Group.

THE PROFESSIONAL NURSING ROLE IN AMBULATORY CARE

22 Clinical Performance Improvement

KATE G. FELIX, PhD, RN, CNAA
REBECCA LINN PYLE, MS, RN

OBJECTIVES

Study of the information presented in this chapter will enable the learner to:

1. Discuss the differences between a quality assurance and a total quality management approach for performance improvement.

2. Explain the appropriate use for the general mechanisms for performance improvement versus the specific mechanisms.

3. Discuss why indicators are integral to the performance improvement process.

4. Describe the multiple factors affecting the development of a reliable and valid process to monitor competencies.

5. Discuss how the presence or absence of critical attributes for collaborative practice impact on a successful collaborative model.

6. Describe the qualities of important change initiatives among a group of highly educated, autonomous professionals.

■■ Continually improving performance is a critical aspect of professional ambulatory nursing practice. The improvement process, a central premise of total quality management programs, can be complex. Improving performance requires the integration of competencies and multiple, interrelated system and interpersonal factors into a cohesive action plan. This chapter is designed to provide nurses with a basic understanding of those factors by providing them with information to develop basis continuous improvement initiatives.

PERFORMANCE IMPROVEMENT

Performance improvement is the systematic analysis of the structure, processes, and outcomes within systems for the purpose of improving the delivery of care.

    A. Performance improvement is one of the most critical endpoints in a quality model.

        1. The ultimate goal of performance improvement is to determine if the care provided makes a difference.

B. Acceptable performance is doing well what needs to be done. The demand to "do the right thing" and "do the right thing well" (Joint Commission on Accreditation of Healthcare Organizations [JCAHO], 1997) increases as resources become increasingly more scarce.
   1. Doing the right thing and doing it well requires us to analyze if the performance is (JCAHO, 1998b):
      a. Effective.
      b. Relevant.
      c. Timely.
      d. Available to those consumers who need it.
      e. Congruent with other providers' services.
      f. Safe.
      g. Efficient.
      h. Respectful.
      i. Delivered in a caring way.
C. Quality definition.
   1. There is no single definition of quality.
      a. Quality depends on who answers the question, how quality is measured, and what is important to those defining the term (Carey and Lloyd, 1995).
      b. What one person may perceive as quality, another person may not.
      c. Regardless of how quality is defined, value is an implicit attribute (Hall, 1996).
         (1) For example, a consumer who does not value prevention will not believe in the need for immunization, or perceive that a health care program that provides immunizations to children is a quality health care program.
   2. Historically, performance improvement initiatives focused on quality assurance (QA).
      a. Attempts to assure quality care were often guided by subjective and anecdotal information that was directed at errors made by individuals.
      b. QA efforts were not linked to causes for performance variation nor consistently considered how variation affected outcomes (Carey and Lloyd, 1995).
   3. Current focus of quality improvement is on problem solving techniques to improve processes and achieve outcomes (Mitchell, Ferketich, and Jennings, 1998), and to subsequently achieve continuous quality improvement (CQI) (Kibbe, Kaluzny, and McLaughlin, 1994).
   4. CQI is the analysis and subsequent management of processes and clinical, financial, and health data to determine the relationship of those factors on health care structures, interventions, outcomes, and costs (Kibbe, et al., 1996).
   5. A classic model that acts as a mechanism to focus our quality efforts is the Donabedian (1966) quality trilogy model: structure, process, and

outcomes. Successful improvement efforts require the *integration* of all three (Williamson, 1991). Within the quality model, structure, process, and outcome can be defined as:

a. Structure.
  (1) Factors within an organization that support the delivery of quality care.
    (a) Staff credentials.
    (b) Staff abilities/competency.
    (c) Staffing ratios.
    (d) Facility design and equipment.
    (e) Administrative structures that support the delivery of care (e.g., policies, procedures, and guidelines).
b. Process.
  (1) The work that supports delivering quality care on behalf of the patient or health care consumer.
    (a) Accurately medicating patients.
    (b) Providing patient education.
    (c) Documenting care in the health care record.
    (d) Complying with evidence that indicates care can be improved if provided a certain way.
    (e) Evaluating clinicians' competency. Competency evaluation may identify a gap or strength in an employee's critical thinking, interpersonal, or technical skills. These data, therefore, can enhance quality improvement efforts.
c. Outcome.
  (1) The result of interventions, such as a clinician's interaction with a patient or organization, to provide care.
  (2) Outcomes can be classified in different ways (Brooten and Naylor, 1995; Flanagan, 1995).
  (3) Four different classifications of outcomes in Benson's (1992) model include:
    (a) Disease specific: physiologic parameters such as temperature, peak flow; biochemical parameters such as $HgA1_c$, Dilantin levels; microbiologic parameters such as GC cultures, etc.
    (b) General health: improvement or deterioration of an individual's health function.
    (c) Patient performance: engagement by the patient in the mutually agreed upon plan of care.
    (d) Patient satisfaction: satisfaction with exam room wait times, access to providers, or clinician interaction.
    (e) Though Benson did not include a financial classification, cost of care is considered an important outcome today.

ESTABLISHING A MECHANISM FOR THE PERFORMANCE IMPROVEMENT PROCESS

Mechanisms provide a structured method of analyzing care delivery structures, processes, and outcomes that result in reliable information that can be used to improve performance.

    A. General mechanisms.

        1. Improving performance by reducing variation is the main focus of the total quality management (TQM) process (Carey and Lloyd, 1995).

        2. Improving every aspect of performance is often not possible because of limited resources.

        3. One general mechanism is to focus quality improvement (QI) efforts by identifying scopes of care, important aspects of care, and indicators of care (JCAHO, 1997).

            a. Scope of care is the organizational or professional reason for being.

                (1) Ask, "Who are you (as an organization/profession)?"

                (2) Ask, "Why are you here?"

                (3) A purpose for being in ambulatory care is to provide continuity of care across the lifespan to maintain and promote health.

                    (a) Examples: continuity of care, health maintenance, and chronic disease management.

            b. An important aspect of care (IAC) is the specific care provided within an organization.

                (1) Ask, "What are the high volume, high risk, or high cost areas of care?"

                    (a) Examples are: appointment accessibility, childhood immunizations, treatment of asthma (corresponding to the continuity of care), health maintenance, and chronic disease management scopes of care, respectively.

            c. Indicators further define the IACs.

                (1) Ask, "What are the processes we deliver and the outcomes of care we want to achieve?"

                    (a) For example, process indicators for the IAC "Treatment of Asthma" may include appropriate medication use, documentation of asthma medications, and develop and implementation of home care plans.

                    (b) For example, outcome indicators might be adequate peak flow levels in asthmatic patients, decreased acute exacerbations, and subsequent decreased emergency department utilization.

                    (c) Once an indicator is identified, data are collected and analyzed for that indicator.

                    (d) If the data indicate care is outside preset goals or thresholds, the problem solving process is initiated and subsequent identified improvement opportunities implemented.

                    (e) The process is then remeasured to determine what improvement outcomes were achieved.

4. A second general improvement mechanism consists of the JCAHO (1997) cycle of four essential activities that support the improvement process.
   a. Designing structures, processes, or services that are viewed as high quality.
   b. Measuring, through routine, ongoing, or focused data collection, those structures, processes, or services and the subsequent outcomes.
   c. Assessing (evaluating) the data to determine if improvement opportunities exist.
   d. Improving the structure or process.
B. Specific mechanisms. Many different specific mechanisms (JCAHO, 1998c) exist to improve quality. Each mechanism serves a different purpose in the QI process. This section discusses three of these mechanisms—benchmarking, flowcharts, and root cause analysis.
   1. Benchmarking (Kobs, 1998) is a continuous and collaborative discipline that involves measuring and comparing the results of key processes with the best performers, and using the information to change/improve practices, resulting in superior performance as determined by measured outcomes. Benchmarking allows the consumer to make informed choices about health care value.
      a. Two types of benchmarking.
         (1) Internal benchmarking: process of examining internal performance and gauging improvement over time.
         (2) External benchmarking: measurement of performance of a given organization with reliable and valid indicators, against that of another similar organization using identical indicator.
      b. Characteristics of benchmarking (Ellis, 1995).
         (1) Benchmarking requires that structures be in place to enable the dissemination of information about practice development and their integration into everyday practice.
         (2) Externally focused: it widens practitioners' horizons of what is realistically achievable.
         (3) Not research dependent: professional consensus is acceptable.
         (4) Evaluated by outcomes that are measurable and client-focused.
         (5) The outcomes or benchmark may be audited locally, but wide comparisons are possible.
         (6) The benchmarks need to be realistic within the clinical setting for which they are being evaluated.
         (7) Benchmark outcomes can be used to develop practice, not just monitor and sustain it.
      c. Outcomes of benchmarking (Ellis, 1995; Jefferies, 1998; Kobs, 1998; Spann, 1997).
         (1) Quality improvement and practice development are accelerated.
         (2) Quality measures are established.
         (3) Motivation and enthusiasm among staff is improved as a result of recognition and reward for achievement and success.

(4) A structured forum for networking is provided.

(5) A systematic process for evaluating and improving care and service delivery to patients is developed.

    d. Potential difficulties (Ellis, 1995).

(1) Benchmarking requires a good relationship between participants.

(2) Requires commitment to the ideal that benchmarking is vital to improve services.

(3) Competition and mistrust may limit the freedom of sharing information.

(4) Benchmarking is limited by the scope of definition, data collection, analysis, and interpretation of the best performers being used for comparison.

(5) Data collection and analysis can be expensive and labor intensive.

    e. Selecting what to benchmark (Kobs, 1998).

(1) Ask the question, "Have the 'best of the best' been identified in any other organization?"

(2) Identify what services, products, and practices have been benchmarked internally and externally.

(3) Decide which services, products, and practices, if improved, would have the most impact within your organization.

(4) Agree on what are the most critical services, products, and practices for quality improvement.

    f. Models and processes for benchmarking (Kobs, 1998).

(1) Follow a simple, logical sequence of activity. Keep process models simple.

(2) Place a heavy emphasis on planning and organization of data collection and analysis.

(3) Use customer-focused benchmarking: identify the customer who will benefit from the improved service, products, or process.

(4) Make benchmarking a generic process. Be consistent throughout the organization.

(5) Utilize characteristics of collaboration and interdisciplinary practices.

2. Process improvement flowcharts provide specific steps to identify opportunities for improvement and develop subsequent solutions to improve the process. Carey and Lloyd (1995) described a process-improvement process that includes the following steps:

    a. Identify the opportunity for improvement.

    b. Organize a team.

    c. Flowchart the process.

    d. Determine if the process is standardized—if not, standardize the process.

    e. If the process is standardized, identify the important aspects of the process.

f. Select the *most* important aspect in the process.

g. Define what is the most important aspect and develop a plan to collect data to study the most important aspect.

h. Analyze the data collected, determine the degree of variation in the data and whether the variation is random (i.e., occurring by chance). If the variation is not occurring by chance, a special reason may be causing the variation.

   (1) Variation that occurs due to chance is called common-cause variation (Carey and Lloyd, 1995). This type of variation is a normal part of every process.

     (a) Example: fluctuating oral/rectal temperatures around a set of normal limits.

     (b) Example: patient satisfaction. Higher or lower values will be seen in some months than other months. Sometimes patients will be satisfied with their care and sometimes they won't be completely satisfied "just because." That is normal variation.

   (2) Variation that occurs due to a special reason is the result of an irregular or unnatural cause that is not a normal part of the process. This type of variation is caused special-cause variation (Carey and Lloyd, 1995).

     (a) Example: a temperature spike that is caused by an infection. A spike significantly higher than most of the values would need to be questioned if something unusual isn't going on to cause the abnormally high temperature.

     (b) Example: patient satisfaction rates drop precipitously following a decrease in the number of clinicians who provide care, therefore causing the waiting room times to skyrocket.

   (3) Different QI actions are taken depending on the type of variation.

     (a) If data indicate common-cause variation is present, then the team must first decide if the degree of variation is acceptable.

       (i) If the data indicate satisfaction varies between 80% to 85%, the team would ask, "is that level acceptable?", or should we attempt to improve our performance by raising the goal to 87% to 90%?

      (ii) The team would also consider what factors have the greatest influence on the process?

     (iii) The most important factor influencing the process is then selected and an improvement strategy is implemented.

     (iv) Data are collected to determine if the intended improvement was achieved.

     (v) If not, another factor is selected, actions are implemented to improve the process, and data are again collected.

(vi) When the action achieves the intended improvement, the action becomes a permanent part of the process.

(b) If data indicate a special cause is present, the team would work to eliminate it. For example, more clinicians would need to be hired in the patient satisfaction special cause example (see h., [2] on previous page).

(4) Root cause analysis is a method to determine the fundamental reason that causes variation in performance (JCAHO, 1998a).

(a) Root cause analysis can be reactive (i.e., analyzing the reason for problems that have occurred).

(b) It can be proactive (i.e., analyzing opportunities for improvement before problems occur).

(c) Key characteristics of root cause analysis include:

(i) A focus on systems rather than individuals. When analyzing systems, the QI team would attempt to design out any flaws that lead to problems.

(ii) Analyzing special causes first, then common causes by repeatedly asking, "can anything be causing this problem," until no further logical answers can be found.

(d) To implement successful root cause analyses, the basic belief must be accepted that clinicians are human and mistakes can be expected, but organizational improvement is achievable.

(e) The steps of a root cause analysis include:

(i) Define the event—what happened?

(ii) Identify the proximate cause—why did this happen? Types of proximate cause may include human error, process deficiency, equipment breakdown, environmental factors.

(iii) Identify the underlying reason for the proximate cause by brainstorming to determine why did the proximate cause happen.

(iv) Collect and assess data on the proximate and underlying causes.

(v) Develop and implement interim changes. If you decide one cause might be broken equipment, the team should not wait to fix the equipment.

(vi) Identify the root cause by asking key questions including:

a) What factors in the environment might have contributed to the errors. For example, was staffing adequate, was the activity level greater than normal, was the equipment working properly, were breaks being taken?

b) How is the flow of communication being managed?

For example, does information flow freely, accurately, clearly? Is the information accessible?

  c) Is staff competent and is a system in place to objectively assess staff competency?

  d) How is competent performance maintained?

C. Evidence-based practice combines research and clinical expertise (Simon, 1999). Evidence-based practice is defined as "the conscientious, explicit, and judicious use of current best evidence in making decisions about the care of individual patients" (Sackett, Richardson, Rosenberg, and Hayes, 1997, p. 5).

 1. Data from health care research suggest a limited relationship between the care we provide and the achievement of specific outcomes (Hall, 1997).

 2. Our clinical judgments and interventions, therefore, have come under increasing scrutiny and questioning (Kibbe, Kaluzny, and McLaughlin, 1994).

 3. Evidence-based practice provides direction for the delivery of care and also establishes a method for evaluating performance. The intent is to provide care based on the best scientific evidence that is supported by expert opinion (ANA, 1995b, Goode and Piedalue, 1999).

 4. Major purposes of evidence-based practice approaches include (National Health Lawyers Association, 1995):

  a. Assisting clinical decision makers.

  b. Educating clinicians.

  c. Providing a framework for evaluating the delivery of care.

  d. Guiding resource allocations.

  e. Reducing risk of liability.

 5. Specific types of evidence-based practice approaches may include (National Health Lawyers Association, 1995):

  a. Clinical practice guidelines.

  b. Critical pathways.

  c. Clinical indicators.

  d. Standards of care.

  e. Clinical policies and procedures.

  f. Care maps.

 6. The degree to which we can trust the validity of the content is driven by the rigor of scientific inquiry on which the evidenced-based practice is founded (McDonald, 1994).

 7. When solid research is not available, then a careful review of expert opinion is included in the development process.

 8. Professional nursing organizations work closely with the Agency for Health Care Policy and Research (AHCPR) and/or other experts to develop solid evidence-based approaches and to influence health care policy (ANA, 1995b).

  a. Nursing leaders recognize developing specific approaches (guidelines, standards, policies, or procedures) has been based on anecdotes, tradition, or cookbook procedures.

  b. If the nurse is to be recognized as a professional team player with a place at the health care table, traditional methods will no longer serve our profession well.

    c. Nursing practice must move toward evidenced-based approaches that are rooted in solid, scientific research, focus on outcomes, and clearly demonstrate the effectiveness of nursing practice (ANA, 1995a).

   9. The AHCPR system for rating the scientific evidence incorporates six levels ranging from the highest level (evidence is based on synthesis of randomized controlled trials) to the lowest level (evidence is based on expert opinions or respected authorities) (ANA, 1995b).

SPECIFICATION OF PERFORMANCE INDICATORS IN AMBULATORY CARE

An indicator is a description of specific performance factors within a particular organization. Identifying and measuring indicators requires a clear understanding of the work of the organization and also identified opportunities for performance improvement.

  A. As health care costs increase, consumers including individuals, employers, and the government will demand to know how an organization is improving performance.

    1. The demand for information about performance is driving a revolution that will profoundly affect health care providers and payers (Ribnick and Carrano, 1995).

    2. Variation in specific indicators will help consumers to determine different values and will help organizations to identify potential opportunities for improvement.

  B. Report cards.

    1. Display collected data on the indicators that affect typical patients such as satisfaction, immunization, and Pap smear rates.

    2. May also display more negative data such as death, disability, and disease rates, etc. (Badger, 1998; Ribnick and Carrano, 1995).

    3. Report cards identify performance measures that include quality indicators (e.g., immunization, Pap smear, and mammogram rates), utilization indicators (e.g., membership, access, finances, hospital, and ER admission), and satisfaction levels.

    4. Consumers use report card data to compare the performance of different organizations against a predetermined standard/best practice.

    5. Report cards support consumers' informed purchasing decisions about which health plan might more closely meet their health care needs.

    6. A challenge in using report cards effectively is to assure the data collection methods are standardized and relevant.

    7. The data contained in report cards may be too broad to explicate the exact factors that make up the data.

      a. Example: high satisfaction scores may not lead to a better understanding of what makes the patient satisfied unless specified. Was a patient satisfied with their care because of the low cost, fast response time to answering questions, or friendliness of staff?

8. Tools that document data on health status, which can be affected by nurses, will begin to illuminate the value nurses add to the health care equation. These data, in turn, will provide recognition for the role nurses can play.

   a. The data must be continually refined in order to determine which nursing structure and processes are linked to nursing outcomes.

9. Report cards are not benchmarks. However, report card data can be used in the benchmark process.

10. Different types of report cards have been created by different organizations to specify what indicators are most important to track or to identify information important to consumers (Lowe and Baker, 1997; Schriefer, Urden, and Rogers, 1997; Spath, 1998).

11. AAACN has begun to identify national nursing indicators for report cards in the ambulatory setting (Mastal, 1999).

12. The ANA (1996) is making significant headway into identifying inpatient indicators.

13. Examples of different ambulatory report cards and their indicators are:

    a. Health Plan Employer Data and Information Set (HEDIS).
       (1) Emphasis is on health plan performance in managed care.
       (2) The indicators are more tangentially then directly linked to nursing (e.g., immunization, Pap smear, and satisfaction rates).
       (3) Data from this report card are used to determine health plan expenditures and performance accountabilities (Ribnick and Carrano, 1995).

    b. Medical Outcomes Trust Short Form (MOS-SF36).
       (1) Originally developed to describe variations in physician practice styles and outcomes (Benson, 1992).
       (2) The newest version (SF-36) includes indicators that can be influenced by nursing interventions including role limitations caused by physical and emotional problems, social functioning, bodily pains, and general health perceptions.

    c. Standardized Outcomes and Assessment Information Set (OASIS) for home health care.
       (1) A lengthy survey that contains predominantly functional criteria required by Medicare-certified home health agencies.
       (2) Examples of some of the functional items are ADL/IADLs, integumentary, sensory, respiratory, elimination status, as well as living arrangements and supportive assistance.
       (3) Most of the items focus on long term rather than short term outcomes such as blood oxygen levels, wound and infusion site infection.

    d. Child Health Questionnaire (CHQ-PF50). Similar to the SF-36 but for use with pediatric patients (Rieve, 1997).

COMPETENCY

Competency is the demonstrated integration of knowledge, skill, and ability in order to perform expected job functions (AAACN, 1996; JCAHO, 1994; Miller, Flynn, and Umadac, 1998). A minimal level of competence is the ability to perform the job safely. Safe performance is expected of all health care clinicians.

A. Aspects of competency.
   1. Competency has three different aspects.
      a. Knowledge: a cognitive foundation for providing work achieved typically through formal and informal education or training.
      b. Skill: the manual dexterity to perform work. Traditional views considered only the skill or technical aspect of competency.
      c. Ability: the capacity or power to perform the expected job functions.
B. Competency model.
   1. Criteria for developing a competency model should include:
      a. Understanding standards of care.
      b. Identifying key strategies for delivering care.
      c. Identifying high-volume, high-cost, high-risk areas in which care is provided.
      d. Including key stakeholders who will be using and benefiting from the delivery of competent care.
   2. A well-developed model should result in a model that staff and managers recognize as realistically depicting the necessary competencies for delivering care within a specific setting. To determine if the model is valid, ask, "Is this what we do?"
   3. del Bueno (personal communication, 1998) provides one conceptual model for understanding competence (Figure 22-1).
      a. del Bueno's model (Anthony and del Bueno, 1993) depicts the importance of integrating three critical competency dimensions: critical thinking, interpersonal skills, and technical skills.
      b. Knowledge, skills, and ability, to integrate within each dimension.
         (1) Example of integration within the critical thinking dimension.
            (a) Competent ambulatory nurses in an internal medicine or family practice department would need to know the signs and symptoms of chest pain in the elderly.
            (b) They would need to demonstrate accurate physical assessment skills.
            (c) They would need to demonstrate the ability to elicit an accurate history to make a clinical judgment about the cause of the patient's signs and symptoms.
         (2) Example of integration within the interpersonal dimension.
            (a) Competent ambulatory nurses would need to know psychosocial dynamics.
            (b) They would need to demonstrate empathic listening skills.
            (c) They would need to demonstrate the ability to alter their therapeutic approach.
         (3) Example of integration within the technical dimension.

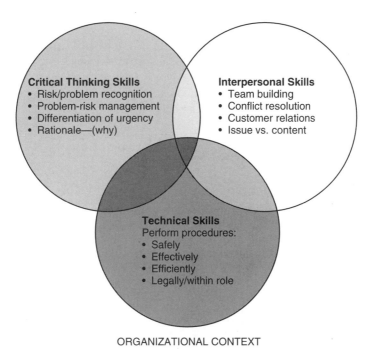

Critical Thinking Skills
• Risk/problem recognition
• Problem-risk management
• Differentiation of urgency
• Rationale—(why)

Interpersonal Skills
• Team building
• Conflict resolution
• Customer relations
• Issue vs. content

Technical Skills
Perform procedures:
• Safely
• Effectively
• Efficiently
• Legally/within role

ORGANIZATIONAL CONTEXT

FIGURE 22-1 ■ Dimensions of Competent Performance (From Anthony CE, del Bueno D [1993]:A performance-based development system. *Nurs Management* 24[6]:32-34.)

(a) Competent nurses would need to know the critical steps in performing the procedure.

(b) They would need to demonstrate the manual skill to perform the procedure.

(c) They would need to demonstrate the ability to modify the procedure within generally accepted standards if unique patient needs require it.

c. Competency dimensions.

(1) Critical thinking is the ability to collect and analyze information in order to arrive at a logical, defendable, conclusion.

(a) Clinical judgment is one form of critical thinking.

(i) Ambulatory care nurses collect and analyze information about the individual, family, group, or community and from the data form clinical judgments to achieve positive outcomes for the client.

(2) Interpersonal is the ability to influence clients and/or team members through verbal and nonverbal skills and behavior.

(3) Technical and manual ability to perform tasks safely.

(4) At times, all three dimensions are equally important and at other times, one dimension may be more important depending on the environment or context.

MONITORING STAFF COMPETENCE

Monitoring competence provides information on how to support performance improvement initiatives and is a key concern in the CQI process (Western, 1994).

- A. Why monitor staff competency?
    - 1. As health care reform rapidly and dramatically changes the workplace, the evaluation of staff competencies will:
        - a. Identify performance improvement opportunities for the individual and the team.
        - b. Support cost effective, safe nursing.
            - (1) RN staff delivering care that medical assistants can competently perform drives more costly staffing models.
            - (2) Training and orientation costs decrease when departments honor and build upon the knowledge, skills, and abilities that staff bring to the work setting rather than training staff on what they already know.
        - c. Provide health care consumers with greater confidence in the qualifications of their health care providers.
        - d. Support effective and efficient educational programs (Nolan, 1998).
- B. Factors affecting competency monitoring.
    - 1. Environment or situational/contextual impact on competency.
        - a. The del Bueno model shows the interrelationships of the different dimensions and also depicts competence occurring within a particular environment or situation/context.
        - b. The context or environment may affect the relative importance of each competency.
        - c. Examples include:
            - (1) Competent scrub nurses in the outpatient surgery setting must demonstrate more technical skills than nurses in a family practice office.
            - (2) Competent nurses working in call centers, performing few technical procedures, must demonstrate more critical thinking skills.
            - (3) In settings, concerned about patient satisfaction, competent nurses would demonstrate highly refined interpersonal skills.
            - (4) In an adult ICU, competent nurses would discontinue and reinsert disconnected IVs that had been contaminated. However, a neonatal ICU nurse exhibiting competent critical thinking would consider all options. Discontinuing the IV may be a greater risk than not having an immediate access.
    - 2. Measurement issues.
        - a. A model provides a foundation for understanding the specific structure processes, or outcomes that we believe should be monitored. Once a competency model is developed, the next step is to develop reliable and valid tools that measure specific competencies within the model.
            - (1) Reliable tools assure the evaluation process will be consistent for every nurse.

      (2) Valid tools assure that the competence dimension (i.e., critical thinking, interpersonal, or technical abilities), is actually being measured.

b. To facilitate buy-in and trust, include staff who will be evaluated and their managers in the tool development process.

c. Specific tools will measure different dimensions. No one tool can be used to measure competence.

d. Examples of competency tools may include:

      (1) Criterion checklists listing the critical steps (measure technical dimension). Criterion checklists are not procedures.

      (2) Troubleshooting exercises using paper and pencil and video-tapes of patient situations (measure critical thinking or interpersonal dimensions).

      (3) Audiotapes of simulated staff-to-staff or staff-to-patient interactions (measure interpersonal dimensions).

e. The multiple, integrated dimensions, the complexity of patient care, and the environmental and contextual impact, precludes developing tools that simply offer multiple choice answers.

f. Valid competency tools require methods that elicit performance similar to that required in the work place.

g. The goal is not only to elicit the employee's description in what action would be taken, but also to validate why the employee would take those actions.

      (1) Responses are analyzed against a predetermined set of criteria developed from the standards of practice and standards of care (del Bueno, personal communication, 1998).

h. Evaluation of competence requires a variety of situations, and, therefore, a variety of tools that sample the universe of what actually occurs in the work setting.

i. Critical thinking is not readily observable.

      (1) A valid tool to evaluate critical thinking might have the nurse view a video of a clinic patient with a problem. The nurse would describe the data she might require to validate or differentiate the problem, and the initial and long-range goals and the immediate and subsequent interventions to achieve these goals.

      (2) A multiple-choice exam would not be an effective way to measure critical thinking, (or any competency), because the patient rarely presents with only a list of four options to choose from in planning care!

      (3) Another tool to evaluate a nurse's critical thinking competence might include a case study that the nurse would review and then outline the care the nurse would provide.

      (4) A chart audit of the nurse's care would also provide data on the nurse's actual management of a patient situation, and, implicitly their critical thinking ability. The nurse's response would be compared against a predefined set of standards that were developed by the team who developed the tool.

3. Competence continuum.
   a. One continuum of competency exists across the inpatient and ambulatory setting.
      (1) Nurses who deliver care in hospital settings provide acute, episodic care that is focused on restoring health. The goal of inpatient nursing care is to manage the acute problem and avoid subsequent hospitalization.
      (2) Conversely, nurses in ambulatory settings provide both acute, episodic, and chronic, long-term care to restore health or prevent illness.
      (3) Competent inpatient nurses focus on the identification and management of acute problems.
      (4) Competent ambulatory nurses focus on the identification and management of both acute and chronic lifespan problems.
   b. Another competence continuum is the range of competence across the different levels on the health care team. All members of the health care team must maintain safe care (a minimal level of competence).
      (1) The expanding competence levels will depend on the educational preparation, experience, licenses, and expected performance (del Bueno, personal communication, 1995; Robinson and Barberis-Ryan, 1995).
      (2) Both a medical assistant and an RN must know and correctly perform the critical steps in taking a blood pressure.
         (a) They must both know the normal and abnormal ranges. However, the RN must also demonstrate additional competencies.
            (i) RNs must demonstrate an ability to analyze the data and convert the data into an effective plan of care.
            (ii) The RN may also initiate relevant interpersonal strategies to support the patient in managing their own health.
      (3) At the far end of the continuum, the competent physician would initiate/order specific interventions such as medications, additional diagnostic work-up needed to correct and manage the hypertension.
C. Regulatory/accreditation issues affecting competency.
   1. Regulatory bodies, such as state nurse practice acts, exist to ensure patient safety.
   2. Implicit or explicit in these statutory regulations is the requirement that nurses are competent to provide care.
   3. Accreditation agencies such as the Joint Commission for the Accreditation of Health Care Agencies (JCAHO) and the National Committee for Quality Assurance (NCQA), view competent providers as a critical element in the provision of quality care.
      a. JCAHO *Standards for Ambulatory Care* (1998b) emphasizes technical aspects of delivering care such as new procedures, technology, techniques, or equipment.

    b. NCQA, implicitly addresses competency through the credentialing process (NCQA 2000).

    c. Board certification, education, and experience may imply competence but they are no guarantee or surrogate indicator of actual ability to perform competently.

    d. The Pew Health Professions Commission Taskforce on Health Care Workforce Regulation (1995) has recommended that professional regulatory bodies (e.g., State Boards of Nursing) should base state practice acts on demonstrating initial and continuing competencies.

COLLABORATION WITH OTHER HEALTH DISCIPLINES

Collaboration is critical to achieving the quality improvement necessary because the task is too big and too complex to accomplish with just a few members of one discipline (McCloskey and Maas, 1998).

    A. Recognition of the contribution's of all members of the health care team leads to the need to coordinate and evaluate everyone's effort to maximize performance improvement. Other factors that have led to the need for collaboration are (Hoffman, 1998; Holt, 1997):

        1. Changes in the economy and escalating health care costs have led to organizational mergers, consolidations, and downsizing.

        2. Increased demand for professional services organized around fiscal goals (cost containment).

        3. Changes in the role of primary care in delivery of health and the challenge of caring for an increasing number of geriatric patients.

        4. The need to define and articulate quality of care outcomes so that useful and meaningful comparisons can be made.

        5. Development of highly sophisticated information management and data systems, which monitor patients along the care continuum, track utilization patterns, evaluate compliance with standards of care, and analyze patient outcomes.

        6. Development of health care report cards and accrediting processes.

        7. Development of performance improvement indicators (e.g., practice protocols, critical pathways, shared patient rounds, and joint planning and evaluation).

MAKING CHANGES TO IMPROVE PRACTICE

Today in business and organizations, the word change means several, often contradictory, things. It sometimes refers to external changes in technology, customers, competitors, market structure, or the social and political environment. Change also refers to internal changes: how the organization adapts to changes in the environment. The term profound change is used to describe organizational change that combines inner shifts in people's values, aspirations, and behaviors with outer shifts in processes, strategies, practices, and systems (Senge, et al., 1999).

    A. Senge and colleagues (1999) has identified a set of forces or challenges that oppose profound change. They are incorporated in the following three broad categories.

1. Challenges of initiating change develop as soon as any group begins to conduct its work in unfamiliar ways. These challenges include the following:
   a. The challenge of control over one's time.
   b. The challenge of inadequate coaching, guidance, and support for innovating groups.
   c. The challenge of relevance: making a case for change.
   d. The challenge of management clarity and consistency.
2. The challenges of sustaining momentum take place within a group as it achieves early success, and between the team and the larger organizational culture. These challenges include:
   a. The challenge of fear and anxiety.
   b. The challenge of negative assessment of progress.
   c. The challenge of isolation and arrogance.
3. The challenges of redesigning and rethinking appear when change initiatives gain broader credibility and confront the established internal infrastructure and practices of the organization. These challenges include:
   a. The challenge of the prevailing governance structure and the conflicts between groups seeking greater autonomy and managers concerned about autonomy leading to chaos and internal fragmentation.
   b. The challenge of diffusion, the inability to transfer knowledge across organization boundaries.
   c. The challenge of the organization's strategy and purpose.

B. At least three fundamental reinforcing processes exist that sustain profound change by building upon each other (Senge, 1999).
   1. Enhancing personal results.
   2. Developing networks of committed people.
   3. Improving business results.

C. The most important change initiatives seem to have these qualities (Senge, et al., 1999).
   1. They are connected with real work goals and processes.
   2. They are connected with improving performance.
   3. They involve people who have the power to take action regarding these goals.
   4. They seek to balance action and reflection, connecting inquiry and experimentation.
   5. They afford opportunities for people to think and reflect without pressure to make decisions.
   6. They are intended to increase people's capacity, individually and collectively.
   7. They focus on learning about learning in settings that matter.

D. The rate of change in the economic environment has become exponential. How can companies prepare to meet the business issues of the next decade if they're unpredictable? They can accommodate the forces of change only by creating and institutionalizing a capacity for changing themselves. The need for change should be treated as seriously as the real work of the organization. A company's business systems (jobs and structure, business processes, values and beliefs, management and measurement systems), must change as the demands upon it change (Hammer, 1996). Hammer identifies two business systems in every organization (Hammer, 1996).

1. The surface system comprises the organized tasks of the business processes, with their attendant jobs, structures, systems, and values.
2. Accomplishing change in the surface system is the job of the deep system. The deep system monitors, governs, adjusts, and reforms the surface system.
   a. A deep system is responsible for detecting external changes, determining what those changes mean, and intervening to modify or transform the surface system accordingly.
   b. The deep system, working beneath the surface, embodies the capacity to change.
   c. The deep system ensures that the appropriate internal change takes place to take account of ongoing external change.
   d. The primary processes of the deep system are learning, redesign, and transition.

E. Using the above information, a process for making changes to improve practice can be articulated (Hammer, 1996).
   1. The learning process: a decision to create new ways of working.
      a. The need for major change to the surface system is recognized, communicated, and accepted.
      b. Important information is identified, understood, evaluated, and spread throughout the organization.
      c. The specific output is the decision to change and concrete objectives for this change.
   2. The redesign process: invents the new ways of working.
      a. Uses the output of the learning process as its input.
      b. Creates a new design for the surface system that better fits the new external realities.
   3. The transition process: translates ideas into realities.
      a. The organization's old surface system is replaced by a new one.
      b. Takes as input a new surface system design, and its result is the new system in actual operation.
      c. Uses such disciplines as change management and implementation.

REFERENCES

American Academy of Ambulatory Care Nursing and American Nurses' Association (1996): *Nursing in ambulatory care: the future is here.* Washington, DC: Author.

American Nurses' Association (ANA) (1995a): *Implementation of nursing practice standards and guidelines.* Washington, DC: Author.

ANA (1995b): *Manual to develop guidelines.* Washington, DC: Author.

ANA (1996): *Nursing quality indicators: definitions and implications.* Washington, DC: Author.

Anthony CE, del Bueno D (1993): A performance-based development system. *Nurs Management* 24(6):32-34.

Badger KA (1998, Jan-Mar): Patient care reports: an analysis. *Outcomes Management Nurs Practice* 2(1):29-36.

Benson DS (1992): *Measuring outcomes in ambulatory care.* Chicago, IL: American Hospital Association.

Brooten D, Naylor MD (1995): Nurses' effect on changing patient outcomes. *Image J Nurs Sch* 27(2):95-99.

Carey RG, Lloyd RC (1995): *Measuring quality improvement in health care: a guide to statistical process control applications.* New York: Quality Resources.

Donabedian A (1966): Evaluating the quality of medical care. *Milbank Q* 44:166-203.

Ellis J (1995): Using benchmarking to improve practice. *Clinical Quality Assurance* 9(35):25-28.

Flanagan A (1995): Ambulatory outcomes management. *AAACN Viewpoint* 17(2):1,6.

Goode C, Piedalue F (1999): Evidence-based clinical practice. *J Nurs Adm* 29(6):15-21.

Hall J (1996): The challenge of health outcomes. *J Qual Clin Pract* 16:5-15.

Hammer M (1996): The process of change. *Beyond reengineering.* New York: Harper Collins, pp. 207-225.

Hoffman S (1998): The three new C's for nursing: collaboration, cooperation, and coalition. *J Prof Nurs* 14(4):194.

Holt FM (1997): Do we need a report card for interdisciplinary collaboration? *Clinical Nurse Specialist* 11(3):133.

Jefferies E. (1998): Sharing good practice: developing network forums. *Nursing Standard* 12(50):33-34.

JCAHO (1994): *Organization-wide competency assessment: mapping out success.* Oakbrook, IL: Author.

JCAHO (1997): *Performance improvement in ambulatory care.* Oakbrook, IL: Author.

JCAHO (1998a): *Sentinel events: evaluating cause and planning improvement,* ed 2. Oakbrook, IL: Author.

JCAHO (1998b): *Standards for ambulatory care.* Oakbrook, IL: Author.

JCAHO (1998c): *Using performance improvement tools in ambulatory care.* Oakbrook, IL: Author.

Kibbe DC, Kaluzny AD, McLaughlin CP (1994): Integrating guidelines with continuous quality improvement: doing the right thing the right way to achieve the right goals. *J Quality Improvement,* 20(4):181-191.

Kobs AEJ (1998, Jan-Mar): Getting started on benchmarking . *Outcomes Management Nursing Practice* 2(1):45-48.

Lowe A, Baker J (1997, Nov): Measuring outcomes: a nursing report card. *Nurs Management* 38:40-41.

Mastal P (1999): New signposts and directions: indicators of quality in ambulatory nursing care. *Nurs Econ* 17(2):103-104.

McCloskey JC, Maas M (1998): Interdisciplinary team: the nursing perspective is essential. *Nurs Outlook* 46(4):157-163.

McDonald CJ (1994): Guidelines you can follow and trust. *JAMA* 271(11):872-873.

Miller E, Flynn JM, Umadac J (1998): Assessing, developing, and maintaining staff's competency in times of restructuring. *J Nurs Care Quality* 12(6):9-17.

Mitchell PH, Ferketich S, Jennings BM (1998): Quality health outcomes model. *Image J Nurs Sch* 30(1):43-46.

National Health Lawyers Association (1995): *Colloquium report on legal issues related to clinical practice guidelines.* Washington, DC: Author.

National Committee for Quality Assurance (NCQA) (2000): *Surveyor guidelines for the accreditation of MCO.* Washington, DC: Author.

Nolan P (1998): Competencies drive decision making. *Nurs Management* 29(3):27-29.

Pew Health Professions Commission (1995): *Reforming health care workforce regulation: policy considerations for the 21st century.* UCSF San Francisco: University of California: Author.

Ribnick PG, Carrano VA (1995): Understanding the new era in health care accountability: report cards. *J Nurs Qual* 10(1):1-8.

Rieve JA (1997, Nov/Dec): Quality management tools, part I. *TCM* 38-41.

Robinson SM, Barberis-Ryan C (1995): Competency assessment: a systematic approach. *Nurs Management* 26(2):40-44.

Sackett DL, Richardson WS, Rosenberg WMC, Haynes RB (1997): *Evidence-based medicine: how to practice and teach EBM.* Edinburgh: Churchill Livingstone.

Schriefer J, Urden L, Rogers S (1997, Jan-Mar): Report cards: tools for managing pathways and outcomes. *Outcomes Management Nurs Practice* 1(1):14-18.

Senge P, Kleiner A, Roberts C, et al. (1999): *The dance of change: the challenges of sustaining momentum in learning organizations.* New York: Doubleday.

Simon JM (1999): Evidence based practice in nursing. *Nurs Diagnosis* 10(1):3.

Spann K (1997): Bench marking best practice. *Medsurg Nursing* 6(1):5-8.

Spath P (1998, Jul-Sep): Nursing performance measurers go public. *Outcomes Management Nurs Practice* 2(3):124-129.

Western P (1994): QA/QI and nursing competence: a combined model. *Nurs Management* 25(3):44-46.

Williamson JW (1991): Medical quality management systems in perspective. In Couch J, editor: *Health care quality management for the 21st century.* Tampa, FL: American College of Physician Executives, pp. 23-72.

23 Ethics

CARROL GOLD, PhD, RN

OBJECTIVES

Study of the information presented in this chapter will enable the learner to:

1. Define nursing ethics.
2. Differentiate ethical issues from legal issues.
3. Identify the essential requirements for ethical practice stated in the ANA Code for Nurses.
4. Discuss the principles that guide ethical decision-making.
5. Discuss two philosophical theories used in ethical decision-making.
6. Identify the critical elements in an ethical dilemma.
7. List the essential steps in the process of ethical decision-making.
8. Identify ethical problems of particular concern to ambulatory nursing.
9. Appreciate the role of the nurse as advocate for patient and family in ethical dilemmas.
10. Discuss the role of the nurse in working with an ethics committee.

■■ Nursing practice is founded on and sustained by adherence to ethical principles. Ethical decision-making involves choosing from two or more options, none of which may be entirely satisfactory or unsatisfactory. The expansion of the scope of nursing practice as well as technologic advances and a wider range of options for patients and families have resulted in nurses' involvement with an increased number of situations in which an ethical conflict is central. These situations require that nurses develop an understanding of ethical decision-making and action processes, either as individuals or as a part of the health care team or ethics committee. The nurse in the ambulatory setting is challenged by many of the same ethical concerns as are inpatient nurses. However, managed care, changes in skill mix and increased use of nonlicensed personnel, less direct supervision, the physical settings in which care occurs, the conflicts between the need for shared information across ambulatory units and patient confidentiality, the increased use of telephone practice (triage), and the need to treat sicker and more frail patients in ambulatory settings, present additional challenges that may result in ethical dilemmas for ambulatory nurses.

DEFINITION OF NURSING ETHICS

A. Ethics attempts to answer the question, "What ought one to do in a given situation?" (Burkhardt and Nathaniel, 1998). Ethics involves an examination of how one ought to act.

B. Nursing ethics involves choosing from two or more options, none of which may be totally desirable, to guide actions within the nurses' scope of practice.

DIFFERENCES BETWEEN ETHICAL ISSUES AND LEGAL ISSUES

A. Ethical principles are not legally binding, although some laws are supported by ethical precepts (Hall, 1996).

  1. The patient's right to confidentiality is supported by law and by the ethical principle of confidentiality. It is an ethical violation to breech confidentiality; a patient can bring a lawsuit over violations of confidentiality.

  2. Giving preferred appointment times to patients with private insurance or who are private pay may be ethically questionable, but does not necessarily violate law.

B. Laws and those things that are legally binding may or may not be considered ethical, based on an individual's ethical stance.

  1. Abortion and withdrawal of life support are supported in law, but may or may not be considered ethical.

  2. Denial of access to certain treatments or medications by managed care companies is, in some cases, legal, but subject to ethical concerns.

THE ANA CODE FOR NURSES

This code has specific statements regarding the nurse's duty to:

A. Respect the dignity of the individual, whatever the socioeconomic status, personal attributes, or type of health problem.

B. Safeguard patient's right to confidentiality.

C. Protect patient and public from unsafe or unethical practices.

D. Exercise responsibility and accountability for nursing actions.

E. Maintain own practice competencies.

F. Exercise professional knowledge and judgment in accepting and carrying out own assignments and in delegating to others (ANA, 1988).

PRINCIPLES THAT GUIDE ETHICAL DECISION-MAKING

A. Autonomy: self-determination, the freedom to choose one's own course of action.

  1. Implies that one is cognitively able to exercise this right.

  2. Implies that no coercion has taken place.

B. Beneficence: doing good.

  1. Requires that what is meant by good in the situation be defined.

  2. Requires an understanding of what is in the best interest of the patient.

C. Nonmaleficence: acting in such a way that avoids harms, either intentional harm or harm as an unintended outcome.

1. Consideration must be given to the need to sometimes do harm in order to do good. For instance, chemotherapy may have serious systemic consequences; the treatment may be as life threatening as the illness.
2. Consideration must be given to the benefits vs. the burden of action, which may result in unintended or secondary harm.

D. Justice: fair, equitable distribution of resources.
   1. Requires recognition that resources and services are not limitless and that a system for decision-making about how resources are used must be in place.
   2. Requires that distribution of resources is based on the belief in the importance and value of each person, because each person has innate value as a human being, not because they have some particular attribute, such as intelligence or creativity or because they hold a particular station in life.

E. Veracity: truth-telling.
   1. Truth is the foundation of the development of trust between patient and nurse. All patients and/or their families, if families are acting as surrogates, are owed the duty of being informed about health conditions, treatments, and prognoses, with as much completeness and accuracy as possible.
   2. Immediate attention, without prejudgment, must be given to situations in which a family or individual does not wish to know about a diagnosis or prognosis, in an effort to understand why a family or individual would take such a stance.
      a. Such situations should be referred for consultation with the institutional ethics committees.
      b. In the absence of such a committee, staff may seek consultation with clergy, with ethics consultants from outside the system (university ethicist, for instance) or with ethical resource persons from specialty or professional organizations.

F. Confidentiality: to protect the patient's and family's right to privacy regarding information that the nurse or institution hold regarding the patient.
   1. Sharing of information must occur only between those parties who require access in order to fulfill obligations to provide care, consultation, or referral.
   2. Attention must be given to electronic patient records and databases that are transferred between numerous care-delivery locations. Technology and the movement of patients through a number of ambulatory care delivery units add new burdens to the protection of confidentiality.

G. Fidelity: faithfulness.
   1. Involves the duty owed to patients, families, and colleagues to do what one says one will do and to consistently act in accordance with the

requirements of the nurse practice act in the state in which the nurse practices and the ethical standards of the profession.

2. Requires an understanding that the privilege of using the protected title, RN, through state licensure, implies a duty owed to the citizens of the state or commonwealth issuing the license to practice. Those duties are stated in the nurse practice acts of each state (Gibson, 1993).

PHILOSOPHICAL THEORIES USED IN ETHICAL DECISION MAKING

Although there are a number of philosophic theories underlying ethical decision-making, the two approaches most commonly used involve assessment of the consequences of an action by weighing the benefits to be gained with the resulting burden; or the selection of an action based on some accepted duty. In concert with the ethical principles, the philosophic approaches structure understanding of dilemmas and assist in clarification of possible solutions to these dilemmas.

A. Utilitarianism (also known as consequence based ethics) is the theory that seeks to choose the thing that will offer the most good to the greatest number of people, increase pleasure, and avoid pain.
1. It is also characterized by the belief that the end justifies the means.
2. An act or decision is judged as a desirable choice based on its outcome. According to this theory, an act is ethical that brings the greatest benefit for the greatest number of people (Edge and Groves, 1994).
   a. Example: Based on the principle of beneficence or doing good, it is permissible to administer morphine for pain relief in a terminally ill patient even though the drug may depress respirations.
   b. This involves weighing the benefit (relief from suffering) from the burden (possible hastening of death).

B. Deontology (also known as duty based ethics) is based on the belief that there are duties to which one must be faithful and which one is obligated to carry out because these duties are owed to all human beings and because of the expectations implied by one's professional role (Edge and Groves, 1994).
1. Decisions are made based on what are considered universally accepted rules, and every person is owed the same duty.
2. People are ends in and of themselves and cannot be used to produce a specific end.
3. Nurses are bound by their professional codes to uphold duties that honor patient autonomy, mandate truth telling, protect patient confidentiality, extend justice and fairness to all, do no harm, seek to do good, and promote well-being.
4. Examples of deontology or duty based ethics:
   a. The use of placebos violates the duty to be truthful. Principle: veracity.
   b. Patient must receive the same quality of care and be offered the same services, regardless of their ability to pay or payer source. Principle: justice.

  c. It is a duty to report incidents of incompetent nursing or medical care. Principles: veracity, fidelity, nonmaleficence.

DISCUSS THE COMPONENTS OF AN ETHICAL DILEMMA

  A. Ethical dilemmas exist because no clear right or wrong answers exist for the question of what one ought to do or how one ought to act in certain situations.
  1. There may be conflicts of duty or a conflict in principles.
  2. Duties of beneficence and nonmaleficence (to do good and avoid harm) can be in conflict with the duty to protect the individual's autonomy (self-determination) when a patient is restrained against his or her will.
  B. Ethics differs from morals in that, for the individual, moral decisions have a clear yes/no, right/wrong answer. If an individual is very clear about what they consider right or wrong and there is no sense of a conflicting possibility, an ethical dilemma does not exist for that person.

ESSENTIAL STEPS IN THE PROCESS OF ETHICAL DECISION-MAKING

  A. Gather relevant information and facts, including a narrative describing the situation. The narrative should include an identification of conflicting duties, rights, beliefs, and cultural, religious, and societal values of the parties involved (Burkhardt, and Nathaniel, 1998).
  B. Identify the stakeholders.
  1. Who are the people involved in the deliberations and decision-making process?
  2. Who holds the authority for making the final decision?
  3. How will the decision be made?
  4. When will the decision be made?
  C. Determine the abilities of the stakeholders to make a decision.
  1. What are the developmental, cognitive, and psychologic states of the individuals who will engage in the decision-making process?
  2. Are these individuals able to engage in a deliberative, reflective process about the issues at stake?
  D. Identify the desired outcome(s).
  1. Which outcomes are acceptable and which are not acceptable?
  2. What are the consequences of each alternative?
  E. Decide upon what action will be taken.
  1. Who will implement the action?
  2. How will the action be implemented?
  3. When will the action be implemented?
  F. Evaluate and reassess the effect of the action taken.
  1. Was the dilemma resolved to the satisfaction of the stakeholders?

2. Has the first action resulted in a situation in which another ethical decision has arisen?

ETHICAL PROBLEMS OF PARTICULAR CONCERN TO AMBULATORY NURSING

A. Maintaining and adhering to standards of care.
   1. Observe for instances of poor judgment and incompetence of caregivers. These may be more difficult to observe in ambulatory care because of the physical design of ambulatory areas, mobility of the patient group, brief length of patient interactions, and the inability to observe the actions of other professional and nonlicensed personnel.
   2. Encourage daily walking rounds through ambulatory areas.
   3. Schedule care conferences on selected groups of patients.
   4. Distribute, analyze, and provide feedback to staff on patient satisfaction surveys.
   5. Perform ongoing chart audits and quality improvement activities.
   6. Designate professional nurse as quality control coordinator.
   7. Educate and expect staff to engage in quality improvement activities.
B. Assess for the delivery of differences of care or treatment, based on the patient's reimbursement sources.
   1. Advocate for necessary equities within patient care system.
   2. Collaborate and network with other health care resources to provide for patient care needs.
C. Protect confidentiality of patient records.
   1. Create system to protect privacy of records that are transferred from one division to another.
   2. Orient and monitor staff to the need for telephone privacy when discussing patients.
   3. Provide for private areas in which to conference with patients, engage in patient education, or discuss treatment plans.
D. Provide for staff mix appropriate to the intensity level of patients by instituting evidence- or research-based staffing pattern designed for ambulatory settings (Haas and Hackbarth, 1995).

THE ROLE OF THE NURSE AS ADVOCATE FOR PATIENT AND FAMILY IN ETHICAL DILEMMAS

In assisting patients and families with ethical dilemmas, the nurse is acting on the principles of beneficence, justice, and fidelity.
A. Educate patients and families about patient rights.
B. Provide a voice for patients and families, especially those unable to articulate their own needs.
C. Identify and articulate ethical concerns as they occur in practice.
D. Assume responsibility to move ethical concerns through to a resolution,

either with the unit or through involvement of an institutional ethics committee.

E. Monitor and evaluate the outcome of actions taken.

ROLE OF NURSE IN WORKING WITH AN ETHICS COMMITTEE

A. Ethics committees serve two major functions within health care organizations.

  1. Education of care providers within institutions regarding the ethical rights of patients, the ethical position of the institution, and the function of the ethics committee.
  2. Consultation on issues brought to the committee.
     a. Inform staff about process for bringing issues to the attention of the committee.
     b. Distribute written documents describing the work and availability of committee to staff and patients.
     c. Select appropriate members for committee, to include nursing, from across all professional caregiver groups.
     d. Observe confidentiality in considering patient issues.

B. Some sources for ethics consultation when an ethics committee does not exist within an organization are:

  1. The *ANA Ethics in Nursing: Position Statements and Guidelines* (1988) (available from the ANA, state nurses' associations, college and university nursing libraries).
  2. Value statements/ethics codes developed and published by specialty organizations, such as AAACN, AACN, AONE and/or colleague consultants from such organizations.
  3. Colleagues in college and university nursing and/or ethics programs with expertise in health care ethics.
  4. Consultants from state nursing organizations.
  5. Colleagues from organizations with ethics committees to advise on how to institute such committees in one's own organization.

REFERENCES

American Nurses' Association (1988): *Ethics in nursing: position statements and guidelines.* Kansas City, MO: Author.

Burkhardt MA, Nathaniel AK (1998): *Ethics & issues in contemporary nursing.* Albany, NY: Delmar.

Edge RS, Groves JR (1994): *The ethics of health care: a guide for clinical practice.* Albany, NY: Delmar.

Gibson C (1993): Underpinnings of ethical reasoning in nursing. *J Adv Nurs* 18:2003-2007.

Haas S, Hackbarth D (1995): Dimensions of the staff nurse role in ambulatory care: part III—using data to design new models of nursing care delivery. *Nurs Econ* 13(4):230-241.

Hall JK (1996): *Nursing ethics and law.* Philadelphia: WB Saunders.

24 Leadership, Inquiry, and Research Utilization

DIANA P. HACKBARTH, PhD, RN

OBJECTIVES
Study of the information presented in this chapter will enable the learner to:

1. Discuss transformational leadership concepts for ambulatory care nursing.

2. Appreciate ongoing inquiry and research utilization as the basis for ambulatory care nursing practice.

3. Describe the planning process for ambulatory care nursing interventions and programs.

4. Explain needs assessment methodologies.

5. Outline the steps for designing ambulatory care nursing interventions and programs.

6. Describe the evaluation process for ambulatory care nursing interventions and programs.

■■ Ambulatory care nurses use leadership skills as they care for individual patients and families, supervise the work of others, and when they use the inquiry and research process to plan and evaluate ambulatory care programs. Nurses must provide leadership within organizations to effect positive change in patient care practices based on scientific evidence. This chapter is designed to provide the ambulatory care nurse with an outline of the specific knowledge and skills needed to understand leadership concepts; value ongoing inquiry and research utilization; and describe needs assessment, program planning, and evaluation methodologies appropriate for ambulatory care nursing. Emphasis is placed on research utilization through the use of evidence-based practice and evaluation of ambulatory care. References include many on-line sources of data that are available through the World Wide Web.

TRANSFORMATIONAL LEADERSHIP IN AMBULATORY CARE

A. Ambulatory care nurses use leadership skills as they care for individual patients and families, supervise the work of others, when they develop programs for patient populations, and when they initiate change in organizations. As pointed out in Chapter 1, ambulatory care nursing is characterized by rapid responses to high volumes of patients in a short time span while dealing with clinical and organizational issues that are not always predictable.

B. Because of the rapidly changing organizational environment, classic transactional theories of leadership that focus on hierarchical structures, personality traits or the status of the leader, or exchange relationships between leaders and subordinates, may have limited usefulness.

C. Newer leadership theories assume situational instability and focus on a process of human relationship-building to provide stability.

   1. Transformational leadership is process-oriented and aimed at congruence between the vision and agenda of both the leader and followers. The role of the leader is to develop people. The leader and followers grow and develop together with a shared vision (Hein, 1998).

   2. No formula or one prescribed set of "right actions" exists for transformational leadership. Rather, the focus is on goals. The proper actions to achieve goals may change from day to day.

   3. A successful leader is able to interpret the situation to others and work collaboratively and creatively to respond to change.

   4. Trust is one constant in transformational leadership. This includes trust in the organization and the trust of the followers in the leader and in themselves.

   5. In order to institute change in ambulatory care organizations, ambulatory care nurses must work collaboratively with many different constituencies/people at different levels of the organization. Desired change will most likely occur when there is consensus in vision.

D. Leadership by nurses is necessary in order to maintain quality, enhance practice, and plan and evaluate ambulatory care nursing interventions and programs.

INQUIRY AND RESEARCH UTILIZATION

A. Inquiry is an ongoing activity of the ambulatory care nurse in which critical thinking skills are developed and used; and in which knowledge is created and transmitted.

B. Inquiry includes the continuous acquisition of disciplinary knowledge, use of a framework to guide ambulatory practice, participation in and conducting clinical and health systems research, and using research findings to guide clinical practice.

C. Design, implementation, and evaluation of ambulatory care nursing interventions are based on scientific evidence from nursing and health care literature and are important components of inquiry and research utilization.

D. Ambulatory care nurses may use inquiry and participate in research in a variety of ways. Nurses ask questions, participate in the research team, and utilize research findings as part of the professional role.

   1. Nurses may serve on boards, committees, or task forces that identify problems/researchable questions within the ambulatory care organiza-

tion, affiliated academic settings, or the community. These questions may be clinical or concerned with the organization and delivery of services.

2. Nurses may serve on institutional review boards (IRBs) for the protection of human subjects.

   a. All institutions that receive federal funds and carry out research must have a formal committee to review research proposals to make sure that the proposed research is conducted ethically and within federal guidelines for the protection of human subjects and the humane treatment of animals. This committee is usually called an Institutional Review Board (IRB), or Human Subjects Committee.

   b. Smaller ambulatory organizations may not have their own IRB or human subjects committee. Nonetheless, nurses should not participate in any research that has not been approved by an authorized IRB (see Chapter 23).

3. Nurses may participate in the research of others either as a subject or as a data collector on the ambulatory research team.

4. Nurses are often the health care provider who are closest to the patient and family and who have the most insight into the day-to-day operations of the ambulatory care organizations. Therefore, nurses often identify researchable clinical questions, point out areas for health services research, and/or come up with suggestions to modify practice, which can be tested in their ambulatory care setting.

5. Nurses prepared at the masters or doctoral level may design and implement ambulatory care nursing and health systems research.

6. All nurses should utilize research findings in clinical practice and use research-based evidence as the basis for designing or modifying ambulatory care nursing interventions and programs.

E. Accessing and using research in ambulatory care.

1. Research utilization: "A process of using research findings as a basis for practice. It encompasses dissemination of scientific knowledge, critique of studies, synthesis of findings, determining applicability of findings, application/implementation of scientific findings in practice, and evaluating the practice change" (Titler, 1998).

2. Evidence-based medicine: "A way of caring for patients, making decisions, and teaching that values being explicit about the integration of high-quality research evidence with pathophysiologic reasoning, caregiver experience, and patient preferences" (Cook, 1998, p. 20).

3. Evidence-based practice (EBP): conscientious and judicious use of current best evidence to guide health care decisions. Levels of evidence range from randomized clinical trials to case reports and expert opinion (Titler, 1998).

4. Rationale for basing ambulatory care nursing interventions on research evidence.

   a. Increased availability and accessibility of research reports, including on-line full text articles from nursing, medicine, and health care.

   b. Refined criteria for appraising research findings.

     c. Risk management concerns; an assumption of decreased risk when ambulatory interventions are supported by research.

     d. Increased interest in improving health care quality.

     e. Increased potential for better outcomes.

     f. Reduction in uncertainty and variability in health care decision-making.

     g. Potential to reduce costs.

     h. Demonstration of the value of ambulatory care nursing.

     i. Potential to increase professional satisfaction.

     j. Increased competitive edge.

5. Key assumptions in evidence-based practice (EBP).

     a. Clinicians directly involved in delivering patient care influence, either positively or negatively, patient outcomes.

     b. Clinicians assume full responsibility for their practice. (In the case of nursing, some aspects of practice are dependent, interdependent, or independent.)

     c. Clinicians draw on, and contribute to, a body of knowledge elucidating best evidence and optimum effectiveness (Kitson, 1997).

6. Levels of evidence: the Agency for Healthcare Research and Quality (AHRQ) is a federal agency that promotes evidence-based practice. AHRQ has developed guidelines to rate the quality of research studies and to develop clinical practice guidelines at www.ahcpr.gov

     a. Rating system used by AHRQ: Level I is the highest level of research that provides the most valid evidence on which to base practice. Level V, case reports and clinical examples, provides the least valid information on which to base practice.

        (1) Level I: meta-analysis of multiple studies.

        (2) Level II: experimental studies.

        (3) Level III: well-designed quasiexperimental studies.

        (4) Level IV: well-designed nonexperimental studies.

        (5) Level V: case reports and clinical examples (Titler, 1998).

7. The National Guideline Clearinghouse (NGC).

     a. The AHRQ, in partnership with the American Association of Health Plans (AAHP) and the American Medical Association (AMA), sponsors a World Wide Web-based National Guideline Clearinghouse (NGC). The NGC is a publicly available electronic repository for clinical practice guidelines and related materials that provides on-line access to guidelines at http://www.guidelines.gov

     b. Criteria for inclusion of guidelines in the NGC.

        (1) The guideline contains systematically developed statements including recommendations, strategies, or information that assists physicians and/or other health care practitioners and patients to make decisions about appropriate health care for specific clinical circumstances. This is in accord with the definition of clinical practice guidelines as set forth by the Institute of Medicine in 1990 (www.nationalacademies.org or www.IOM.edu/).

(2) The guideline was produced under the auspices of medical specialty associations; relevant professional societies; public or private organizations; government agencies at the federal, state, or local level; or health care organizations or plans.

(3) Corroborating documentation can be produced, verifying that a systematic literature search and review of existing scientific evidence published in peer-reviewed journals was performed during the guideline development process.

(4) The guideline is in English, current, and the most recent version (i.e., developed, reviewed, or revised within the last 5 years).

F. Sources of research data to utilize in ambulatory care practice.

1. Nurses who are members of professional organizations such as the American Association of Ambulatory Care Nursing (AAACN) receive peer-reviewed journals and newsletters as a member benefit. These journals are usually specific to the practice area of the nurse and are an excellent source of current information.

2. Ambulatory care organizations, hospitals, and medical centers usually maintain both print libraries and access to on-line databases. On-line databases are available to organizations that have paid for a subscription. Others may be free to the public. Sample databases useful to ambulatory care nurses include:

   a. AIDSLine: a National Library of Medicine database of bibliographic citations focusing on research, clinical aspects, and health policy issues related to AIDS.

   b. Article 1st: index of articles from nearly 13,000 journals in science, technology, medicine, social science, business, the humanities, and popular culture.

   c. BioethicsLine: includes more than 47,000 records of English language materials on bioethics selected from the disciplines of medicine, nursing, biology, philosophy, religion, law, and the behavioral sciences. Selections from popular literature are also included.

   d. CancerLit: covers all aspects of cancer therapy, including experimental and clinical cancer therapy.

   e. CINAHL: provides comprehensive coverage of the English language journal literature for nursing and allied health disciplines.

   f. Dissertation abstracts: dissertation abstracts from a complete range of academic subjects appearing in dissertations accepted at accredited universities.

   g. EBM reviews—Best Evidence: Best Evidence screens the top clinical journals, identifying studies that are both methodologically sound and clinically relevant, and provides an enhanced abstract of the chosen articles, providing a commentary on the value of the article for clinical practice.

   h. EBM reviews—Cochrane Database of Systematic Reviews (COCH): includes the full text of the regularly updated systematic reviews of the effects of health care prepared by The Cochrane Collaboration (www.cochrane.delcc/cochrane/index.htl).

  i. Health and Psychosocial Instruments: a database of evaluation and measurement tools in health and psychosocial studies. Instruments available include questionnaires, checklists, index measures, rating scales, project techniques, tests, and interview schedules.

  j. Health Reference Center—academic: provides access to the full text of nursing and allied health journals, plus a wide variety of personal health information.

  k. Health Reference Center: designed especially for the lay researcher, Health Reference Center is a multi-source, mostly full-text database for health and wellness research.

  l. HealthStar: citations to the published literature on health services, technology, administration, and research. Covers patient outcomes, treatment effectiveness, administration, and many other topics.

3. World Wide Web sample sites with health care information.

 a. Federal government websites.

  (1) National Institutes of Health: www.nih.gov

  (2) Centers for Disease Control: www.cdc.gov

  (3) Department of Health and Human Services: www.dhhs.gov

  (4) Morbidity and Mortality Weekly Report: www.edu.gov/mmwr

  (5) Health Finder: www.healthfinder.gov

 b. Professional associations.

  (1) American Nurses' Association: www.ana.org or www.nursingworld.org

  (2) American Academy of Ambulatory Care Nursing: www.aaacn_assn.org/

  (3) American Medical Association: www.ama.org

  (4) American Academy of Pediatrics: www.aap.org

 c. Voluntary health organizations.

  (1) American Lung Association: www.ala.org or www.lungs.org

  (2) American Heart Association: www.americanheart.org

  (3) American Cancer Society: www.cancer.org

PLANNING AMBULATORY CARE NURSING INTERVENTIONS AND PROGRAMS

A. The goal of planning is to produce the best possible practical plan that will achieve organizational goals and specific program objectives *and* has the support of all the stakeholders (Posavac and Carey, 1997).

B. Strategic planning is the continuous process of systematically evaluating the nature of the ambulatory care organization, defining its long-term objectives, identifying quantifiable goals, developing strategies to reach these objectives and goals and allocating resources to carry out these strategies (Airedale Group, 1998). Strategic planning begins by addressing the following three questions:

 1. Where are we today?

 2. Where are we going?

    3. How do we get there?
- **C.** Situation analysis answers the question: Where are we today?
  - **1.** Do an *external analysis* and analyze ambulatory care as a whole and predict future direction for your particular product or services (i.e., what's the future of pain clinics? Nurse-run anticoagulation clinics? Smoking cessation programs?)
  - **2.** *Analyze internal organization* (i.e., what ambulatory care programs/services are now offered? Are they used? Successful?)
  - **3.** Look at *partners and competitors* who are or could offer similar ambulatory programs (Veney and Kaluzny, 1998).
- **D.** Program planning answers the question: Where are we going?
- **E.** Implementation plans answer the question: How do we get there?
- **F.** Program evaluation answers the question: Have we achieved desired outcomes?
- **G.** General considerations in planning health care programs for ambulatory care.
  - **1.** Proposed program must be consistent with mission of organization and strategic plan.
  - **2.** Proposed program must be consistent with values of all stakeholders (i.e., Board of Directors, regulators, accreditors, administrators, patients, providers, community, general public). For example, genetic testing program may be inconsistent with values of some religious-based ambulatory care institutions.
    - **a.** Various stakeholders often have different values, wants, and agendas.
      - (1) Board of Directors often interested in promoting the mission, image/prestige of an organization as well as its financial vitality.
      - (2) Regulators are mandated to protect safety of public; assure all laws/regulations are followed. They want things "done right."
      - (3) Administrators and managers in ambulatory care want to accomplish the work on time and within budget.
      - (4) Health care providers usually value quality care, servicing needs of clients, autonomy, recognition, job satisfaction, pleasant work environment. They want to do the "right thing for the patient," often regardless of cost.
      - (5) Patients and families want quality care that is accessible, affordable, respectful.
      - (6) Community wants ambulatory services that meet needs of population and are accessible to all in need.
      - (7) Payers want high quality care at low cost (Posavac and Carey, 1997).
    - **b.** Must conduct a stakeholder analysis to be sure proposed intervention or program addresses wants and needs of all stakeholders. Unless stakeholders can come to consensus on a shared vision for the program, conflict may result.
  - **3.** Plan must include consideration of resources needed to support the program (i.e., money, time, staff, space, goodwill of the community, etc.).

4. There should be a theory base to link perceived need, proposed intervention, and clinical outcomes.
5. Proposed program must be evidence-based and include latest clinical practice guidelines as standard of care.
6. Plan should include a monitoring system for both day-to-day management as well as the collection of data to evaluate outcomes.
7. Data captured should be sensitive to nursing inputs (see Chapter 7).
8. Plan should include evaluation criteria and standards to judge success/failure based on program goals and measured outcomes.

NEEDS ASSESSMENT

A. Needs assessment is the first step in planning ambulatory care nursing interventions and programs. It is useless to plan programs that nobody wants, needs, or will utilize.
   1. The impetus to explore the need for new ambulatory care nursing interventions and programs may be triggered by perceived deficits in existing programs, changes in standards and guidelines from national organizations, or the availability of innovations or approaches to care in the literature.
   2. The need for programs that are likely to have significant clinical impact, high fiscal benefit, and are congruent with the organization's mission and strategic plan is worth exploring (McKillip, 1987).
B. Multi-trait/multi-method assessment is the most comprehensive approach to needs assessment for health and human service programs.
   1. Use multiple sources of information.
   2. Use both quantitative and qualitative data from a variety of sources.
   3. Assume each source of data has strengths and weaknesses.
   4. Keep collecting data about need until data sources corroborate each other.
C. Sources of data for needs assessment in ambulatory care.
   1. Census data, vital statistics, and statistical information on population health status is often cheapest and easiest to use because data is regularly collected by local, state, and federal government and regulatory agencies.
      a. Local library, local or state health department, local or state government, special reports, annual statistical information (often available on-line).
      b. Federal government compiles census and health data; most data available on-line. For example, see National Center for Health Statistics at www.cdc.gov/nchs
      c. Problem is that readily available population and health data may be reported for a large area (state or county) and not for the smaller service area of your ambulatory organization. Data may also not be specific to your population characteristics (i.e., pediatric population with diabetes; Hispanic pregnant women; residents within a 20-mile

radius of your clinic). Nurse may need help of expert statistician/ consultant to interpret data for a particular service area or target population.

2. Epidemiologic studies provide information on patterns of health, disease, and injury in populations.

a. Epidemiologic information may be helpful in estimating population health problem and needs in your service area, providing the characteristics of the persons included in the epidemiologic studies (age, race, gender, risk factors, lifestyle, socioeconomic status, access to health care, etc.) are similar to people in your service area.

b. A review of current epidemiologic studies relevant to your current or potential patient population is an important component of needs assessment. Epidemiologic studies may be accessed through the on-line databases listed in section F of the Inquiry and Research Utilization section on pp. 441-442.

3. The Healthy People 2010 Objectives for the Nation (2000) is another source of information on national health priorities and needs.

a. This U.S. government document, available at www.health.gov/ healthypeople, lists two main goals and 26 specific prevention-oriented objectives that could be catalysts for the development of ambulatory care nursing interventions and programs.

b. Goals and objectives point out areas for health promotion, disease and injury prevention, and risk management to promote quality of life. This document can help in assessing needs and planning ambulatory programs for the population groups served by ambulatory organizations.

c. Guidelines for federal funding of health care programs require that organizations address Healthy People 2010 goals and objectives.

d. The levels of prevention model, which is part of the conceptual framework for ambulatory care nursing, underpins our nation's health promotion agenda.

e. Healthy People 2010 goals for the nation.

(1) Increase quality and years of healthy life.

(2) Eliminate racial and ethnic disparities in health, and disparities in health of gender groups, socioeconomically disadvantaged people, disabled people and people of specific age groups.

f. Healthy People 2010 health promotion and disease prevention objectives.

(1) Promote healthy behaviors.

(a) Physical activity and fitness.

(b) Nutrition.

(c) Decrease tobacco use.

(2) Promote healthy and safe communities.

(a) Educational and community-based programs.

(b) Environmental health.

(c) Food safety.

(d) Injury/violence prevention.

> > > (i) Injuries that cut across intent (intentional and unintentional).
> > > (ii) Unintentional injuries.
> > > (iii) Violence and abuse.
> > (e) Occupational safety and health.
> > (f) Oral health.
> (3) Improve systems for personal and public health.
> > (a) Access to quality health services.
> > > (i) Preventive care.
> > > (ii) Primary care.
> > > (iii) Emergency services.
> > > (iv) Long-term care and rehabilitation services.
> > (b) Family planning
> > (c) Maternal, infant, and child health, including the prevention of low birth weight and infant mortality.
> > (d) Medical product safety.
> > (e) Public health infrastructure.
> > (f) Health communication.
> (4) Prevent and reduce diseases and disorders.
> > (a) Arthritis, osteoporosis, and chronic back conditions.
> > (b) Cancer.
> > (c) Diabetes.
> > (d) Disability and secondary conditions.
> > (e) Heart disease and stroke.
> > (f) HIV.
> > (g) Immunization and infectious diseases.
> > (h) Mental health and mental disorders.
> > (i) Respiratory diseases.
> > (j) Sexually transmitted infections.
> > (k) Substance abuse (www.health.gov/healthypeople).

4. A resource inventory documents what ambulatory programs and services already exist in your service area and within competitor/partner organizations. A resource inventory helps determine if there are gaps in ambulatory services your organization could fill (McKillip, 1987).
   a. Sources of data on existing programs include the telephone book; community guides and fact books; existing reports from local governments, voluntary agencies, insurance companies, or the state agency that licenses health facilities. Much of this information is available on-line at your state, county, or community website.
   b. Surveys of providers in area might also be done by telephone or mail to see what services are currently being offered.
5. Client or consumer surveys question people you are already serving in order to get data on how ambulatory services can be modified/improved. Client surveys also help to determine what additional services are desired by current patients/clients and their families.
   a. May collect client data routinely on all clients or a sample of clients annually.

b. May be conducted by mail or telephone survey.

c. Only provides information on the needs/wants of those already served, not potential clients who might use your ambulatory care services.

6. Citizen surveys seek data on the need for a program from the community/people living in your service area who might potentially use the program.
   a. Mail or telephone survey to sample of households. Select by zip code or telephone area code within service area.
   b. Need a high level of skill and assistance of experts in survey research to select sample, design questionnaire, conduct survey, analyze and weigh results.
   c. Expensive, time consuming.
   d. Often the most educated, informed persons respond to surveys, so could leave out the most needy, potential users of ambulatory care services (McKillip, 1987).

7. Key informants are people who have the knowledge and ability to report on community needs. They are an excellent source of data about both the need for services and potential acceptability of various types of programs (McKillip, 1987).
   a. Health care providers, community leaders, social service providers, police, government officials, teachers, business people, clergy, often have unique knowledge of the needs of people in your service area.
   b. Interview in person, telephone, or mail survey.

8. Forming structured groups to find out about perceived needs for ambulatory services can be very helpful in assessing needs and acceptability of proposed programs.
   a. Could include clients, key informants, citizens.
   b. Focus groups: 6 to 10 people, homogenous; tape record, 1 to 2 hours, to query about both perceived needs and the acceptability of possible programs (i.e., would pregnant women use nurse-midwifery services? How far would senior citizens travel for cardiac rehabilitation services?)
   c. Nominal groups are highly structured groups that use a set format of procedures to gain information. Can use varied participants to get a variety of viewpoints using nominal group techniques (McKillip, 1987).
   d. Delphi panels are another type of group that does not meet in person. Rather, use mail or e-mail contact with a panel of experts to get input on needs and potential solutions (McKillip, 1987).

9. Public forums are open meetings to discuss needs and possible interventions.
   a. May be required by law (i.e., certificate of need regulations; required meetings under state or local "open meetings" legislation).
   b. Can be used to facilitate communication and good public relations.
   c. Need to plan/structure so both fair and orderly. Set up sign-in sheets, time frame for speaking, accept written testimony, plan for crowd

control/maintain order if program may generate controversy. For example, would residents around your ambulatory care clinic support an outpatient drug treatment program?

    d. May raise expectations that something will be done. Can produce ill will if organization does not follow through with implementing a program.

D. Using data generated by needs assessment, identify gaps in ambulatory services and needs that could potentially be filled by a new intervention or program. Only after a need has been identified can the planning process proceed.

DESIGNING AMBULATORY CARE NURSING PROGRAMS AND INTERVENTIONS

A. Write program goals and objectives based on mission of organization, strategic plan, results of needs assessment, and documentation from the literature on best practices and evidence-based practice. This is usually best accomplished by a small group of stakeholders working collaboratively with a shared vision of needs and desired outcomes.

B. Consider a small-scale pilot project if organization has time/resources before committing to a full-scale program.

C. Enumerate the things that must get done in order for the program to be operational. Examples include:

    1. Securing agreements and contracts, exploring legal aspects of proposed program, licensing, permits, certificate of need.

    2. Developing a budget and securing funding.

    3. Securing space, purchasing equipment and supplies.

    4. Establishing policy and procedures, designing forms.

    5. Developing accounting, budgeting, and management information systems.

    6. Set standards and criteria for evaluation.

    7. Hiring and training of personnel.

    8. Plan marketing, etc. (DiLima and Schust, 1997).

D. Determine what needs to be done first and what items or processes must be in place before others can start.

E. Develop timeline charts. Several computer programs allow the user to list tasks in order and then print out a timeline.

F. Carry out tasks outlined in timeline; make corrections as needed.

G. Implement the ambulatory care program when all components are in place.

EVALUATING AMBULATORY CARE PROGRAMS

A. Program evaluation is an applied social science aimed at the improvement of human services. Program evaluation is a systematic collection and analysis of information using various methods in order to determine:

    1. Whether an ambulatory service is needed.

2. Whether an ambulatory service is being provided as planned (i.e., monitoring program operations. Do activities occur on time, in the manner expected, at the budgeted cost?)
3. Whether the ambulatory service is meeting identified needs of the target population.
4. Whether desired health outcomes are achieved (i.e., impact).
5. Whether the service is cost effective and sustainable (Posavac and Carey, 1997).

B. Why evaluate ambulatory care interventions and programs?
1. Accountability to funders, providers, and public.
2. Fulfill accreditation requirements.
3. Obtain information to improve the program.
4. Help administrators make decisions about how best to use resources.
5. To assure the quality of care.
6. Good outcomes can be used for marketing the program and attracting new clients.
7. To justify costs and use of resources.
8. To learn about unintended consequences, both positive and negative.
9. To see if health outcomes are achieved.
10. To contribute to the scientific knowledge base on ambulatory care nursing effectiveness.

C. Types of program evaluation (Posavac and Carey, 1997).
1. Evaluation of need: needs assessment.
2. Evaluation of structure: evaluating the extent to which necessary components/resources are available to support the program and safe patient care.
3. Evaluation of process: evaluating the extent to which the program has been implemented as planned.
   a. Formative evaluation (process evaluation) is ongoing during program operation. The objective is to provide feedback so the program can be modified in its early stages.
   b. Monitoring is the comparison between program operation and expectations. It is a continuous process of collecting and analyzing data to learn about program processes and improve operations.
   c. Case reports, qualitative studies, clinical examples, nonexperimental and quasiexperimental designs can be used in process evaluation.
   d. Sources of information for evaluating program processes can include: management information systems; chart reviews; existing reports; observations of program operation; checklists; interviews of clients, staff, providers; questionnaires; and quality assurance (QA) or total quality management/ continuous quality improvement (TQM/ CQI) data.
   e. Most national accrediting agencies, such as the Joint Commission on Accreditation of Healthcare Organizations (JCAHO) and the National Commission on Quality Assurance (NCQA) consider monitoring of program processes extremely important in assessing quality.

    f. Evidence that the program has been implemented as planned, or its modification documented, must be established *before* attempts are made to link the program as implemented with outcomes.

4. Evaluation of outcomes: impact. Evaluation of what has occurred as a result of the program.

    a. Outcome or impact evaluation seeks to determine what changes in knowledge, attitudes, behaviors, risk factors, health status, morbidity, or mortality can be linked to the ambulatory care intervention in a cause-and-effect relationship.

    b. Most evaluations done in ambulatory care as part of routine management or QA functions do not have the rigorous research designs to reach the level of evaluation research or Levels I, II, or III of the AHRQ guidelines to the quality of research studies and to develop clinical practice guidelines. However, these program evaluations are useful in providing managers and practitioners information to update, modify, or change programs to better serve clients.

    c. Rigorous evaluation research involves experimental designs, clinical trials, and field trials that include randomization of program participants into intervention and control groups and strict control over program implementation, data gathering, etc., so that true differences, if they exist, can be detected.

        (1) Internal validity: did the intervention as implemented cause the effect that was measured for the specific persons observed in this particular setting?

        (2) External validity: can the results of this ambulatory intervention be generalized to similar patient populations in other settings?

    d. Rigorous research designs must be used in order to validly link ambulatory care interventions with observed outcomes/impacts. Program evaluation designs that have the potential to demonstrate a causal link between an intervention and outcomes include:

        (1) Certain types of quasiexperimental designs (AHRQ Level III).

        (2) Experimental designs, randomized clinical trials (AHRQ Level II).

        (3) Field trials.

    e. Impact evaluation is increasingly included in NCQA and JCAHO accreditation. Policy makers, funders and the general public want to know the impact of ambulatory programs. Outcome data will be increasingly important to funders and consumers in the future.

    f. Data used to determine best practices, evidence-based medicine, and clinical practice guidelines is based on meta-analysis of program evaluations using experimental designs, randomized clinical trials, and field trials whenever possible.

5. Evaluation of efficiency: what is the cost of outcomes achieved in terms of time, money, resources, etc.? For example, a successful ambulatory care nursing program that requires a great amount of resources may simply not be a good choice if similar outcomes can be achieved with less resources.

   a. Costs of programs can be determined by examining the program budget and adding up the value of all input/resources used in the program. This is usually not as simple or straightforward as it sounds, especially if personnel, space, resources are shared with other programs. It is also difficult if accounting systems cannot generate accurate cost data at the program level.

   b. Cost-effectiveness analysis is a methodology for estimating program productivity under different scenarios.

      (1) Assume amount of money to be spent is fixed; choose among alternative ambulatory programs with different benefits for the same cost. Example: A program has $15,000 to spend on smoking-related programs. What is a better use of money, a smoking prevention program in the schools or a smoking cessation clinic at the Senior Center?

      (2) Assume goal (outcome) desired is fixed; examine different ambulatory programs with different costs to achieve desired outcome. Example: Should we staff our primary care clinic with three nurse practitioners and one doctor or two doctors and an LPN?

      (3) Assume fixed ambulatory program; examine outcomes at various levels of the program. Example: Should our family practice clinic stay open three or five nights per week?

   c. Cost-benefit analysis—answers question: Should we? Ought we? Cost benefit analysis attempts to provide a scientific process to make judgments based on values under conditions of uncertainty.

      (1) Cost-benefit analysis is extremely complex both conceptually and methodologically because it requires the identification of all possible impacts of an activity—current and future, direct and indirect, probable/possible, intended and unintended.

      (2) Also requires the monetization of possible benefits, including such intangibles as feelings of well-being, a healthy baby, long life, etc.

      (3) For health care, cost-benefit analysis may require putting a price on human life, something some people consider priceless. Example: How should we ration organs in our transplant program?

6. Program evaluation data may be used internally within an ambulatory care organization to modify, strengthen, or improve a program or to justify discontinuation of a program that does not achieve desired processes or outcomes. Well-designed evaluation studies that meet AHRQ standards for scientific research may be published and shared with others and contribute to the scientific knowledge base on ambulatory care nursing effectiveness.

REFERENCES

Airedale Group. (1998). *Handbook of strategic planning.* Sydney: The University of Sydney. www.oac.usyd.edu

Cook D (1998): Evidence-based critical care medicine: a political tool for change. *New Horizons* 6(1):20-25.

DiLima S, Schust C (1997): *Community health education and promotion.* Gaithersburg, MD: Aspen.

Hein E (1998): *Contemporary leadership behavior,* ed 5. Philadelphia: JB Lippincott.

Kitson A (1997): Using evidence to demonstrate the value of nursing. *Nursing Standard* 11(28):34-39.

McKillip J (1987): *Need analysis: tools for human services and education.* Beverly Hills, CA: Sage.

Posavac E, Carey R (1997): *Program evaluation methods and case studies,* ed 5. Upper Saddle River, NJ: Prentice Hall.

Titler M (1998): Evidence-based practice and research utilization . . . one and the same? Unpublished. 1998 Pre-Convention Research Utilization Conference. Evidence Based Nursing Practice. June 26, 1998.

US Department of Health and Human Services (2000): *Healthy People 2010 Conference Edition.* Washington, D.C.: Author.

Veney J, Kaluzny A (1998): *Evaluation and decision making for health services,* ed 3. Chicago: Health Administration Press.

25 Regulatory Compliance and Risk Management

CANDIA BAKER LAUGHLIN, MS, RN, Cm

OBJECTIVES
Study of the information presented in this chapter will enable the learner to:

1. Describe regulatory standards that apply to the practice of ambulatory care nursing, including federal and state statutes, and accreditation standards of the Joint Commission on Accreditation of Healthcare Organizations (JCAHO), the National Committee for Quality Assurance (NCQA), and the Accreditation Association for Ambulatory Health Care (AAAHC).

2. Discuss key principles of risk management in the ambulatory care setting.

■■ The quality of the services provided in the ambulatory health care setting are subject to external monitoring by government agencies, third party payers, consumer groups, and the legal system of our society. The ambulatory care nurse is accountable to these groups and to individual patients/families to monitor performance and measure outcomes of care delivery against standards; exercise processes for ongoing improvement; and maintain a system of checks and balances for prevention, detection, and management of problems and errors in care delivery. Additionally, health care organizations and nurses who work for them are responsible for self-assessment to reduce risks to patients, visitors, and staff; to ensure high quality of care; and to minimize potential legal and financial liability.

REGULATORY REQUIREMENTS

Regulatory requirements are generated by federal and state legislative acts, by requirements of official agencies representing the public and the purchasers of health care services, and by standards of professional organizations.

    A. Occupational Safety and Health Administration (OSHA) has a set of federal workplace statutes that are monitored by compliance inspections. The following are some of the more significant statues that apply to the ambulatory care setting.

1. The employer is responsible for ensuring safety of employees and the public from blood-borne pathogens (OSHA, 1996).
   a. Standard Precautions will be observed to prevent contact with blood or other potentially infectious materials.
   b. Personal protective equipment will be provided and the employer will ensure that employees use it appropriately.
   c. Contaminated work surfaces will be decontaminated with an appropriate disinfectant after completion of procedures.
   d. Containers for contaminated sharps will be readily accessible and not overfilled.
   e. Regulated medical waste will be placed in containers that are closable, leak-proof during transport, and color-coded or labeled for ready identification.
   f. Hepatitis B vaccine will be available at no cost to all employees with occupational exposure.
   g. Postexposure medical evaluation and follow-up will be provided at no cost to all employees.
   h. Following an exposure, the identified source of the exposure will have his/her blood tested as soon as feasible to determine hepatitis B and HIV infectivity. (If the source is known to be infected with hepatitis B or HIV, tests need not be repeated). If consent for testing cannot be obtained, many states permit testing of the source individual's blood without consent.
   i. Warning labels will be affixed to containers of regulated waste, refrigerators, and freezers containing blood or other potentially infectious material.
2. Measures are taken to prevent the transmission of *Mycobacterium tuberculosis* (OSHA, 1996).
   a. When feasible, occupational exposure to aerosolized *M. tuberculosis* should be prevented by accepted engineering measures (e.g., ventilation).
   b. When effective engineering controls are not feasible, respiratory protection equipment or devices will be provided and employees trained in their use.
   c. The respiratory protective equipment must meet specific standards, and may require fit testing.
3. The employer is responsible for communication about hazards—employees' "right to know" the hazards and identities of chemicals, and the protective measures to prevent exposure (OSHA, 1996).
   a. All hazardous materials must be labeled with identifying information that will link with the Material Safety Data Sheet (MSDS) for the material, either the common/trade name or a chemical name. Also, a brief statement of the hazardous effect of the chemical (e.g., "flammable," "causes lung damage") is required. (Note that this requirement also applies to materials transferred to a secondary container.)
   b. Material Safety Data Sheets provided by the manufacturer must be readily accessible to employees in their work area.

      c. Each employee who may be exposed to hazardous chemicals at work must be provided information and training at the time of assignment and whenever there is a change in the hazards. The training includes the potential risks, safe handling, and what to do in the event of an exposure or spillage.

      d. Potential carcinogens are subject to specific OSHA regulations and may require special handling, environmental monitoring, and health screening of employees (e.g., formalin, ethylene oxide).

   4. The employer will provide medical services and first aid to employees for consultation and advice on matters of occupational health.

   5. The employer will maintain a log and summary of recordable occupational injuries and illnesses and make it available within 6 working days after receiving information that a recordable injury or illness has occurred.

B. Americans with Disabilities Act (ADA) of 1990 prohibits discrimination in the rendering of health care services or the process of employment based on a disability (42 USCA section 12182).

   1. Individuals may not be denied full access to goods, services, facilities, privileges, advantages, and accommodation by any place considered an organization of public accommodation or public services because of a handicap (USCA 12182[a]).

      a. Handicap includes any disability.

      b. Physical barriers must be removed from facilities.

      c. Communication barriers must be resolved for patient instructions and informed consent.

   2. If the rendering of care poses sufficient risks to both the patient and provider, eligibility requirements may be necessary to determine the appropriateness of a patient receiving a particular treatment or procedure (e.g., transplantation of organs) (42 USCA 12182[b]2).

   3. *Disability* means:

      a. a physical or mental impairment that substantially limits one or more major life activities,

      b. a record of such impairment, or

      c. being regarded as having such an impairment (42 USCA 12102 [2]).

   4. Individuals with HIV infection were intended to be regarded as disabled under the ADA legislation, and this interpretation has been upheld by federal courts.

C. State legislation and regulations. State government agencies have a variety of policy approaches for regulating the health care provided to the public.

   1. Licensing and regulation.

      a. State practice acts define the scope of practice of health professionals, including physicians, nurses, and pharmacists.

      b. Misconduct by health professionals must be reported to the state and may result in disciplinary action, including restrictions of an individual's license.

      c. States regulate the storage, prescribing, and dispensing of medications, including federally regulated scheduled substances.

  d. Hospitals and other health facilities are licensed by the state. Some states require a Certificate of Need for health facilities to expand or add major capital equipment.

 2. State regulation of managed care (Hackey, 1998).

  a. Many states have been authorized by the federal government to enroll their Medicaid beneficiaries in managed care plans.

  b. The internal operations of managed care organizations have a number of statutory requirements to ensure continuity and quality of health services (Aspen, 1998), including:

   (1) Quality assurance.

   (2) Utilization review.

   (3) Marketing of the managed care plan.

   (4) Changes in corporate structure (e.g., mergers, dissolutions).

   (5) Open enrollment.

   (6) Protection of enrollees against financial insolvency of the plan.

   (7) Liability.

D. Joint Commission on Accreditation of Healthcare Organizations (JCAHO) is an independent, not-for-profit organization that establishes and assesses compliance with standards of quality for health care services (JCAHO, 1998).

 1. JCAHO provides accreditation of health care organizations and produces a Joint Commission Performance Report, which is a public summary of accreditation findings.

 2. JCAHO surveys and accredits health care organizations using one of several sets of standards, such as the Comprehensive Accreditation Manual for Ambulatory Care Organizations, the Comprehensive Accreditation Manual for Health Care Networks, and the Comprehensive Accreditation Manual for Hospitals.

 3. JCAHO reviews the organization's activities in response to medical errors (sentinel events) to promote root cause analysis and learning across organizations to reduce the risk of occurrences. A sentinel event is an unexpected occurrence involving death or serious physical or psychologic injury, or risk thereof. Examples may include infant abductions, surgery on the wrong patient or body part, hemolytic transfusion reaction, and suicide of an inpatient. The organization has some latitude in setting the specific parameters around sentinel events.

 4. Most sets of JCAHO standards are organized into the following functional areas (some sets have additional specific standards, such as Health Promotion and Disease Prevention standards for Health Care Networks) (JCAHO, 1996):

  a. Patient rights and organization ethics (RI).

  b. Assessment of patients (PE).

  c. Care of patients (TX).

  d. Education of patients and families (PF).

  e. Continuum of care (CC).

  f. Improving organizational performance (PI).

  g. Leadership (LD).

    h. Management of the environment of care (EC).

    i. Management of human resources (HR).

    j. Management of information (IM).

    k. Surveillance, prevention, and control of infections (IC).

5. The ambulatory care nurse should be aware of the following JCAHO standards commonly assessed in an ambulatory care setting.

    a. Informed consent is obtained for invasive or high-risk procedures (RI).

    b. Patients with advance directives have that information on their medical record (RI).

    c. Patient care and information management protect confidentiality, verbal, auditory, and written (RI).

    d. Patients undergoing an operative or other procedure are monitored physiologically (e.g., national standards for monitoring with conscious sedation are applied) (PE).

    e. Training and orientation demonstrate staff competence in performance of tests and use of equipment (PE).

    f. Suspected victims of abuse and neglect are identified and assessed, and their special care needs are addressed (PE).

    g. Medications are ordered, procured, stored, and dispensed according to law and regulation (e.g., sample drugs are labeled when dispensed, controlled substances are counted and secured, and cytotoxic drugs are safely stored and prepared) (TX).

    h. A medication recall system is in place, including a system for recalling sample drugs (TX).

    i. Patients and families receive education tailored to address the patient's needs, abilities, learning preferences, and readiness to learn, and documentation reflects this (PF).

    j. Patients are educated about pain management.

    k. Patient care and patient education are coordinated among health professionals and across settings (CC) (PF).

    l. Interdisciplinary and collaborative performance improvement is conducted in a planned and systematic method, and leadership is involved (PI).

    m. Data is collected about the appropriateness of care; quality control activities; risk management; and significant events, including adverse drug reactions, medication errors, and transfusion reactions (PI).

    n. Outcomes of care are monitored. The Oryx™ data is collected and analyzed and the organization responds appropriately to the findings, both with clinical and administrative actions (PI).

    o. Management plans are in place for safety and security, control of hazardous materials, disasters and emergencies affecting the environment of care, and maintenance of medical equipment (EC).

    p. Fire drills are conducted at least quarterly in all buildings where patients are housed or treated, and staff are knowledgeable about their roles in the event of fire (EC). Free-standing buildings classified as business occupancies need participate in only one drill annually.

q. Licensed independent practitioners are credentialed and privileged (this may include advanced practice nurses, depending upon the state practice act recognition of these practitioners as independent and the role they are employed to exercise) (HR).

r. The competence of all staff to do their work is continually assessed, maintained, and improved (HR).

s. Orientation and ongoing development is provided to staff (HR).

t. Staffing is adequate for the volume and intensity of the work (HR).

u. Data and information are maintained in a confidential and secure manner (IM).

v. A summary list of significant diagnoses, procedures, drug allergies, and medications is maintained for patients receiving continuing care and is initiated by the third visit (IM).

w. Endemic and epidemic nosocomial infection risks are managed and minimized (e.g., tuberculin testing program, segregation of potentially communicable patients from others in the waiting areas) (IC).

x. Staff follow policies and procedures for infection control, including the separation of clean and dirty materials, the application of body substance precautions, and the cleaning and disinfection of equipment and work areas (IC).

E. National Committee for Quality Assurance (NCQA).

1. NCQA is a not-for-profit, independent organization that assesses, evaluates, and publicly reports on the quality of managed care organizations (MCOs).

2. NCQA accreditation program provides performance-based evaluations of how well an MCO manages all parts of its delivery system—their administrative offices, physicians and other providers, hospitals, ambulatory care settings, and other sources of service.

3. The MCO may delegate authority for performing some NCQA-required functions to another entity, such as the ambulatory care facility or physician group.

4. The NCQA standards (NCQA, 1998) fall into the following categories:

a. Quality improvement (QI).

b. Utilization management (UM).

c. Credentialing and recredentialing (CR).

d. Members' rights and responsibilities (RR).

e. Preventive health guidelines (PH).

f. Medical records (MR).

5. The ambulatory care nurse should be aware of the following standards commonly assessed in the ambulatory care setting.

a. Access standards are monitored for improvement opportunities, including preventive appointments, routine primary care appointments, urgent care appointments, emergency care, after-hours care, and telephone service (QI).

    b. Member satisfaction is assessed and improvement strategies are implemented (QI).

    c. Members with chronic conditions are identified and services and programs are offered to assist in management of these conditions (QI).

    d. Clinical practice guidelines for acute and chronic care are adopted and disseminated, and performance is measured against guidelines (QI).

    e. At least three meaningful clinical issues are assessed, evaluated, and improved as indicated, to detect problems related to utilization and/or continuity and coordination (QI).

    f. If the MCO has a restricted drug formulary, an exception policy exists for prescription drugs not included (UM).

    g. Qualified health professionals assess the clinical information used to support utilization management decisions (UM).

    h. The MCO credentials and recredentials MDs, DOs, DDSs, DPMs, DCs, and other licensed independent practitioners with whom it contracts or employs who treat members outside the inpatient setting (CR).

    i. Members' rights to dignity and privacy are protected (RR).

    j. Members are involved in decision-making and the full discussion of options (RR).

    k. Prevention, early detection, and frequency of services are identified for each age group, and are based on scientific evidence (PH).

    l. Procedures for handling medical information protect confidentiality (MR).

    m. Critical criteria are present on the member's medical record, including problem list, allergies, history, diagnoses, treatment plans, and appropriate treatment (MR).

6. NCQA sponsors and maintains Health Plan Employer Data and Information Set (HEDIS).*

7. HEDIS is a set of standardized performance measures designed to assure that purchasers and consumers have the information they need to reliably compare the performance of MCOs.

8. In 1999, NCQA incorporated HEDIS measures into the accreditation process.

9. HEDIS assesses the quality of health plans across eight categories or domains.

    a. Effectiveness of care.

    b. Access to/availability of care.

    c. Satisfaction with experience of care.

    d. Cost of care.

    e. Stability of the health plan.

    f. Informed health care choices.

---

*HEDIS® is a registered trademark of the National Committee for Quality Assurance (NCQA).

    g. Use of services.

    h. Health plan descriptive information.

  10. Examples of performance measures in HEDIS important to the ambulatory care nurse include the following (NCQA, 1998):

    a. Vaccination rates for children and adolescents.

    b. Well child visits.

    c. Frequency of ongoing prenatal care.

    d. Utilization of services and readmissions for mental health and chemical dependency.

    e. Outpatient medication usage (e.g., asthma).

    f. Influenza vaccines for older and high-risk adults.

    g. Telephone access.

F. Accreditation Association for Ambulatory Health Care (AAAHC) (AAAHC, 1997).

  1. The AAAHC offers voluntary non-governmental, peer-based review of the quality of health care services of organizations such as ambulatory care clinics, physician and dental group practices, HMOs, procedure centers, and similar facilities.

  2. Accreditation is based on a careful assessment of the organization's compliance with applicable standards.

  3. AAAHC does not release information to the public about accreditation survey findings, but may release information about an ambulatory surgery center to Health Care Financing Administration (HCFA) if required for Medicare reimbursement.

  4. Core standards will be applied to all types of organizations being surveyed, and adjunct chapters will apply to specific types of services provided (e.g., urgent care centers, radiation oncology centers, and occupational health providers). The core standards include:

    a. Rights of patients (RP).

    b. Governance (G).

    c. Administration (A).

    d. Quality of care provided (QC).

    e. Quality management and improvement (QM).

    f. Clinical records (CR).

    g. Professional improvement (PI).

    h. Facilities and environment (FE).

  5. The ambulatory care nurse should be aware of the following standards commonly assessed in the ambulatory care setting:

    a. Information is available to patients regarding their rights, their responsibilities, the services offered, the provisions for after-hours care, fees, and payment procedures (RP).

    b. Patients have the right to privacy and to confidentiality in the management of their information (RP).

    c. Patients have the right to participate in decisions regarding their health care (RP).

    d. The governing body appoints and reappoints, assigns, or curtails clinical privileges for practitioners. The process has characteristics similar to those required by NCQA (mentioned earlier) and also requires peer evaluation (G).

e. Personnel policies define responsibilities of staff, require qualifications related to the responsibilities, and require periodic performance appraisals, including current competence (A).

f. Patient satisfaction with services and facilities is periodically assessed and acted upon by the governing body, as indicated (A).

g. Patients are contacted appropriately about significant problems or test results (QC).

h. Health care services are accessible, appropriate, and timely, and include treatment and testing appropriate to the working diagnosis (QC).

i. Referrals and consultations are appropriate and timely, and provide for continuity (QC).

j. Provisions are made for communication with patients in the patient's primary language (QC).

k. An organized process of peer review is conducted as part of the quality management program (QM).

l. Important aspects of care are monitored in an ongoing manner, and data are evaluated to identify trends that influence outcomes of patient care (QM).

m. The organization has a quality improvement program for identifying problems and improving processes (QM).

n. A risk-management program is maintained to protect the welfare of the organization's patients and employees (QM).

o. Patients' clinical information is accessible to authorized practitioners during hours of operation (CR).

p. Patient information is protected from unauthorized disclosure (CR).

q. If the patient's record is complex and lengthy, a summary will list past surgical procedures and past and current diagnoses or problems (CR).

r. Absence or presence of drug reactions or allergies are recorded prominently (CR).

s. Staff receive adequate orientation and training and access to reference and educational materials and programs (PI).

t. The facilities comply with local and state fire regulations, as well as applicable federal regulations (e.g., ADA, OSHA) (FE).

u. Staff have training and appropriate equipment to address internal and external emergencies (FE).

v. Facilities are clean and procedures minimize the risk of transmission of infections (FE).

RISK MANAGEMENT

Risk management in ambulatory care is an organized set of activities designed to assess and reduce risks to patients, visitors, and staff; to ensure high quality of care; and to minimize potential liability (Kavaler and Spiegel, 1997).

A. The risk management process has five progressive steps (Kavaler and Spiegel, 1997).

1. Identifying potential risks of exposure to accidental loss to the institution, analyzing past experiences and current exposure, considering:
   a. Severity of harm.
   b. Number that may be harmed.
   c. Likelihood or frequency of occurrence.
2. Examining feasible options for managing the potential exposures.
3. Selecting risk management options.
4. Implementing the chosen techniques.
5. Monitoring the chosen techniques to determine effectiveness.

B. Health care organizations generally commit resources to risk management personnel to advise and educate, generate policy, monitor data, oversee credentialing and analyze adverse events.

C. The nurse can minimize the risk of safety, legal, and ethical concerns of patients, families, and others in many ways, including:

1. Respecting the dignity and worth of individuals, and applying ethical and moral concepts to promote care (American Academy of Ambulatory Care Nursing, 2000).
2. Assuring that patients have information about their rights and responsibilities in the health care system.
3. Practicing within the acceptable standards of practice.
   a. Applying up-to-date knowledge in care delivery.
   b. Documenting completely and accurately.
   c. Knowing the limits of one's scope of practice and expertise and referring appropriately.
4. Using due care in maintaining equipment and facilities.
5. Delegating appropriately to others.
6. Assuring the patient and family understand the diagnosis and treatment process, and their role in the process.
7. Avoiding making statements that could be interpreted as an admission of negligence or malpractice.
8. Providing the patient and family with information about the cost of care.
9. Avoiding using the medical record as a place to reflect conflicts.
10. Responding to complaints in a timely manner.
11. Promptly reporting incidents and adverse patient occurrences (APOs) to line managers and to the risk management officials.
    a. Some states and third parties require reporting of specific lists of APOs, including sentinel events (refer to Regulatory Requirements, D,4).
    b. Inconsistencies in operations or care that may or do result in an accident or injury should be documented.
    c. Incident report documentation provides an informational base from which corrective or preventive action can be taken.
12. Providing patients a mechanism to voice opinions without recrimination, and to have the issues reviewed and resolved, to the extent possible.

13. Participating in quality improvement and other corrective actions to reduce sources of risk.
  D. Health care organizations must manage risks of potentially violating laws or regulations or standards of professional organizations, such as the regulatory standards described previously in this chapter.
  E. Health care organizations must also manage risks as an employer, including worker's compensation, sexual harassment, affirmative action, and Americans with Disabilities Act.
  F. Health care organizations evaluate potential financial losses and determine the appropriate insurance options as part of the risk management plan.

REFERENCES

Accreditation Association for Ambulatory Health Care (1997): *Accreditation handbook for ambulatory health care.* Skokie, IL: Author.

American Academy of Ambulatory Care Nursing (2000): *Ambulatory care nursing administrative and practice standards.* Pitman, NJ: Jannetti.

Aspen Health Law Center (1998): *Managed care state regulation.* Rockville, MD: Aspen.

Hackey R (1998): *Rethinking health care policy: the new politics of state regulation.* Washington, DC: Georgetown University Press.

Joint Commission on Accreditation of Healthcare Organizations (JCAHO) (1996): *Comprehensive accreditation manual for ambulatory care.* Oakbrook Terrace, IL: Author.

JCAHO (1996): *Comprehensive accreditation manual for health care networks.* Oakbrook Terrace, IL: Author.

JCAHO (1998): *Comprehensive accreditation manual for health care networks.* Oakbrook Terrace, IL: Author.

JCAHO (2000): *Comprehensive accreditation manual for hospitals.* Oakbrook Terrace, IL: Author.

Kavaler F, Spiegel A (1997): *Risk management in health care institutions.* London: Jones and Bartlett.

National Committee for Quality Assurance (1997): *HEDIS 3.0: Health plan employer data and information set, Version 3.0.* Washington, DC: Author.

National Committee for Quality Assurance (1998): *Standards for the accreditation of managed care organizations.* Washington, DC: Author.

Occupational Safety and Health Administration, US Department of Labor (1996): *OSHA Regulations (Standards—29 CFR).* Washington, DC: Author.

US Congress (1990): *Americans with Disabilities Act of 1990, S.933.*

26 Staff Development

LINDA BRIXEY, RN
CATHERINE TURNER, MSN, FNP, RN
JANE W. SWANSON, MS, RN, CNAA

OBJECTIVES

Study of the information presented in this chapter will enable the learner to:

1. Discuss self-care barriers and resources.
2. Describe professional growth and development needs.
3. Explain professional organization membership benefits.
4. Discuss continuing professional education using traditional and distance learning methods.

■■ Staff development for the professional nurse entails a broad arsenal of tools. Nurturing and developing of the professional nurse utilizes knowledge and use of self-care skills. Many educational avenues are available to the nurse. Inservices, professional books and journals, continuing nursing education (CNE) programs, and mentoring by more experienced nurses are a few options available. These all work to improve skills and develop a broader knowledge base. One must recognize the importance of continual learning to meet the constantly changing demands of the ambulatory care setting in which one works. Active involvement in professional organizations can facilitate professional growth and expertise. Professional organizations provide a forum for the introduction of new benchmarks for changes and promote networking opportunities. Continuing professional education, whether in the traditional classroom setting or through distance learning, permits the professional nurse to expand his or her role in nursing.

SELF-CARE PRACTICES AND BARRIERS

Self-care practices used by the nurse promote harmony in mind, body, and spirit. They also aid in the prevention of illness related to depletion of energy from stressors. Skills in making rapid decisions on what must be fixed, nurtured, or jettisoned to remove patient-care barriers and pressures from self are essential. These decisions enhance holistic care to others and self, providing harmony.

    A. Levels of balance.
        1. Harmony: maximum potential of wellness and balance in the mental, physical, and spiritual dimensions of self-care (Dossey, et al., 1995).
        2. Stressed or out-of-balance.

      a. Eastern philosophy definitions: absence of inner peace.

      b. Western culture: loss of control or harmony between mind, body, or spiritual well-being (Seaward, 1997).

    3. Wound healer: term used to describe individual who has recognized strengths and weaknesses and able to assist with greater self-knowledge (Achterberg, 1990).

B. Self-discovery of traits that can sabotage balance.

    1. Rushed or hurried lifestyle (sometimes called Type A personality).

      a. Extended work hours.

      b. Time urgency: preoccupied with time and impatient regarding waiting.

      c. Polyphasia: engaged in multiple thoughts or activities at one time.

      d. Ultra-competitiveness: comparing self with others to the point that peers considered a threat.

      e. Rapid speech pattern: often finish sentences for other people.

      f. Manipulative control: influences others or promotes one-upmanship.

      g. Hyperaggressiveness and free-floating hostility: need to dominate others, free-floating anger erupts at trivial occurrences.

      h. Low self-esteem and perception of self-worth based on other's perceptions.

    2. Codependent traits: individuals dependent on making others dependent on them as a means of self-validation.

      a. Traits developed in early childhood in a lifestyle or environment that is chaotic, unpredictable, or threatening.

      b. Ardent approval seekers: seeking approval or feedback to validate efforts.

      c. Perfectionist: extremely well organized and in the habit of going beyond the requirements in every task.

      d. Super-overachievers: involvement in an abundance of activities and obligated to do it all well.

      e. Crisis manager: thrive on crisis and constantly trying to make order out of chaos.

      f. Devoted loyalist: extreme loyalty to friends and family possibly from fear of rejection or abandonment.

      g. Self-sacrificing martyr: puts everyone else first to the point of sacrificing own time, values, property, and even life goals.

      h. Manipulator: manages through generosity and favors.

      i. Victim: in tandem with repeated acts of martyrdom, perceives that they never receive enough credit.

      j. Inadequate: "black cloud" of inferiority over their heads.

      k. Reactionaries: tend to overreact rather than respond to situations.

C. Traits that enhance balance and self-care.

    1. Hardy personality traits: an individual who despite stressful circumstances appears resistant to the psychophysiologic effects of stress and has the following three traits.

      a. Commitment: dedication to oneself, one's work, and one's family that provides the individual with a sense of belonging and life purpose.

    b. Control: empowerment or self-control that helps one overcome elements in the environment so one does not feel victimized.

    c. Challenge: ability to see change and even problems as opportunities for growth rather than threats to one's existence.

2. Self-esteem factor: a critical indication of individual's stress response (Branden, 1994).

    a. Focus on action and achievement of highest potential.

    b. Living consciously or living in the present moment.

    c. Self-acceptance or refusal to be in an adversarial relationship with self.

    d. Self-responsibility or choosing to acknowledge responsibility for one's feelings.

    e. Self-assertiveness or honoring one's wants, needs, and values and seeking appropriate ways to satisfy them.

    f. Living purposefully or taking action to make one's goals happen.

    g. Personal integrity or working to achieve congruence between values and actions.

D. Self-care activities provide form and guidance for behaviors during times of regeneration and growth for our minds, bodies, or spirits.

1. Self-care activities for the mind.

    a. Dreaming.

    b. Active imagination.

    c. Journaling.

        (1) Gain perspective.

        (2) Allows safe venting of emotions.

    d. Self-forgiveness.

    e. Affirmations.

    f. Using humor.

    g. Time alone.

    h. Reading and continual learning.

2. Self-care activities for the body.

    a. Nutritious diet.

    b. Exercise (e.g., yoga, aerobics, walking).

    c. Massage.

    d. Rest and relaxation.

    e. Baths.

    f. Deep breathing.

    g. Routine check-ups, screening exams, and physical examinations.

3. Self-care activities for the spirit and emotions.

    a. Time in nature.

    b. Meditation or prayer.

    c. Travel.

    d. Cherish solitude.

    e. Journaling.

      f. Reflection.

      g. Crying.

      h. Sabbaticals.

  E. Presence: concept has significant implications for nursing education, practice, research, and self-care. Watson (1999) defines presence as the "being" or essence of the individual and delineates three levels.

      1. Physical presence: "being there" for another, as nursing interventions and providing routine tasks.

      2. Psychologic presence: "being with" as the nurse uses self as an intervention tool to create a therapeutic psychologic environment that meets need for comfort and support.

      3. Therapeutic presence: "being whole" nurse relates to client as whole being to whole being, using all of their body, mind, emotion, and spiritual resources.

      4. Presence is a state achieved when one moves oneself to an inner reference of balance.

      5. To be present implies a quality, an essence of being in the moment.

  F. Benefit of self-care.

      1. Improved health.

      2. Improved job satisfaction.

      3. Improved job performance.

      4. Ability to balance personal and work life.

  G. Interrelationships.

      1. Mentoring.

         a. Choosing a mentor.

         b. Goals of the relationship.

         c. Time required/invested for relationship.

         d. Communication: criticism/praise, confidence-building.

      2. Networking.

         a. Collaboration: nurses use informed judgment, individual competencies, and qualification when seeking consultation.

         b. Accepting care responsibilities, and delegation of nursing care.

PROFESSIONAL MANDATES FOR CONTINUING DEVELOPMENT

Today's practice settings demand definable competency of care providers. Whether mandated by the Joint Commission on Accreditation of Healthcare Organizations (JCAHO), Health Plan Employer Data and Information Set (HEDIS), the National Committee for Quality Assurance (NCQA), the insurance carriers, or the patient, the quality of care is equated to the continual development and learning by the care provider. Although education can occur in a variety of formats all have value in meeting the many needs of the learner.

  A. Governmental and regulatory agency directives (see Chapter 25).

      1. Occupational Safety and Health Administration (OSHA).

         a. Blood-borne pathogens.

      b. TB program.
   2. JCAHO.
      a. Staff competency.
      b. Abuse recognition training.
      c. Age-specific training.
      d. Process improvement initiatives.
   3. State laws: some states require 20 or more continuing education hours be obtained to be eligible for relicensure. Choosing programs not applicable to the current practice and practice setting defeats the intent of these mandates.
  B. Facility-specific directive inservices.
   1. New equipment inservices.
   2. Change policy and procedure of inservices.
   3. Review of low-frequency, high-risk skills.
   4. Orientation: this is a program provided to new staff allowing smooth assimilation into a new position (Alspach, 1995).
      a. Environment.
      b. Culture.
      c. Policies and procedures.
      d. Promote learning and functioning within the setting.
      e. Equipment and safety issues.
  C. CNE programs targeting development of skills used in the ambulatory care setting.
   1. Patient education issues.
   2. New trends in care management.
   3. Drug updates.
  D. Challenges and goal setting.
   1. Short and long-term goals and objectives.
   2. Realistic.
   3. Measurable.
   4. Writing and sharing to legitimize.
   5. Establishing the stretch or reach.
   6. Facing and overcoming fears.
   7. Building confidence and self-esteem.

MEMBERSHIP IN PROFESSIONAL ORGANIZATIONS

Organizations have many common components. They provide a sense of belonging, peer recognition, educational opportunities, service opportunities, and mentoring from professional experts.
  A. Benefit of membership.
   1. Remain current with contemporary issues.
   2. Sense of belonging.
   3. Awareness of changes in practice standards.
   4. Opportunity for peer recognition.
   5. National issues balanced with local focus.

6. Sharing of best practice standards.
- **B.** What professional organizations provide.
  - **1.** Role development.
    - **a.** Active participant can participate and contribute to the profession's ongoing body of knowledge development.
    - **b.** Inactive participant can obtain knowledge.
  - **2.** Effective means for influencing policies and shaping trends.
    - **a.** Develop and improve standards of nursing practice.
    - **b.** Work to protect patients from misinformation and substandard care.
    - **c.** Establish benchmarks and levels of nurse competence.
  - **3.** Set standards for clinical competency.
    - **a.** Collaborate with multi-discipline groups of care providers.
    - **b.** Promote community and national initiatives to meet the changing health needs of the public.
- **C.** Choosing an organization.
  - **1.** Goals of organization fit your interests and work setting.
  - **2.** Services and information provided by organization assist in practice.
  - **3.** Scope of benefits provided with membership.
    - **a.** Newsletters and journals.
    - **b.** Local and national conferences.
    - **c.** Networking opportunities.
    - **d.** Specialty practice standards.
    - **e.** Consultation services.
    - **f.** Membership directory with specialty experts.
    - **g.** Internet communications.

CONTINUING PROFESSIONAL EDUCATION/DISTANCE LEARNING

Traditional classroom settings have been the standard educational model. Recent advances in technology allow creative educators to offer alternative methods for learning. Video programs, teleconferencing, and on-line interactions provide new resources for meeting educational needs of the professional nurse. In an age when information growth is expanding at an accelerated speed, it is difficult to keep pace. Readily available, easily accessed educational opportunities are a priority. New graduates as well as experienced professionals benefit from continuation of their education. Opportunities must meet the varied learning needs of the professional nurse. Education for the professional nurse is an ongoing process of reflection, discovery, and adaptation that is based on beliefs, experiences, and research.

- **A.** Identify learning needs.
  - **1.** Personal/self-knowledge/individual learning.
  - **2.** Practice/organizational needs/group learning.
  - **3.** Presentations, lectures, readings, classroom on-line.
- **B.** Key factors to how we learn.
  - **1.** Willingness to learn.
  - **2.** Observation.

3. Doing.
4. Repetition.
5. Questioning.
6. Validating.
7. Emotions (e.g., feelings, hope, desire).
8. Pattern identification.
9. Evaluations.
10. Re-doing.
11. Personal attributes.
   a. Motivation for learning.
   b. Interest in subject matter.
   c. Availability of time.
   d. Resources/cost.
C. Learning and professionalism is enhanced by:
   1. Critical thinking.
   2. Confidence.
   3. Positive relationships.
   4. Appropriate timing.
D. Distance learning.
   1. Purpose: access to learning modalities.
      a. Initially designed to reach/include persons in rural/isolated areas.
      b. Bring educational opportunities/resources to isolated areas.
      c. Correspondence-type courses.
         (1) Individuals enrolled in a correspondence course.
         (2) Worked on material at own pace.
         (3) Submit results for grading/credit as applicable.
      d. E-mail and Internet have allowed for interchange with a quicker turn-around and increased teacher/learner feedback.
      e. Video capabilities.
      f. Video-interactive capabilities.
      g. Internet access to references, persons, knowledge bases.
   2. Era of information/knowledge explosion and instant communications.
      a. "Increasingly, viewing a college education as mastery of a body of knowledge or a complete preparation for a lifetime career is becoming outmoded. Instead, we recognize that graduates need to have acquired skills, such as critical thinking, quantitative reasoning, and effective communication, along with abilities, such as the ability to find needed information and the ability to work well with others" (Twigg, 1994, p. 2).
      b. Increased need for learning environments and systems integration of learning.
   3. Who, when, where needed?
      a. Once, the cost of technology was the limiting factor.
      b. Tools now available: do learners have the skills to use them?
      c. Learning once occurred in a "place": the environment is changing and information can be sought wherever the tools are readily

available, by those with the critical thinking skills to put the tools to use.

4. How and cost.

    a. Self-initiated learning, not for credit.

    b. Formalized learning: a clear objective/purpose established by a traditional institution of learning.

    c. Formalized distance learning for credit.

    d. Universities with distance programs offer credit and even degrees via distance learning.

    e. Cost (e.g., program cost, materials, mailing costs, computer access/cost, video/audio capability).

    f. Medium: Internet, correspondence (mail), video, audio interactive capability, e-mail.

5. Future considerations.

    a. Language assimilation.

    b. Limits potentially placed on the Internet and access.

    c. Capabilities of learners to use the tools effectively.

    d. Cost implications of updates to software that are incompatible with older versions of the software.

    e. Changing structure of educational environments.

    f. Establishing standards.

    g. Evolving purposes for education tools.

    h. How to validate learning and effectiveness.

    i. Maintaining cost effectiveness.

    j. Changing criteria for workers, leaders.

        (1) Skill sets.

        (2) Communication abilities.

        (3) Power.

    k. Multiple skill sets.

    l. Integration of learning and competency.

    m. Utilization of method based on learner needs/requirements/time.

REFERENCES

Achterberg J (1990): *Woman healer.* Boston: Shambhala.

Alspach JG (1995): *The educational process in nursing staff development.* St. Louis: Mosby.

Branden N (1994): *The six pillars of self-esteem.* New York: Bantam.

Dossey BM, Keegan L, Guzzetta GE, Kolkmeir LG (1995): *Holistic nursing: a handbook for practice,* ed 2. Gaithersburg, MD: Aspen.

Twigg CA (1994): The need for a national learning infrastructure. 29(5). Educom Review, http://www.educause.edu/pub/er/review/reviewArticles/29516.html

Seaward J (1997): *Managing stress: principles and strategies for health and well-being,* ed 2. Sudbury, MA: Jones and Bartlett.

Watson J (1999): *Postmodern nursing and beyond.* London: Churchill Livingstone.

Glossary*

Advocacy act or process of advocating or supporting (a cause or proposal) on behalf of another.

Ambulatory care personal health care provided to individuals or a population of individuals who are not occupying a bed in a health care institution or at home.

Ambulatory care nursing a specialty practice area that is characterized by nurses responding rapidly to high volumes of patients in a short span of time while dealing with issues that are not always predictable

Ambulatory nursing practice domain the overall scope of nursing practice in the ambulatory arena; it includes attributes of the environment in which practice occurs, patient requirements for care, and specific nursing role dimensions.

Americans with Disabilities Act (ADA) prohibits discrimination in the rendering of health care services or the process of employment based on a disability.

APGs ambulatory patient groups; patient classification system designed to explain amount and type of resource used in ambulatory care visit.

AVGs ambulatory visit groups; single payment for all services provided during an ambulatory visit.

Benchmarking a continuous and collaborative discipline that involves measuring and comparing the results of key processes with the best performers, and using the information to change/improve practices, which results in superior performance as determined by measured outcome.

Capitation method for funding expenses of enrollees in prepaid health plans; pays providers a fixed fee per member regardless of service.

Care coordination a process that seeks to achieve the optimal cost-effective use of scarce resources by helping individuals get health, social, and support services that meet their needs at a given point in time or across the life span.

Case management collaborative process that assesses, plans, implements, coordinates, monitors, and evaluates options and services for meeting an individual's health needs and promoting quality cost-effective outcomes; a method for managing the provision of health care to members/patients with catastrophic or high cost medical conditions.

CHAMPUS (Civilian Health and Medical Program of the U.S.) a federal program providing coverage to families of military personnel, military retirees, spouses, and dependents

Codependent traits individuals dependent on making others dependent on them as a means of self-validation

Collaboration to work together toward a common goal; to pursue a common purpose and a sharing of knowledge to resolve problems, decide issues, and set goals within a structure of collegiality.

Commercial indemnity plans a type of insurance contract in which the insurer pays for care received up to a fixed amount per encounter or episode of illness.

---

*Definitions are taken from the text.

Competency   the demonstrated integration of knowledge, skill, and ability in order to perform expected job.

Computerized patient record (CPR)   an electronic patient record that resides in a system specifically designed to support users by providing accessibility to complete and accurate data, alerts, reminders, clinical decision support systems, links to medical knowledge, and other aids.

Conflict resolution   the use of effective techniques to achieve the desired level of conflict.

Continuity   refers to care that is received over time (delivered or coordinated) by a single provider or team of health care professionals.

Continuous quality improvement (CQI)   the analysis and subsequent management of processes and clinical, financial, and health data to determine the relationship of those factors on health care structures, interventions, outcomes, and costs.

Coordinating   refers to the function that ensures that the care (any combination of therapies and services) occurs to meet the individual's needs holistically.

Copayment   out of pocket expense paid by an individual for a specific service defined in the insurance plan

Corporate compliance   internal review of congruency of practices, including billing, with a variety of laws, regulations, and program requirements.

Cost benefit analysis   a formal financial analysis completed by organizations, to determine the cost of a program, projected revenues, and to identify program benefits.

CPT   the physicians' current procedural published by American Medical Association; the internationally recognized coding system for reporting medical services and procedures.

Critical thinking   the ability to collect and analyze information in order to arrive at a logical, defendable, conclusion.

Delegation   to commit or entrust to another.

Deontology   (also known as duty-based ethics) based on the belief that there are duties to which one must be faithful and which one is obligated to carry out because these duties are owed to all human beings and because of the expectations implied by one's professional role.

Diagnostic related group (DRG)   a system for classifying hospital inpatients into groups using similar quantities of resources according to characteristics such as diagnosis, age, procedure, and complications.

Disease management   method that uses standardized care plans based on evidence and best practices to manage patients with chronic diseases.

Environmental management   the assurance of appropriate management plans to provide a safe, accessible, effective, and functional environment of care.

Equal Employment Opportunity Commission (EEOC)   a federal agency that enforces regulations concerning equal opportunity.

Ethics   a branch of philosophy dealing with the values related to human conduct, with respect to the rightness or wrongness of certain actions; and to the goodness and badness of the motives and ends of such actions; a set of moral principles or values, the principles of conduct governing an individual or a group.

Evidence-based medicine   a way of caring for patients, making decisions, and teaching which values being explicit about the integration of high-quality research evidence with pathophysiologic reasoning, caregiver experience, and patient preferences.

Evidence-based nursing practice   the conscientious, explicit, and judicious use of the current best evidence in making decisions about the care of individual patients.

Evidenced-based practice   the conscientious, explicit, and judicious use of current best evidence in making decisions about the care of individual patients; combines research and clinical expertise.

Family   members are defined by the patient in his/her own terms and may include individuals related by blood or marriage, or in self-defined relationships (this definition is intended to include the family in nursing care as appropriate; it is *not* intended as a legal definition of family).

Fee for service   reimbursement method in which payment is made for each service or item.

HCPCS (Health Care Financing Administration [HCFA] Common Procedure Coding System)   a uniform method for health care providers and medical suppliers to report professional services, procedures, and supplies to health care plans.

Health Care Financing Administration (HCFA)   division within the U.S. Department of Health and Human Services, determines the standard rules and reporting mechanisms for health care services.

Health care team   includes the patient, family, and other members of the health care system who are involved in the development and implementation of the care plan.

Health maintenance organization (HMO)   a health plan that uses physicians as gatekeepers who are responsible for all aspects of care management and must authorize or give permission for referral to other providers; provides comprehensive health care services with an emphasis on preventive care on a prepayment or capitated system to voluntarily enrolled persons within a designated population.

HEDIS   a set of standardized performance measures designed to assure that purchasers and consumers have the information they need to reliably compare the performance of Medical Care Organizations (MCOs).

ICD 9 (*International Classification of Diseases,* 9th revision)   clinical modification published by U.S. National Center for Health Statistics; the internationally recognized system for the purposes of international morbidity and mortality; in the United States used for coding and billing purposes.

Independent practice association (IPA)   a legal entity whose members are independent physicians who contract with the IPA for the purpose of having the IPA contract with one or more HMOs.

Inpatient acute care   hospital-based care in which patients are admitted overnight for diagnosis, treatment of an acute problem, or treatment of an acute exacerbation of a chronic problem.

Inquiry   an ongoing activity of the ambulatory care nurse in which critical thinking skills are developed and used; and in which knowledge is created and transmitted.

Key informants   people who have the knowledge and ability to report on community needs. They are an excellent source of data about both the need for services and potential acceptability of various types of programs.

Managed care   a system of care delivery that influences and measures service utilization, cost, and performance; goals of managed care are quality, cost-effectiveness, and accessible health care; a coordinated system of health care, that achieves outcomes (reduced utilization and improved population health) through preventive care, case management, and the provision of medically necessary appropriate care.

Medicaid   A plan jointly funded by federal and state governments, introduced in 1966 to cover poor individuals and managed by each state.

NANDA (North American Nursing Diagnosis Association)   nomenclature for nursing diagnosis used by nurses to document nursing diagnoses in all settings where nursing care is delivered.

National Institute for Occupational Safety and Health (NIOSH)   a federal agency responsible for research and education; has representatives who perform inspections to ensure compliance.

NCQA   a not-for-profit, independent organization that assesses, evaluates, and publicly reports on the quality of managed care organizations (MCOs).

Nonmaleficence   acting in such a way that avoids harm, either intentional harm or harm as an unintended outcome.

Nursing informatics   the development and evaluation of applications, tools, processes, and structures that assist nurses with the management of data in taking care of patients or supporting the practice of nursing.

Nursing Interventions Classification (NIC)   taxonomy for classifying nursing interventions; used in all settings where care is delivered to document nursing interventions; developed by a team at University of Iowa lead by McCloskey and Bulechek.

Nursing Management Minimum Data Set (NMMDS)   data set developed by Delaney and Hubner for use by managers in all nursing care settings; it contains 17 defined data elements that include environment, nurse resources, nursing care staff, and financial resources.

Nursing services   organized services delivered to groups of patients by nursing staff; includes nursing care as well as services to support or facilitate direct care, such as referral and coordination of care.

Omaha   the Omaha VNA's system for problems, interventions, and outcomes; used by nurses to describe and document care in community settings; contains 40 nursing problems (diagnoses), and a number of associated nursing interventions, and outcomes.

Out-of-pocket expense   refers to the portion of health care cost for which the individual is responsible.

Ozbolt's Patient Care Data Set (PCDS)   taxonomy used by nurses to document care in all settings, but primarily developed for the acute care setting; comprises nursing diagnoses, patient care actions, and nursing outcomes.

Patient   an individual who requests or receives nursing services; also called client, consumer, member, or customer in many settings.

Peer review   a continuous quality improvement activity whereby nurses assess each other's care; reportable situations can be reviewed via an internal organizational system called peer review; peer review activities are generally protected and not discoverable in a court of law.

Perioperative Nursing Data Set (PNDS)   developed by the Association of Operating Room Nurses; used by perioperative registered nurses and surgical service managers in a variety of perioperative settings.

Physician Hospital Organization (PHO)   legal organization often developed for purposes of contracting with managed care plans; links physicians to specific hospitals for hospitalization care.

Point of Service (POS)   a plan that defines service providers in the service area outside of usual preferred provider network.

Precertification   process of obtaining authorization or certification from a health plan for routine hospital admissions, referrals, procedures, or tests.

Preferred provider organization (PPO)   program in which contracts exist between the health plan and care providers, at a discount for services; typically the plan provides incentives for patients to use in-network providers as opposed to nonparticipating providers (independent/noncontracted) through decreased copayments.

Primary care   the provision of integrated, accessible health care services by clinicians who are accountable for addressing a large majority of *personal* health care needs, developing a sustained partnership with patients, and practicing in the context of family and community.

Research utilization   a process of using research findings as a basis for practice. It encompasses dissemination of scientific knowledge, critique of studies, synthesis of findings, determining applicability of findings, application/implementation of scientific findings in practice, and evaluating the practice change.

Resource based relative value system (RBRVS)   a classification system that attempts to assign within a defined setting the resource requirements based on weights according to relative cost of each service.

Risk management   in ambulatory care, an organized set of activities designed to assess and reduce risks to patients, visitors, and staff, to ensure high quality of care and to minimize potential liability.

Root cause analysis   a method to determine the fundamental reason that causes variation in performance.

RVU (relative value unit)   established by HCFA to approximate the work, practice expense, and malpractice expense for delivery of physician services.

Self-esteem factor   a critical indication of individual's stress response.

Standard   an authoritative statement developed and disseminated by a professional organization or governmental or regulatory agency by which the quality of practice, services, research, or education can be judged.

Strategic planning   the continuous process of systematically evaluating the nature of the ambulatory care organization, defining its long-term objectives, identifying quantifiable goals, developing strategies to reach these objectives and goals, and allocating resources to carry out these strategies.

Supervision   the direction and oversight of the performance of others.

Telehealth   use of modem telecommunications and information technology to provide healthcare to individuals at a distance and to transmit information to provide.

The Agency for Healthcare Research and Quality (AHRQ)   in partnership with the American Association of Health Plans (AAHP) and the American Medical Association (AMA), sponsors a World Wide Web-based National Guideline Clearinghouse™ (NGC); the NGC is a publicly available electronic repository for clinical practice guidelines and related materials that provides on-line access to guidelines at www.guidelines.gov

Transformational leadership   process-oriented and aimed at congruence between the vision and agenda of both the leader and followers.

Usual and customary (U&C)   a method used to determine if a fee is usual, customary, and reasonable; customary is the normal fee charged in the geographic area for the same service; usual refers to fees normally charged by a doctor or health care provider for a service.

Utilitarianism   (also known as consequence-based ethics) the theory that seeks to choose the thing that will offer the most good to the greatest number of people, increase pleasure, and avoid pain.

Utilization management   the second process of care coordination across the continuum of care; the management and evaluation of the medical necessity, appropriateness, and efficiency of the use of health care services, procedures, and facilities under the auspices of the applicable health benefit plan.

Wound healer   term used to describe an individual who has recognized strengths and weaknesses and is able to assist with greater self-knowledge.

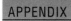

American Academy of Ambulatory Care Nursing Information

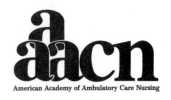
American Academy of Ambulatory Care Nursing

American Academy of Ambulatory Care Nursing (AAACN) Fact Sheet

IDENTITY STATEMENT: The American Academy of Ambulatory Care Nursing is the association of professional nurses who identify ambulatory care practice as essential to the continuum of high quality, cost-effective health care.

MISSION STATEMENT: Advance the art and science of ambulatory care nursing.

VISION: AAACN is the premier nursing organization for ambulatory care.

VALUES: The following values guide each member's and the organization's vision, actions, and relationships: (1) excellence in health care delivery for individuals and communities; (2) visionary and accountable leadership; (3) productive partnerships and alliances; (4) proactive innovation and responsible risk-taking; (5) responsive member services; (6) diverse and committed membership; and (7) continual advancement of professional ambulatory care nursing practice.

GOALS: (1) Be the voice of ambulatory care nursing; (2) Promote professional practice; (3) Stimulate innovative thinking; (4) Build collaborative relationships; (5) Strengthen the AAACN resource base; and (6) Develop AAACN leadership ability and capacity.

ABOUT AAACN: AAACN (formerly the American Academy of Ambulatory Nursing Administration) was founded in 1978 as a not for profit, educational forum. In 1991 AAACN membership was broadened to include nurses in direct practice, education, and research roles as well as those in management and administration. Practice settings include universities, medical centers, HMOs, group practices, urgent care centers, physician office settings, hospital based ambulatory care settings, military, community health, and others. The Academy serves as a voice for ambulatory care nurses across the continuum of health care delivery and has membership in the National Federation for Specialty Nursing Organizations (NFSNO) and the Nursing Organization Liaison Forum (NOLF). These two organizations provide a forum for specialty nursing organizations to dialogue, collaborate, and facilitate policy formulation on professional practice and national health.

MEMBERSHIP BENEFITS: Academy membership benefits include discounted rates to the AAACN National Preconference and Conference, regional programs, and publications; the annual conference includes multiple practice innovations, industry exhibits, research forum, and numerous networking opportunities; the bimonthly newsletter, *Viewpoint*; subscription to **one** of four journals—*Nursing Economic$, Medsurg Nursing, Dermatology Nursing,* or *Pediatric Nursing*; opportunity to join a special interest group in the area of: Case Management; Pediatrics; Staff Education; Telehealth Nursing Practice; Standards; Veterans Affairs; Tri-Service Military; and Informatics; awards and scholarship programs and access to national experts and colleagues through AAACN's membership directory, list serves, and web site **aaacn.org**

AAACN PUBLICATIONS:
- *Ambulatory Care Nursing Administration and Practice Standards* (2000)
- *Nursing in Ambulatory Care—The Future is Here* (1997)
- *Telehealth Nursing Practice (TNP) Administration and Practice Standards* (2001)
- *Examination Preparation Guide for Ambulatory Care Nursing Certification Examination* (1999)
- *Ambulatory Care Nursing Certification Review Course Syllabus* (2000)
- *Ambulatory Care Self Assessment* (2000)
- *Telephone Nursing Practice Resource Directory* (2000)

For more information, call (800)AMB-NURS or (856)256-2350 or fax (856)589-7463
E-mail: aaacn@ajj.com or visit our web site at aaacn.org
Mailing address: East Holly Avenue, Box 56, Pitman, New Jersey 08071-0056

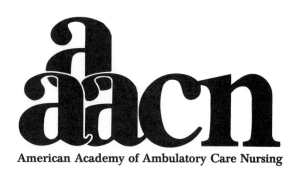

American Academy of Ambulatory Care Nursing

Publication and Merchandise Order Form

Order	Price	Quantity	Total
Ambulatory Care Nursing Administration and Practice Standards (©2000)	$15.00 Member $25.00 Nonmember	_____ _____	$_____ $_____
Ambulatory Care Nursing Certification Review Course Course Syllabus (©2000)	$35.00 Member $40.00 Nonmember	_____ _____	$_____ $_____
Ambulatory Care Nursing Self-Assessment (©2000)	$25.00 Member $30.00 Nonmember	_____ _____	$_____ $_____
Examination Preparation Guide For Ambulatory Care Nursing Certification Examination (©1999)	$15.00 Member $20.00 Nonmember	_____ _____	$_____ $_____
Nursing in Ambulatory Care—The Future is Here (©1997)	$18.95 $13.95 SNA Member	_____ _____	$_____ $_____
Telephone Nursing Practice Administration and Practice Standards (©1997)	$10.00 Member $15.00 Nonmember	_____ _____	$_____ $_____
Telephone Nursing Practice Resource Directory (©2000)	$5.00 Member $7.00 Nonmember	_____ _____	$_____ $_____
AAACN Official Member Pin	$10.00	_____	$_____
AAACN Official Mug	$5.00	_____	$_____

Name _____

Address _____

_____

City   State   Zip

Daytime Phone _____

E-mail Address _____

Method of Payment: Check Cash Credit Card

___ American Express ___ Mastercard ___ Visa

Account # _____

Expiration Date _____

Total $ _____

Signature _____

Make checks payable to AAACN, East Holly Avenue, Box 56; Pitman, NJ 08071-0056

Index

Page numbers in *italics* indicate illustrations; page numbers followed by a "t" indicate tables